Glass-Ionomer Cement

Alan D. Wilson, B.Sc., D.Sc. (London),
D.Tech. (C.N.A.A.), C.Chem., F.R.S.C.
Head
Materials Research and Development
Laboratory of the Government Chemist, London

John W. McLean, O.B.E., F.D.S., R.C.S. (England),
M.D.S., D.Sc. (London), Dr. Odont. (Lund)
Consulting Professor in Fixed Prosthetics and Biomaterials
Louisiana State University Medical Center
School of Dentistry
Senior Research Fellow
Institute of Dental Surgery
Eastman Dental Hospital, London

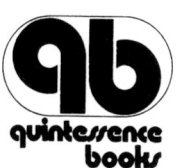

Quintessence Publishing Co., Inc. 1988
Chicago, London, Berlin, São Paulo, Tokyo, and Hong Kong

Library of Congress Cataloging-in-Publication Data

Wilson, Alan D.
  Glass-ionomer cement.

  Includes bibliographies and index.
  1. Dental glass ionomer cements.   I. McLean, John W.
II. Title.   [DNLM: 1. Cementation—methods.   2. Dental
Cements.   WU 190 M4783g]
RK652.8.G55M38   1988   617.6′75   87-35717
ISBN 0-86715-200-1

© 1988 by Quintessence Publishing Co., Inc., Chicago, Illinois.
All rights reserved.

Lithography: JUP Industrie- und Presseklischee, Berlin
Composition: The Clarinda Co., Clarinda, IA
Printing and binding: Franz W. Wesel Druckerei und Verlag GmbH & Co., KG., Baden-Baden

Printed in West Germany

Contents

Preface

Many years have passed since the glass-ionomer cement was first invented at the Laboratory of the Government Chemist. More than a decade has gone by since it was first placed on the market, yet it is only in the last few years that it has become a major restorative material. The first international conference on the material was not held until 1985. This may seem surprising, for glass-ionomer cement is the only restorative material that bonds to untreated enamel and dentine. Now there has been an upsurge of interest in the material, and there have been several causes for this. The cement itself has been improved. Clinical techniques have been developed that are appropriate to the material and exploit its virtues. Its range of application has been extended. Above all, the clinician is now realizing the advantages and uses that this material has in everyday general practice. The pace of research, particularly clinical research, has quickened, and this has been accompanied by a surge in the literature on the topic. Articles have appeared in a wide range of journals from those devoted to practical clinical dentistry, to those concerned with clinical research, to the basic materials science journals. Not surprisingly, the literature at times contains conflicting statements and opinions. It has become increasingly obvious that there is a need for a critical compilation on the materials contained in widely scattered journals.

It is the aim of *Glass-Ionomer Cement* to fill this gap. We the authors, one as a clinician and the other as a materials scientist, feel uniquely qualified to write such a work. Both of us have been associated with the topic since its inception 20 years ago. Indeed, we have seen the subject through its early uncertain days, through the years when there was both scientific and clinical doubt, to these present days when glass-ionomer cement has become accepted as a vital material in the dental clinician's armoury.

We have aimed this book at the general clinician, the research clinician, and the materials scientist. We have sought to unify all the diverse elements of the subject. In particular, we have attempted to relate clinical practice to the science underlying it.

The first eight chapters of this book describe the basic science of the system— its chemistry, physical characteristics, biological behaviour, and performance in service. The remaining chapters give practical instructions for the clinical use of the materials. Points of technique are described and illustrated to enable the clinician to get optimum results from the material.

In order to achieve this the clinician should have a basic understanding of the setting reaction of these cements and how to protect them from the oral environment in the early setting stages. This is the key to success and has, in the past, been a major cause for disappointment when the glass-ionomer cement has failed during short periods of service. We believe that if the clinical techniques described in this book are followed, long-term success with these cements is possible. In addition, every practitioner should realize that glass-ionomer cement's chemical adhesion and ability to leach fluoride make it the material of choice in treating early dental caries.

New concepts for treating both fissure and approximal caries are described that could have a major impact on public health. The replacement of amalgam alloys in treating early carious lesions is now possible, and the preservation of tooth enamel is given great prominence in this book. Indiscriminate cutting of human enamel leads to more and more restorative work. This book attempts to reverse this situation and offers the clinician an opportunity of entering the world of micropreparation using magnification and fibre-optic lighting. We believe that the future for restorative dentistry lies in this area.

The glass-ionomer cement/composite resin laminate restoration is gaining in popularity and could extend the use of composite resins in clinical practice. Porcelain or microfill resin veneers are also receiving great attention, and their limitations as well as advantages are evaluated, particularly in relation to the use of glass-ionomer linings.

Future developments in glass-ionomer cement look promising, and efforts are being made to improve their abrasion-resistance and strength. Disperse-phase glasses have been developed with improved strengths and the introduction of the cermet-ionomer cements may offer a solution to the problem of abrasion under occlusal loading. The new water-hardening glass-ionomer cements could be developed further since higher molecular weight polyacids can be used to improve flexural strengths. The diversity of these new cements offers the researcher many avenues for exploration.

The glass-ionomer cement/composite resin laminate may be the key to future developments in which the dentine is replaced with an adhesive, anticariogenic, and biologically compatible cement and the enamel with a translucent, abrasion-resistant composite material. The dentist may then be offered opportunities of creating a true replica of tooth structure which could survive long periods in the hostile oral environment.

Human enamel still remains our best restorative material and traditional forms of restorative dentistry have often resulted in massive destruction of teeth in order to comply with past teaching, which was based on the use of nonadhesive materials. We hope that this book will encourage a new look at how we should be teaching students in the future and change our approach from macro- to microcutting of teeth where operative dentistry is necessary.

Acknowledgments

The late Dr. John Longwell, C.B.E., Deputy Government Chemist, first induced the Laboratory of the Government Chemist to work in the dental field in the late 50s and early 60s with the introduction of fluoridation of the water supplies in the U.K.

At a time when the road ahead was uncertain and far from clear, research at the Laboratory of the Government Chemist concentrated on the nature and behaviour of the dental-silicate cement, and from these studies the setting mechanism as an acid-base reaction was first elucidated. This was a vital step that opened up a whole new field of exploration.

Mr. Brian Kent was coworker in the dental silicate research which led to the invention of the glass-ionomer cement. He was also a coinventor of the glass-ionomer cement and gave it its name. Dr. Stephen Crisp was a codiscoverer of the effect of tartaric acid on the setting reaction, a discovery which led to the first really practical glass-ionomer cement. Dr. Havard Prosser was a coworker in the studies which unravelled some of the finer details of the chemistry of the system. Throughout, Mr. Brian Lewis gave valuable experimental assistance.

This work has been supported by succeeding Government Chemists, Dr. D. T. Lewis, C.B., Dr. Harold Egan, and Dr. Ronald Colman (now chief scientist at the Department of Trade and Industry).

The pioneering work of Professor Dennis Smith, who developed the zinc polycarboxylate cements which established the cement-forming potential of poly-(acrylic acid), gave encouragement to all of us in the field of polyelectrolyte cements. Professor Ralph Phillips and his coworkers at Indiana University have greatly assisted the general practitioner in understanding the important properties of glass-ionomer cement.

Dr. Geoffrey Knight and Dr. Peter Hunt have stimulated our thinking in the area of microcavity preparation. The initiative of Dr. Peter Hunt and Dr. Joe Simmons in organizing the First International Conference on Glass-Ionomer Cements, which was held in Philadelphia in the autumn of 1985, is greatly appreciated.

Dr. Graham Mount has done more than any other dentist to promote the clinical teaching of glass-ionomer cement—his contribution to our profession has been invaluable.

We are particularly grateful to Dr. Ted Croll for supplying clinical pictures and technical support on treating deciduous dentitions with glass-ionomer cement for chapter 14.

Dr. Edwina Kidd has been kind enough to supply colour diagrams and photographs of the early carious lesion. Her contribution to this area of our knowledge has greatly assisted us in preparing this book.

Mr. Fred Hill has supplied radiographs

of fissure caries, and Mr. Richard Miller-Yardley, O.B.E., and Mr. Reg Dinsdale have kindly allowed us use of radiographs to illustrate the use of silver-cermet ionomer for the treatment of apical infection employing a retrograde filling technique.

Dee McLean has prepared all the colour illustrations. Her skill in devizing diagrams to illustrate new clinical procedures has enhanced the clarity of the text.

We thank Mrs. Margaret Wilson for her help in checking the manuscript and the proofs.

We ask forgiveness from our wives for our inattention to them and our domestic affairs while we were writing the book.

Finally, we would like to give encouragement to all those who work in this difficult field and commend them to inventiveness combined with persistence of effort and an indifference to disappointment.

Chapter 1

Scientific and Clinical Development

During the early and mid-1960s, the science and technology of clinical dental materials—those materials that can be used directly by the dental surgeon—remained where they had been almost 60 years before. For example, the dental silicate cement, the principal anterior restorative material of those days, was recognized as flawed for use in the general dental practice. It had remained essentially the same for 50 years. Even the nature of its setting and structure were but imperfectly understood.

This unsatisfactory state of affairs, however, produced a positive response, and the period of the late 1960s and early 1970s was a most creative one in the development of new materials. There was a general recognition that *(1)* adequate physical properties are not enough by themselves, *(2)* a restorative material should be more than just an inert stopping, *(3)* biocompatibility and adhesion are important, and *(4)* new materials and techniques should be developed with these characteristics. One outcome of these considerations was Smith's (1968) zinc polycarboxylate cement, which utilized the adhesive properties of poly(acrylic acid).

In the realm of restorative materials, Buonocore, in 1955, had advocated an acid-etch technique for bonding resins to enamel; however, his findings were neglected for many years probably because of the inadequacy of simple resins

as restorative materials. Acid etching came into its own with the advent of the composite resins. Much of the success of composite resins is attributable to Buonocore's technique.

The invention of the glass-ionomer cement in 1969 (first reported by Wilson and Kent in 1971) also arose from a general positive and creative response to inadequate materials, in particular from the deficiencies of the dental silicates. This book will describe the development of glass-ionomer cements—both scientific and clinical—relating the science to practical applications, and will demonstrate the correct clinical techniques for obtaining optimum results using glass-ionomer cements.

The glass-ionomer cement is an unusual material with unusual properties. It is neither purely organic nor purely inorganic but a hybrid of both. It is neither a polymer nor a hydraulic cement but sets by chemical gelation as a result of a reaction between an acid and a base. It is one of a number of acid-base reaction cements used in dentistry (Wygant, 1958; Wilson, 1978). The material is a kind of composite resin but one where the filler has taken part in the setting reaction.

Glass-ionomer cements have porcelainlike translucency, adhere to tooth substances, and have favourable bioactive properties. The material lends itself to restorative dentistry, for which it was originally designed (McLean and Wilson, 1977a, 1977b, 1977c). In recent years it has shown promise as a bone cement, where it is demonstrably bioactive and promotes bone growth (Jonck, 1986).

The two components of a glass-ionomer cement are a special alumino-silicate glass (a base) and a polyelectrolyte* (an acid). Translucent properties derive from the glass and adhesive properties from the polyelectrolyte. When mixed together as a water-based paste, the cement forms.

Because both components are materials of wide chemical diversity, the range of glass-ionomer cements is very wide indeed and the material has considerable potential for further development. Significant advances in the technology and clinical applications of glass-ionomer cements can be expected in the future. The development of glass-ionomer cements is difficult, however, because changes in formulation affect more than one property. Therefore, we agree with the wisdom expressed by F.N. Doubleday in 1920 in his article, "The Translucent Filling Cement."

> The first medical aphorism enunciated by Hippocrates is as follows: "Life is Short, Art Long, Opportunity Fleeting, Experiment Slippery, Judgement Difficult." He who attempts to investigate translucent cement fillings learns by experience its truth.

This quotation is as appropriate today as at the time when it was first written.

The progress of the glass-ionomer cement has been one of intertwining scientific and clinical development. It is wrong to suppose that a material is invented and developed purely in the materials laboratory and that the whole of the creative effort lies within the laboratory.

While it is true that the original invention and early development is made in the laboratory, subsequent development is equally divided between the materials scientist and the clinician. Clinical ingenuity in exploiting the properties of a new material becomes just as important as laboratory developments.

Human nature is essentially conservative and tends to treat a new material with techniques that have been developed for traditional materials. Only slowly is it realized that the maximum benefit from a new material can only be obtained by developing new and appropriate technologies. This has been very true of the development of glass-ionomer cements (Table 1-1).

Invention

The invention of the glass-ionomer cement in 1969 (reported in Wilson and Kent, 1971) resulted directly from basic studies on dental silicate cements (Wilson et al., 1972) and studies where the phosphoric acid in dental silicate cements was replaced by organic chelating acids (Wilson, 1968). A significant contribution was also made by D.C. Smith (1968), who used poly(acrylic acid) in his zinc polycarboxylate cements. Glass-ionomer cement (the term was coined by B.E. Kent) has been described as a hybrid of dental silicate cements and zinc polycarboxylates. Formally, this view seems neat, but it is not correct. The problems of controlling the reaction between aluminosilicate glasses and poly(acrylic acid) for a practical cement formation are formidable and were only solved by the invention of novel glasses and the discovery of the importance of tartaric acid as a reaction-controlling additive in the system.

---

*A polyelectrolyte is an electrolyte where either the cation or the anion is a polymer bearing a multiplicity of electrical charges. Poly(acrylic acid) is an example of an anionic polyelectrolyte.

Table 1-1 Scientific and clinical development of glass-ionomer cement*

Scientific	Clinical
Original invention, ASPA I: 1969 (Wilson & Kent, 1971, 1972, 1973)	First clinical trials: 1970 (McLean)
First practical material: ASPA II: 1972 (Wilson & Crisp, 1976)	
First marketable material, ASPA IV: 1973 (Crisp & Wilson, 1977) (Europe 1975, Australia 1976, USA 1977)	Class I restorations, fissure sealing, preventive dentistry (McLean & Wilson, 1974)
Luting agent, ASPA IVa: 1975 (Wilson et al., 1977)	Erosion lesions, deciduous teeth, lining, luting, composite/ionomer laminates (McLean & Wilson, 1977a, 1977b, 1977c)
Improved translucency, ASPA X: 1977 (Crisp, Abel, & Wilson, 1979)	Improved clinical techniques: 1976–1977 (Mount & Makinson, 1978)
	Approximal lesions, minimal cavity preparation (buccal approach) (McLean, 1980)
Silver-tin alloy, metal oxide and carbon-reinforced cements: 1977 (Sced & Wilson, 1980; Simmons, 1983)	
Cermet ionomer cements: 1978 (McLean & Glasser, 1985)	
Water-activated cements, ASPA V: 1982 (Prosser et al., 1984)	Water-activated luting agent (McLean et al., 1984; Prosser et al., 1984)
	Tunnel Class I and II preparations (Hunt, 1984; Knight, 1984; McLean, 1986)
	Double-etch ionomer/composite-resin laminates (McLean et al., 1985)

*Dates given after colon indicate when a development or technique was first introduced; names and dates in parentheses refer to when it was first reported or when it was published as a patent.

Early development

Scientific development of glass-ionomer cement has been in two steps. First, effort was devoted to improving properties to make it a fully practical material for anterior restorations. And second, properties were modified in order to extend its range of applications.

In early studies carried out in 1965 and 1966, A.D. Wilson examined cements prepared by mixing dental silicate glass powder with aqueous solutions of various organic acids, including poly(acrylic acid). The polyacrylate cement pastes were almost unworkable, set slowly and sluggishly, and were not hydrolytically stable. They were not reported in the published paper (Wilson, 1968). Later, however, in the years 1968 and 1969, in collaboration with Kent and Lewis, he found that by employing novel glass formulations, hydrolytically stable cements could be produced (Wilson and Kent, 1971, 1972, 1973). A key observation had been made by Kent in 1968 during the course of unpublished studies on dental silicate cements. He found that setting of these cements was controlled by the Al_2O_3/SiO_2 ratio in the glass. This discovery enabled more reactive glasses to be prepared suitable for forming rapid-setting cements with poly(acrylic acid), which is a weaker acid than phosphoric acid used in dental silicate cements.

The first glass-ionomer cements lacked workability and hardened slowly. Eventually, Kent et al. (1973, 1979) found a glass that was high in fluoride (G-200*) that gave a usable cement, ASPA I.†

However, this cement still had a sluggish set, working time was minimal, and post-set hardening was slow. The time that cements were sensitive to water was considerable because of flow hardening. McLean found that good clinical results could only be obtained with the greatest of care. Also, the high-fluoride, almost opaque G-200 glass gave a cement with a translucency well below that required by cosmetic dentistry and was not suitable for general clinical use.

The key discovery was made in 1972 by Wilson and Crisp (reported in Wilson and Crisp, 1976), who found that tartaric acid modified the cement-forming reaction, thus improving manipulation, extending working time, and greatly sharpening the setting rate (Crisp et al., 1975b; Wilson et al., 1976). This refinement of ASPA I was termed ASPA II and constituted the first practical glass-ionomer cement. Even by today's standards its properties were excellent.

Over the years research workers have further improved glass-ionomer cements in terms of setting rate, translucency, and strength. The discovery of the benefits of tartaric acid was, perhaps, equal in importance to the original concept in the development of the glass-ionomer cement.

Even before ASPA II was developed, McLean had investigated its clinical possibilities and found it suitable for Class III restorations. Great care had to be taken in using the material, however, because it hardened very slowly and during this stage was vulnerable to water. The advent of ASPA II eased this problem. Its set was still sluggish by present standards and the use of the rather opaque G-200 glass, because it is very high in fluoride, resulted in poor aesthetic properties. But in other respects it was a fine material and its physical properties have only recently been equalled. The disadvantage for general practice was that its

*G-200 is a designation of the Laboratory of the Government Chemist (LGC) (London).
†ASPA is an acronym for aluminosilicate polyacrylates, a series of experimental glass-ionomer cements developed by the LGC.

liquid tended to gel (Crisp et al., 1975a). This problem was solved by Crisp and Wilson, who developed a copolymer of acrylic and itaconic acid that did not gel at high (50%) concentrations in aqueous solution (Crisp et al., 1975a; Crisp and Wilson, 1977). However, this cement, ASPA IV, was inferior to ASPA II in other properties.

Meanwhile, McLean and Wilson (1974), pursuing studies on applications for the adhesive properties of glass-ionomer cements, used the cement for fissure sealing and filling. It had the obvious advantages of truly bonding to enamel and releasing fluoride. Sadly, this idea has not prospered and composite resins, which have neither of these advantages, have dominated the field. McLean and Wilson (1977c) also found that the material was ideal for the restoration of Class V erosion lesions. These call for an adhesive filling, to avoid the clinically doubtful technique of extending such cavities by mechanical preparation. Good clinical results were obtained. In three years ASPA X, with excellent translucency, was developed (Crisp et al., 1979). The need for a luting version became pressing, and in 1977 a fine-grain version, ASPA IVa, was developed for the purpose (Wilson et al., 1977).

Also in 1977, a review of the state-of-the-art and forecast of future clinical developments was made by McLean and Wilson in three papers (1977a, 1977b, 1977c). In retrospect, these papers were prophetic and anticipated many of the subsequent clinical developments. The authors described a variety of clinical applications; in addition to the applications already mentioned, they suggested use in pediatric dentistry and as a liner in composite-resin/ionomer laminates, a technique which has only recently been generally adopted. Perhaps only tunnel preparations were omitted from this list, although the concept of minimal cavity preparations was clearly enunciated. Unfortunately, the findings of these papers, which are still valid today, were ignored for many years and have only recently been rediscovered.

Later development

In a search for further improvement it was realized that the best way to solve the problems associated with the instability of poly(acrylic acid) solutions lay not in developing special copolymers, which although stable in water might not yield the best cements, but in an alternative approach described many years before by Wilson and Kent (1973). These authors reported the use of poly(acrylic acid) in dry powder form blended with the glass powder. The cement was formed by mixing this powder with water or tartaric acid solutions. This approach was re-examined in greater depth and resulted in the development of ASPA V (Prosser et al., 1984).

A number of problems were solved. For example, even ASPA IVa, a luting cement with a low-viscosity polyacid liquid, lacked the mobility of the traditional zinc phosphate cement. But ASPA Va, a water-hardening luting agent, proved to have the mixing qualities and mobility of the zinc phospate cement. Another advantage is that higher molecular weight polyacids can be used at higher concentrations, which results in cements of higher strength.

The original 1977 idea of using a composite-resin/ionomer laminate was revived in a modified form (McLean et al., 1985). In the improved technique the glass-ionomer cement, as well as the enamel, was etched—a double-etch technique, in effect. Thus, the composite resin was attached, micromechanically, to both tooth enamel and to the glass-ionomer cement. It was also bonded indirectly to dentine.

The concept of minimal cavity preparations has undergone steady development over the years. The first application of this concept was the simple opening up of early Class I carious lesions (McLean and Wilson, 1974). In 1980, McLean proposed treating early approximal lesions by a minimal-preparation technique involving a buccal or lateral marginal ridge approach (McLean, 1980). This idea has been extended using "tunnel" preparations for Class II carious lesions (Hunt, 1984; Knight, 1984; McLean, 1986). The object of this approach is to remove caries but at the same time preserve the maximum amount of surface enamel. The reasoning behind this technique is that the glass-ionomer core bonds the enamel shell together, preventing its fracture. This technique has been fully described by Hunt (1984) and McLean (1987).

Attempts to improve the strength of glass-ionomer cement by incorporating metallic oxide and metal alloy fillers have been reported by Sced and Wilson (1980) and Simmons (1983). Although of high flexural strength, their resistance to wear is suspect. A major advance in improving wear resistance was made by McLean and Gasser (1985), who fused silver particles onto the ionomer glass, giving the cement radio-opacity, burnishability, and a smoother surface, with concomitant advantages. Moore et al., (1985) have reported that resistance to abrasion is improved considerably. These new cermet cements have been subsequently developed for clinical use (McLean, 1986). Two excellent reviews of the glass-ionomer cement have recently appeared: Mount (1984) and Walls (1986).

The future

The glass-ionomer cement has come a long way since it was first introduced. Its properties have improved, and there are now many versions for various applications. Can it be developed still further? Although stronger and more aesthetic materials with improved handling characteristics are now available, lack of toughness remains a problem. There are problems in finishing, for current materials do not have the amalgamlike, carvable stage during setting that the first glass-ionomer cement, ASPA I, had. Nor have the problems of early moisture contamination and desiccation been entirely solved. Varnishing of the restoration is still required. Most of these problems will be overcome as development proceeds. The most intractable problem is likely to be lack of strength and toughness.

References

Buonocore, M.G. (1955) Simple method of increasing the adhesion of acrylic filling materials to enamel surfaces. J. Dent. Res. 34:849–853.

Crisp, S., and Wilson, A.D. (1977) Polycarboxylate cements. Br. Pat. 1,484,454, August 1973.

Crisp, S., Abel, G., and Wilson, A.D. (1979) The quantitative measurement of the opacity of aesthetic dental filling materials. J. Dent. Res. 58:1585–1596.

Crisp, S., Lewis, B.G., and Wilson, A.D. (1975a) Gelation of polyacrylic acid aqueous solutions and the measurement of viscosity. J. Dent. Res. 54:1173–1175.

Crisp, S., Ferner, A.J., Lewis, B.G., and Wilson, A.D. (1975b) Properties of improved glass ionomer cement formulations. J. Dent. 3:125–130.

Doubleday, F.N. (1920) The translucent filling cement. Dent. Record 40:551–562.

Hunt, P.R. (1984) A modified Class II cavity preparation for glass ionomer restorative materials. Quintessence Int. 15:1011–1018.

Jonck, L.M. (1986) Personal communication.

Kent, B.E., Lewis, B.G., and Wilson, A.D. (1973) The properties of a glass ionomer cement. Br. Dent. J. 135:322–326.

Kent, B.E., Lewis, B.G., and Wilson, A.D. (1979) Glass ionomer cement formulations. I. The preparation of novel fluoroaluminosilicate glasses high in fluorine. J. Dent. Res. 58:1607–1619.

Knight, G.M. (1984) The use of adhesive materials in the conservative restoration of selected posterior teeth. Aust. Dent. J. 29:324–331.

McLean, J.W. (1980) Aesthetics in restorative dentistry: The challenge for the future. Br. Dent. J. 149:368–373.

McLean, J.W. (1986) New concepts in cosmetic dentistry using glass-ionomer cements and composites. J. Calif. Dent. Assoc. April: 20–27.

McLean, J.W. (1987) Limitations of posterior composite resins and extending their use with glass ionomer cements. Quintessence Int. 18:517–529.

McLean, J.W., and Gasser, O. (1985) Glass-cermet cements. Quintessence Int. 16:333–343.

McLean, J.W., and Wilson, A.D. (1974) Fissure sealing and filling with an adhesive glass-ionomer cement. Br. Dent. J. 136:269–276.

McLean, J.W., and Wilson, A.D. (1977a) The clinical development of the glass-ionomer cement. I. Formulations and properties. Aust. Dent. J. 22:31–36.

McLean, J.W., and Wilson, A.D. (1977b) The clinical development of the glass-ionomer cement. II. Some clinical applications. Aust. Dent. J. 22:120–127.

McLean, J.W., and Wilson, A.D. (1977c) The clinical development of the glass-ionomer cement. III. The erosion lesion. Aust. Dent. J. 22:190–195.

McLean, J.W., Wilson, A.D., and Prosser, H.J. (1984) Development and use of water-hardening glass-ionomer luting cements. J. Prosthet. Dent. 52:175–181.

McLean, J.W., Powis, D.R., Prosser, H.J., and Wilson, A.D. (1985) The use of glass-ionomer cements in bonding composite resins to dentine. Br. Dent. J. 158:410–414.

Moore, B.K., Swartz, M.L., and Phillips, R.W. (1985) Abrasion resistance of metal reinforced glass-ionomer cements. J. Dent. Res. 64:371(abstr. 1766).

Mount, G.J. (1984) Glass ionomer cements: Clinical considerations. chapt. 20A In J. W. Clark (ed.) Clinical Dentistry. Philadelphia: Harper & Row.

Mount, G.J., and Makinson, O.F. (1978) Clinical characteristics of a glass-ionomer cement. Br. Dent. J. 145:67–71.

Prosser, H.J., Powis, D.R., Bryant, P., and Wilson, A.D. (1984) The characterisation of glass-ionomer cements. 7. The physical properties of current materials. J. Dent. 12:231–240.

Sced, I.R., and Wilson, A.D. (1980) Poly(carboxylic acid) hardenable compositions. Br. Pat. Appl. GB 2,028, 855A, 1978.

Simmons, J.J. (1983) The miracle mixture glass ionomer and alloy powder. Texas Dent. J. October (10) 6–12.

Smith, D.C. (1968) A new dental cement. Br. Dent. J. 125:381–384.

Walls, A.W.G. (1986) Glass polyalkenoate (glass-ionomer) cements: A review. J. Dent. 14:231–246.

Wilson, A.D. (1968) Dental silicate cements. VII. Alternative liquid cement formers. J. Dent. Res. 47:1133–1136.

Wilson, A.D. (1978) The chemistry of dental cements. Chem. Soc. Rev. 77:265–296.

Wilson, A.D., and Crisp, S. (1976) Poly(carboxylate) cement. Br. Pat. 1,422,337, April 1972.

Wilson, A.D., and Kent, B.E. (1971) The glass-ionomer cement: A new translucent dental filling material. J. Appl. Chem. Biotechnol. 21:313.

Wilson, A.D., and Kent, B.E. (1972) A new translucent cement for dentistry: The glass ionomer cement. Br. Dent. J. 132:133–135.

Wilson, A.D., and Kent, B.E. (1973) Surgical cement. Br. Pat. 1,316,129, December 1969.

Wilson, A.D., Crisp, S., and Ferner, A.J. (1976) Reaction in glass-ionomer cements. IV. Effect of chelating co-monomers J. Dent. Res. 55:489–495.

Wilson, A.D., Crisp, S., Lewis, B.G., and McLean, J.W. (1977) Experimental luting agents based on the glass-ionomer cements. Br. Dent. J. 142:117–122.

Wilson, A.D., Kent, B.E., Clinton, D., and Miller, R.P. (1972) The formation and microstructure of dental silicate cements. J. Mater. Sci. 7:220–238.

Wygant, J.F. (1958) Cementitious bonding in ceramic fabrication. pp. 171–188 In W.D. Kingery (ed.) Ceramic Fabrication Processes. Cambridge, Mass.: MIT Press.

Chapter 2

Composition

The compositions of glass-ionomer cements are complex and varied. No two commercial examples are chemically identical, and they may even differ qualitatively. Nevertheless, there are several chemical features common to all.

Glass-ionomer cement is an acid-base reaction cement as defined by Wilson (1978) and Wygant (1958). This class of cement sets, as the name implies, as a result of a reaction between an acid and a base; the product of the reaction, a hydrogel salt, acts as a binding matrix. A simple example of an acid-base reaction cement used in dentistry is the traditional zinc phosphate cement. The base, powdered zinc oxide, and the acid, an aqueous solution of phosphoric acid, combine to form a zinc phosphate matrix. Excess zinc oxide powder acts as the filler. Such a simple system allows no variation in the basic chemical formulation, so that the development potential of the material is limited. Indeed, since the system was optimized—at the turn of the century—no further development has taken place.

The glass-ionomer cement is much more complex and varied in nature. The basic component is a calcium aluminosilicate glass containing fluoride. The compositional range of useful glasses is wide. Many hundreds of glasses have been prepared in the U.K.'s Laboratory of the Government Chemist by A.D. Wilson and his coworkers.

The acid is a polyelectrolyte, which is a homopolymer or copolymer of unsaturated carboxylic acids known scientifically as alkenoic acids. Many are known, but poly(acrylic acid) is the one most commonly used.

Since both glasses and polyelectrolytes are chemically diverse materials, the number of possible combinations of the two is immense. The materials scientist has much scope when devising new formulations for specific applications.

Glasses

The composition of the glass can be varied greatly, although those based on ion-leachable calcium aluminosilicates are the only ones, so far, to have found practical applications (Wilson and Kent, 1973; Kent et al., 1979; Wilson et al., 1980). Ionomer glasses used in dentistry also contain fluoride. The composition of the original ionomer glass, G-200, is given in Table 2-1.

Fluoride is an essential constituent of glass-ionomer dental cements. It lowers the temperature of fusion, improves the working characteristics of the cement paste, increases markedly the strength of the set cement, in moderate amounts enhances translucency, and contributes to

Table 2-1 Chemical composition of the original ionomer glass, G-200*

Species	Composition(%)
SiO_2	30.1
Al_2O_3	19.9
AlF_3	2.6
CaF_2	34.5
NaF	3.7
$AlPO_4$	10.0

*Modified from Barry et al. (1979).

the therapeutic value of the cement by releasing fluoride over a prolonged period.

The ionomer glasses are unusual ones, for unlike most silicate glasses they are decomposed by acids—an essential property, as we shall see, for cement formation. This property arises because the glasses contain aluminium. Aluminium can enter the silica network, replacing silicon, thus conferring a negative charge on the network, which becomes basic and susceptible to attack by hydrogen ions from the acid.

The three essential constituents of dental ionomer glasses are silica (SiO_2), alumina (Al_2O_3), and calcium fluoride, or fluorite (CaF_2). When fused together they form a glass suitable for cement formation. In practice other components, such as cryolite and aluminium phosphate, are added, for reasons that will be given later.

The types of calcium fluoroaluminosilicate glasses that may be employed in glass-ionomer cement formulations are listed below in order of increasing complexity:

SiO_2-Al_2O_3-CaF_2
SiO_2-Al_2O_3-CaF_2-$AlPO_4$
SiO_2-Al_2O_3-CaF_2-$AlPO_4$-Na_3AlF_6

Glasses are prepared by fusing the components between 1,100°C and 1,500°C (the exact temperature of fusion depends on the chemical makeup of the fusion mixture), then pouring the melt onto a metal plate or into water. The glass is then ground to a fine powder (maximum particle size 50 μm for restorative cements and 20 μm for luting cements) for mixing with the polyacid. The finer the particle size the more rapid the setting and the stronger the cement will be.

For the sake of simplicity, we will discuss only the simple three-component SiO_2-Al_2O_3-CaF_2 system. The triangular compositional diagram in Fig. 2-1 shows that the visual appearance of the glass—that is, whether it is clear, opal, or opaque—depends on its chemical composition. Glasses high in silica (greater than 40%) are transparent, whereas glasses high in calcium fluoride or alumina are opaque (Figs. 2-1 and 2-2). This opaqueness arises from the presence of dispersed crystalline phases of fluorite or corundum; such a composition might better be described as a glass ceramic rather than a glass.

Cement formation is also related to glass composition (Fig. 2-3). The Al_2O_3/SiO_2 ratio of the glass is crucial, and is required to be 1:2 or more by mass for cement formation (Wilson et al., 1980; Kent et al., 1979). Only then is there sufficient replacement of silicon by aluminium to render the network susceptible to acid attack. Further increases in the Al_2O_3/SiO_2 ratio give rise to glasses ever more basic and reactive, with corresponding reductions in the setting times of the cements. However, a limit is reached when the Al_2O_3/SiO_2 ratio reaches 0.75:1.0 by mass (Fig. 2-3). Subsequent increases in this ratio have little effect on setting time—if anything, they prolong it slightly. But the nature of the glass itself changes, and it goes from

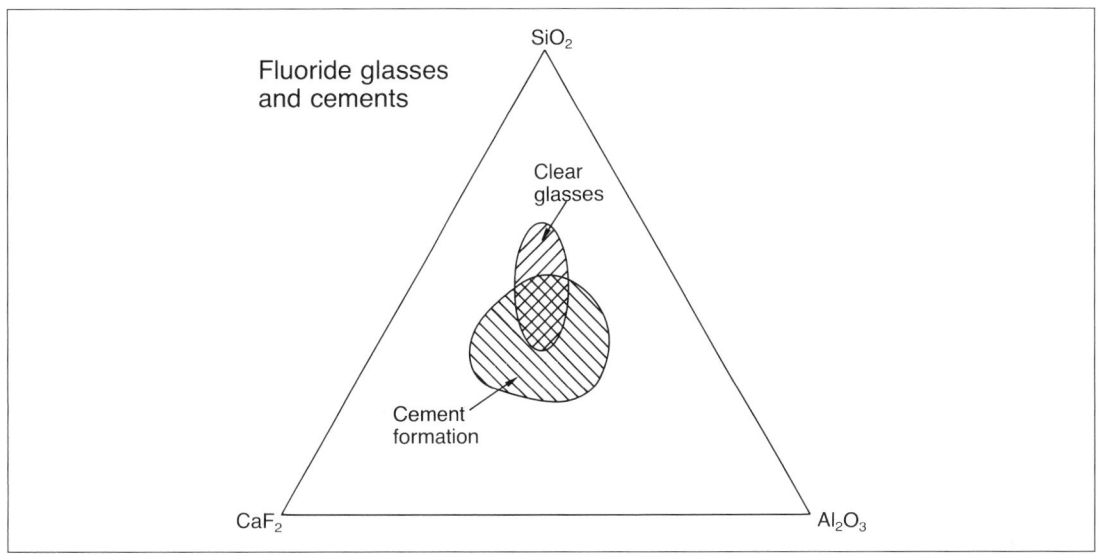

Fig. 2-1 Compositional diagram of the basic SiO_2-Al_2O_3-CaF_2 glasses showing areas of cement formation.

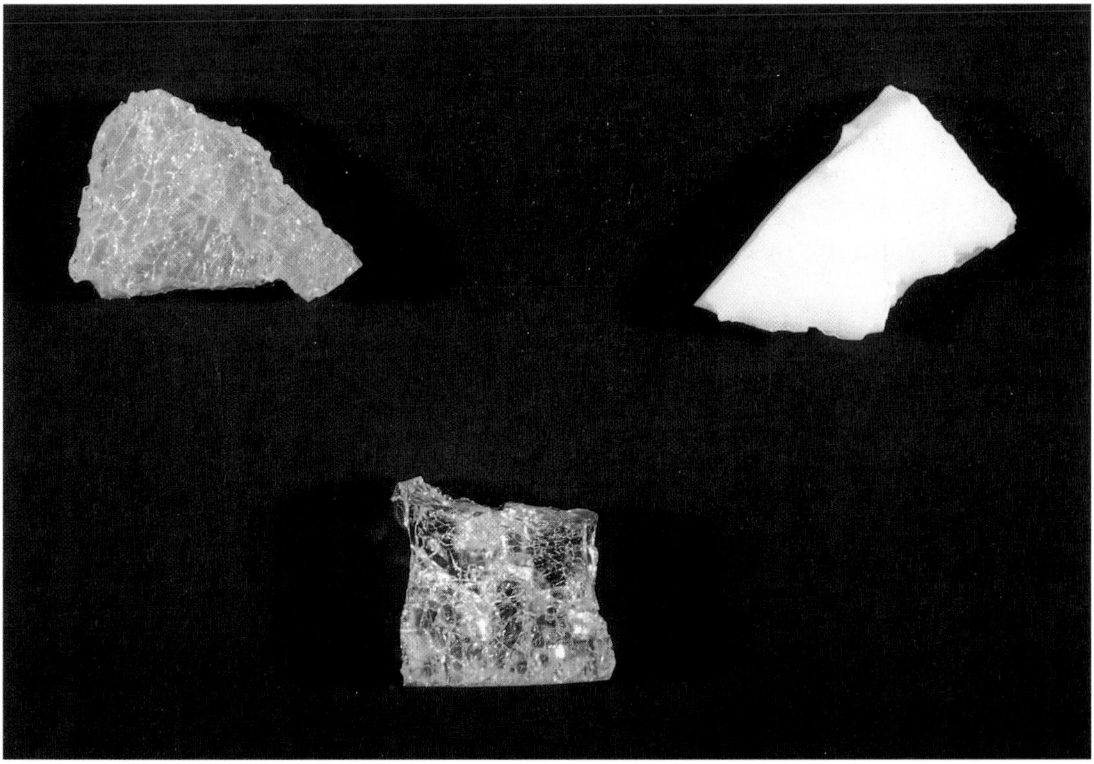

Fig. 2-2 Appearance of ionomer glasses. *(top left)* Opal; *(top right)* opaque; *(bottom)* clear.

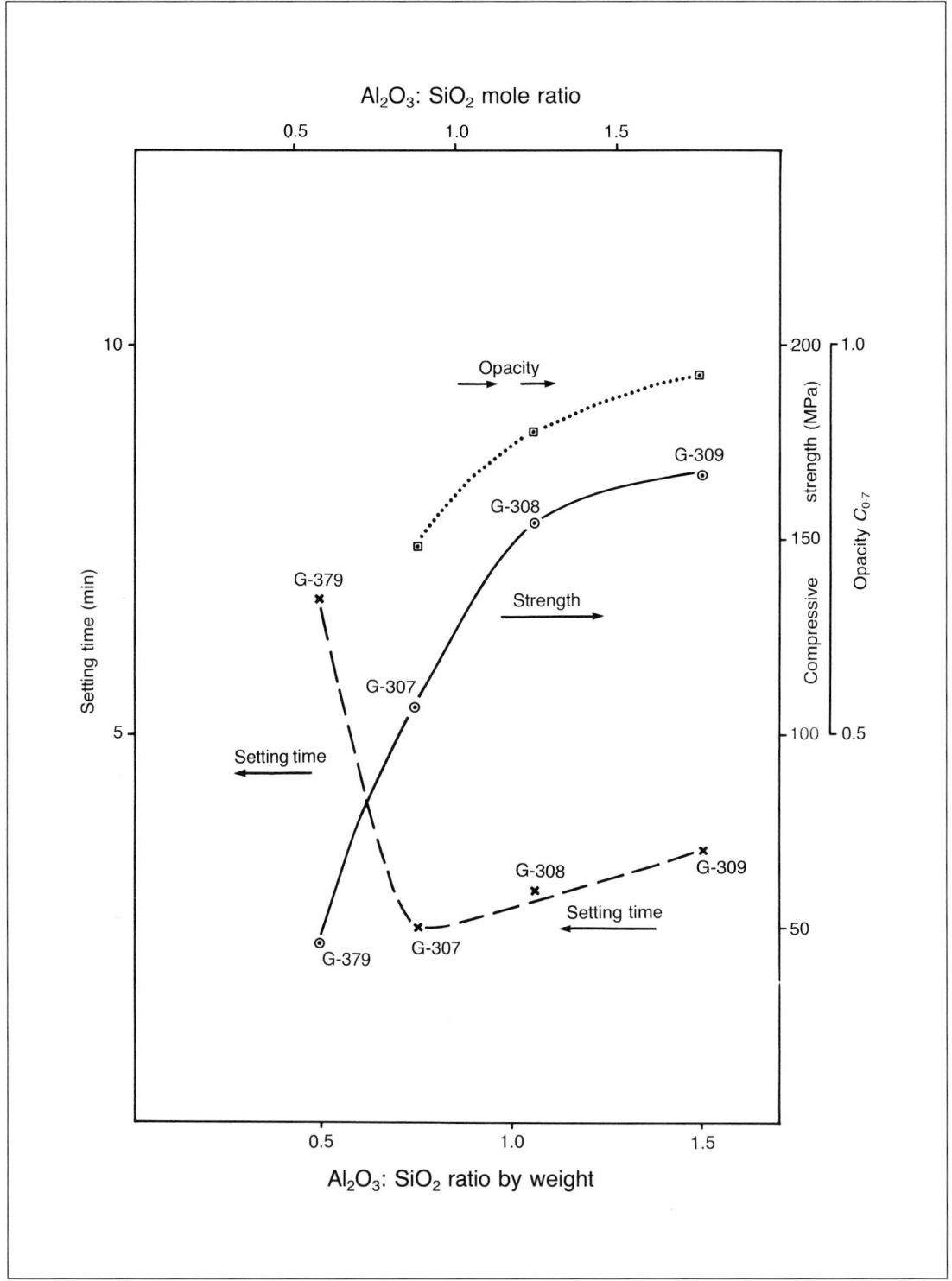

Fig. 2-3 Effect of the Al₂O₃/SIO₂ mass ratio in glasses (generic composition: xSIO₂, 100Al₂O₃, 100CaF₂) on glass appearance and cement properties: setting time, composite strength, and opacity.

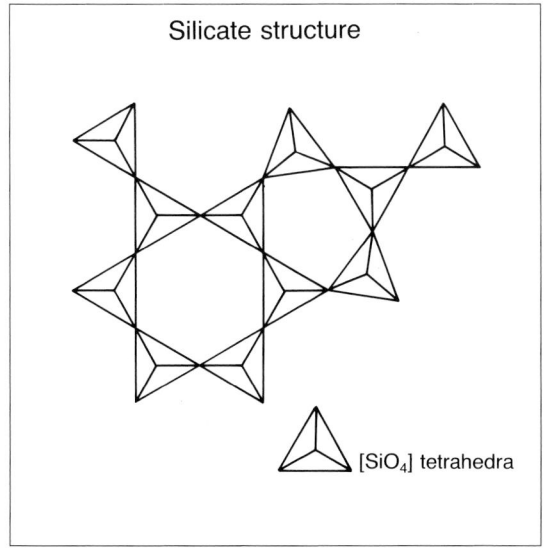

Fig. 2-4a Structure of silica—a neutral network.

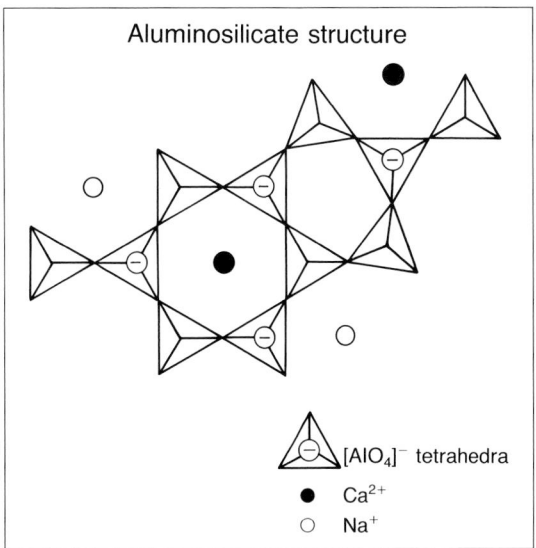

Fig. 2-4b Structure of an aluminosilicate—an electrically charged network.

being clear to becoming opaque as corundum separates out from the glass structure.

Setting time and opacity are not the only properties affected by the alumina/silica ratio: compressive strength increases with increasing alumina content (Fig. 2-3). But, although strength may be increased by these means it is achieved at the expense of translucency.

Why does the cement-forming propensity of dental ionomer glasses derive from their decomposition in the presence of acids? The reason lies in the structure of the glass. A silica glass is a highly crosslinked network of connected silicon and oxygen atoms (Fig. 2-4a). It does not carry an electric charge, and is impervious to acid attack. By contrast, the ionomer glass is an ionic polymer—the network is similar to that of silica, but it contains negative sites because aluminium has partly replaced silicon in the glass network (Fig. 2-4b). These negative sites are vulnerable to attack by the positive hydrogen ions of the acid. If

there are enough aluminium atoms in the network, all of the connecting links in the network will be broken down and the glass will be completely decomposed (Fig. 2-5). Such a glass has cement-forming potential.

From this discussion it is apparent that the Al_2O_3/SiO_2 ratio of the glass is crucial as it determines whether the glass network will break down at all when exposed to acids, and the rate at which the breakdown occurs.

Glasses used in practice are generally more complex than the simple three-component systems we have described. And the fluxing action of calcium fluoride is generally supplemented by the addition of cryolite (Na_3AlF_6). This flux reduces the temperature at which the glass will fuse and increases the translucency of the set cement. Aluminium phosphate is also often included in the glass fusion mixtures; it too improves translucency and apparently adds body to the cement paste.

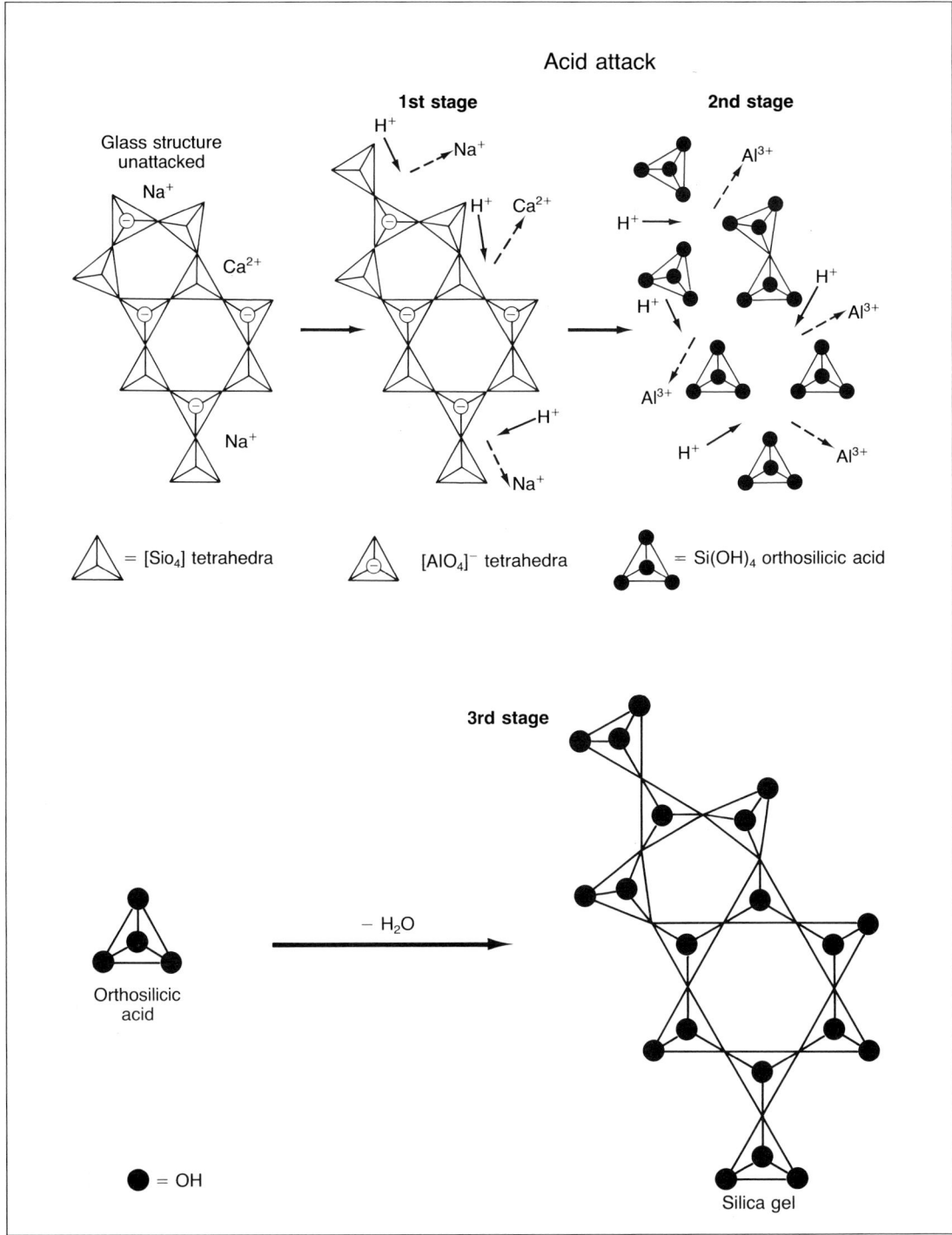

Fig. 2-5 Decomposition of an aluminosilicate by acids. *(1st stage)* Hydrogen ions attack the network-dwelling ions, Ca^{2+} and Na^+. *(2nd stage)* Hydrogen ions attack the charged aluminosilicate network itself, destroying the glass network and liberating aluminium ions. *(3rd stage)* Silicic acid formed condenses to form silica gel.

Glass structure

Little attention has been paid in the literature to the structure of ionomer glasses. Research appears to be confined to the studies of Barry and coworkers (1979). The reader is also referred to an earlier, very comprehensive study by Wilson and coworkers (1972) on the similar dental silicate cement glasses.

The glass studied by Barry et al. was G-200, the basis of the first practical glass-ionomer cement, but not typical of present-day ionomer glasses. The G-200 contains phase-separated glass droplets of complex structure, as well as massive inclusions of fluorite (Fig. 2-6). More recently, unpublished studies (Hill and Wilson, 1986) indicate that other opal glasses, while not containing inclusions of fluorite, do contain droplets similar to those in G-200. These phase-separated droplets are calcium-rich (compared with the continuous-phase) and contain a crystalline core of calcium and fluoride surrounded by an amorphous phase rich in calcium but containing some aluminium and silicon (Fig. 2-7). This amor-

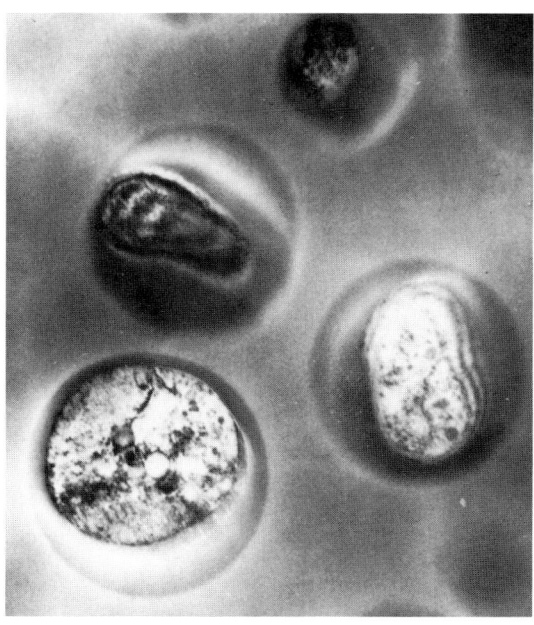

Fig. 2-6 Micrograph of an opal aluminosilicate glass showing phase-separated droplets. Reprinted with permission from Barry et al. (1979).

phous phase is selectively leached by acids. Thus, calcium is preferentially leached from the glass, as will be discussed in chapter 3.

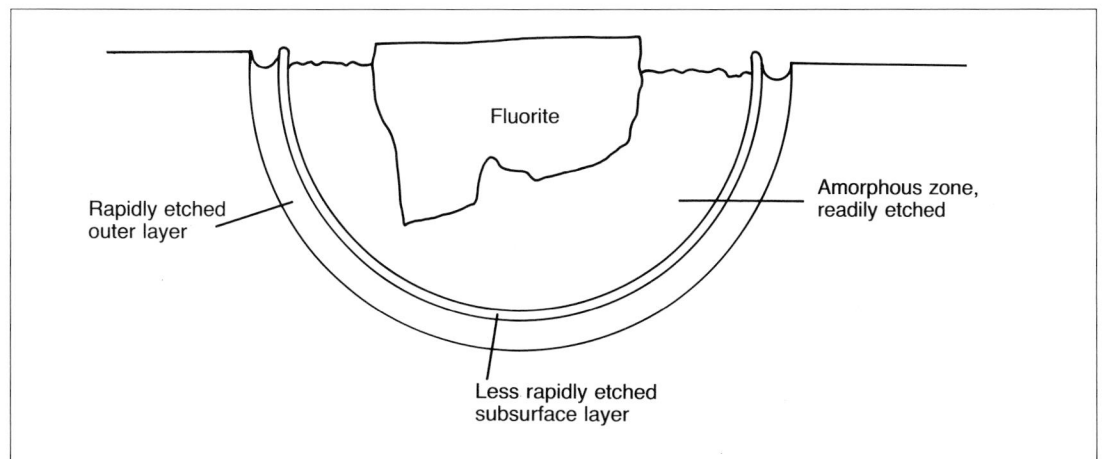

Fluorite

Rapidly etched outer layer

Amorphous zone, readily etched

Less rapidly etched subsurface layer

Fig. 2-7 Structure of a phase-separated droplet. Reprinted with permission from Barry et al. (1972).

Treatment of glasses

Washing glasses with mineral or organic acids has been advocated in order to reduce the concentration of calcium at the surface of phase-separated droplets in the glass. This process reduces the amount of calcium extracted during the early stages of the reaction, and so prolongs working time (Schmitt et al., 1981a).

Effect of particle size on cement properties

From the previous discussion it can be seen that glass composition has a considerable effect on cement properties. Indeed, for a glass to have cement-forming properties at all, it must fulfill certain basic requirements. Glass composition affects working characteristics, setting time, resistance to erosion, aesthetics, and cement strength. In addition, the presence of phase-separated droplets will affect both cement translucency and strength.

Another important factor is the particle size of the glass powder. It is obvious that, other things being equal, the finer the particle size (i.e., the greater the specific surface of the powder), the faster the setting reaction will be. Data are not available for the glass-ionomer cements, but the research of Kent and Wilson (1971), who studied the effect of particle size on dental silicate cement properties, confirms this observation. These researchers also found that, other things being equal, fine-grained glasses produced the strongest cements. To achieve the film thickness of 20 μm demanded of a luting agent, a fine-grained glass has to be used (Wilson et al., 1977b). The tendency over the years has been for finer-grained powders to be used in restorative materials.

Variations on the basic glass composition

Calcium may be replaced wholly by strontium which is another alkaline earth metal, and partly by barium, also an alkaline earth metal, or lanthanum, a rare earth metal, to give a radio-opaque glass. Strontium, which has a similar ionic radius to that of calcium ($Sr^{2+} = 1.13$Å, $Ca^{2+} = 0.99$Å), can replace calcium without disrupting the glass structure, and so does not cause loss of translucency. The same is not true of barium and lanthanum, which have significantly greater ionic radii than calcium does ($La^{3+} = 1.35$Å, $Ba^{2+} = 1.35$Å).

Disperse-phase glasses

Glasses may be modified by phase separation. Wilson and coworkers (1980) observed that clear glasses yielded weaker cements than glasses containing droplets of a disperse phase. This observation led Prosser and coworkers (1986) to increase deliberately the amount of the disperse phase in a glass; they found that when this was done the flexural strength of the cements was increased (Table 2-2, Fig. 2-8). Suitable disperse phases were found to be corundum, rutile (TiO_2), baddeleyite (ZrO_2), and tieilite (Al_2TiO_5). Baddeleyite has been found in one commercial core material.

Fibre reinforcement

The incorporation of alumina fibres and other fibres (Sced and Wilson, 1980) has been used to improve flexural strength of glass-ionomer cements—50 MPa can be obtained (Table 2-3, Fig. 2-9)—but apparently abrasion resistance is poor.

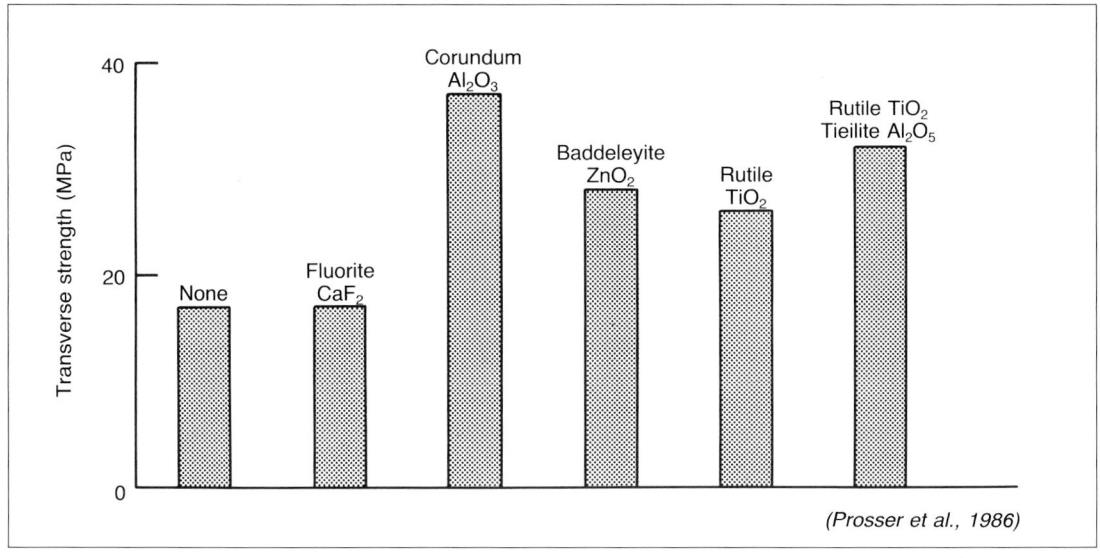

Fig. 2-8 Effect of disperse phase in glasses on the flexural strength of glass-ionomer cements.

Table 2-2 Effect of phase-separated crystallites on cement strength*

Glass	Phase-separated crystallites	Flexural strength (MPa)
G-228	None	21
G-309	Fluorite (CaF$_2$) Corundum (Al$_2$O$_3$)	33
G-385	Rutile (TiO$_2$) Tieilite (Al$_2$TiO$_5$)	30
G-381	Baddeleyite (ZrO$_2$)	28

*Modified from Prosser et al. (1986).

Table 2-3 Effect of reinforcing fillers on flexural strength of glass-ionomer cements*

Filler	Filler/ glass ratio (by mass)	Flexural strength (MPa)
None	—	10
Silica fibre	1:2	26
Glass fibre	1:2	21
G-200 glass fibre	1.4:1	30
Carbon fibre	1:4	53
Alumina fibre	1:3	44
Ag$_3$Sn	4.5:1	40
Ag$_3$Sn$_5$	4.5:1	13

*Glass-ionomer cement, De Trey Chem-Fil, Dentsply International Inc., Weybridge, England, and York, Pa. Modified from Sced and Wilson (1980).

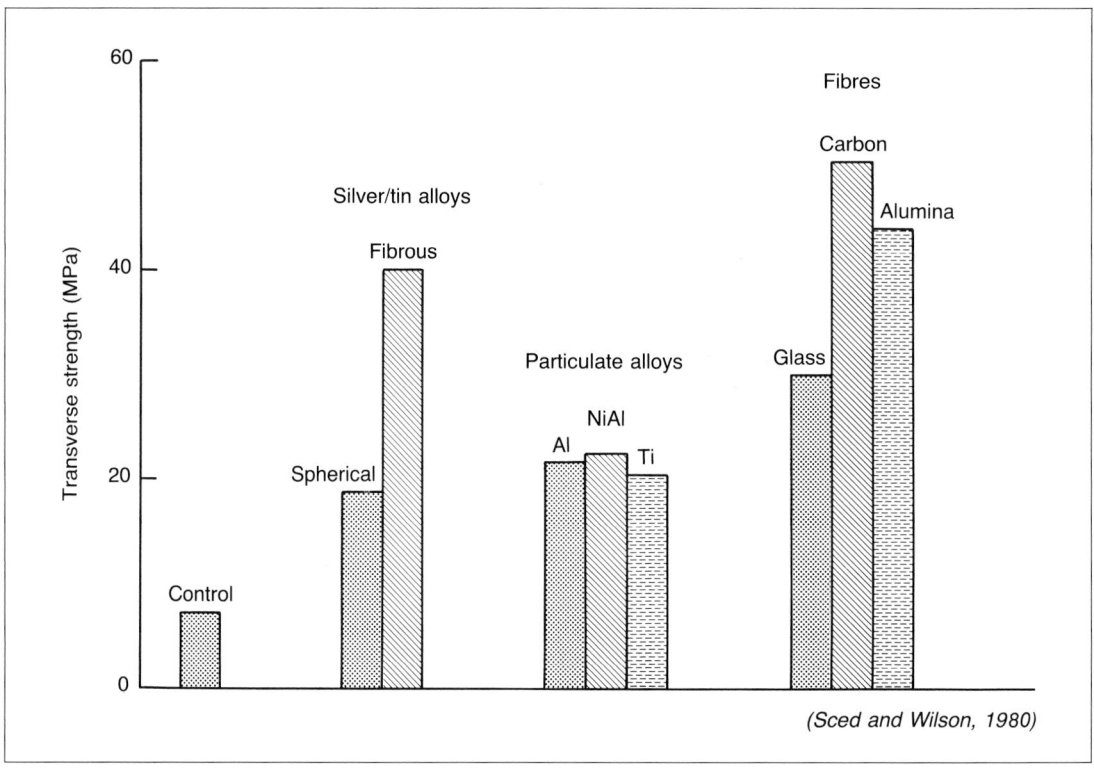

Fig. 2-9 Effect of filler reinforcement on the flexural strength of glass-ionomer cements.

Metallic inclusions

Sced and Wilson (1980) found that the amalgam alloys could be incorporated into glass-ionomer cements and that these served to increase the flexural strength. These systems have been used clinically by Simmons (1983) and are available commercially.* However, their aesthetics are poor and they do not take burnish. Their resistance to abrasion is also less than that of regular glass-ionomer cements (Moore et al., 1985).

*Miracle Mix, G-C International Corp., Tokyo, and Scotts-dale, Ariz.

Cermet-ionomer cements

In an attempt to improve the abrasion resistance and strength of glass-ionomer cements, McLean and Gasser (1985) developed the cermet-ionomer cements. These cements, unlike simple mixtures of alloy particles or metal fibres, contain glass-metal powders sintered to high density that can be made to react with poly-acids to form a cement. Ion-leachable calcium fluoroaluminosilicate glasses are used in the preparation of the glass powder. The set cement can be burnished or polished to produce a metal finish (Fig. 2-10a), but the surface will not be comparable to the typical Beilby veneer of metals (Fig. 2-10b).

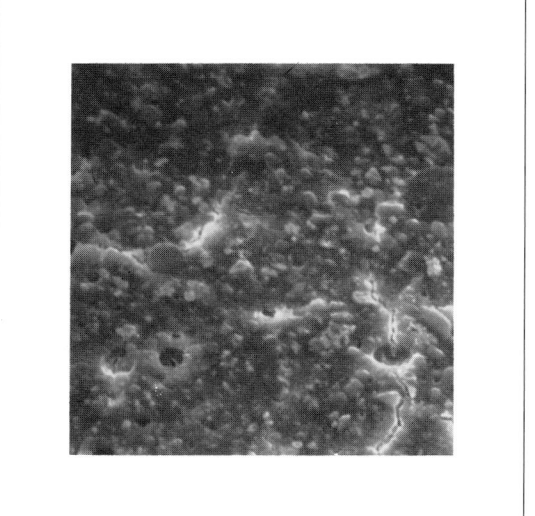

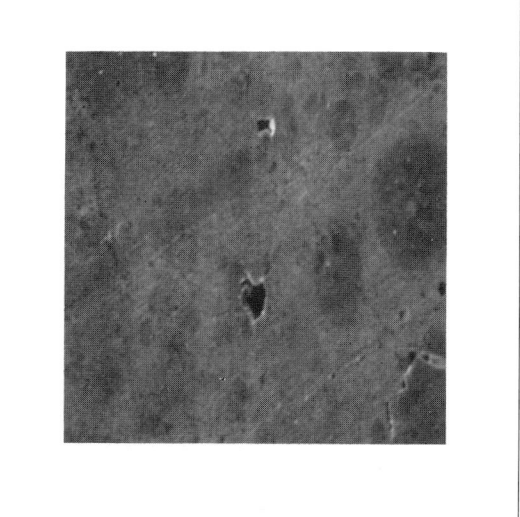

Fig. 2-10a Electronmicrograph of a polished surface of silver-cermet-ionomer cement. Slight cracking is due to dehydration during specimen preparation. Note the small amount of porosity with the silver particles embedded firmly in the glass surface after polishing (original magnification × 1,400). Courtesy of N. Sarker, Ph.D., Louisiana State University Medical Center.

Fig. 2-10b Electronmicrograph of a polished surface of amalgam alloy (original magnification × 1,400).

Any of the precious metals well known in dentistry may be used in the preparation of these cements, but gold and silver are the most suitable. The glass-metal powder is compressed in a pelletizer; pelletizing is preferably carried out at high pressures in a hydraulic press (usually at pressures above 300 MPa). It is favourable to evacuate the pelleting chamber during pelletizing at pressures around 100 MPa. The compressed pellets are then fused at around 800°C: The sintered metal-glass composite, when ground to a fine powder, retains its characteristics because the metal powder remains firmly bonded in the glass (Fig. 2-11). It is interesting to note that the ground powder is more rounded than a conventionally ground glass powder, which imparts to the cement the excellent handling properties of high packing density and low porosity.

At present a commercial cermet-ionomer cement is available that contains fine silver powder particles of less than 3.5 μm in size. Colour has also been improved by the addition of up to 5% titanium dioxide.

Physical properties

By fusing silver powder into the glass, very strong bonding of the metal has been achieved, allowing the surface to be burnished (Fig. 2-12), which in turn has dramatically improved abrasion resistance. McKinney and coworkers

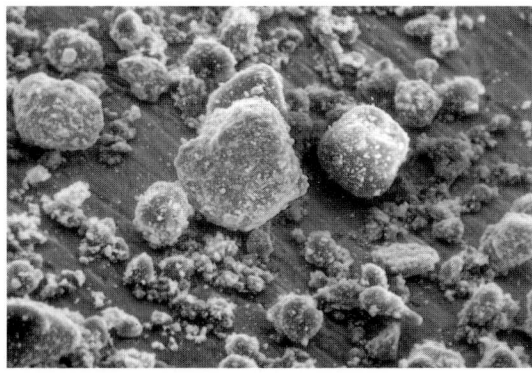

Fig. 2-11 Surface of cermet silver particles fused to glass, showing the rounding of particles after grinding and the silver powder firmly attached to the glass surface (original magnification × 400).

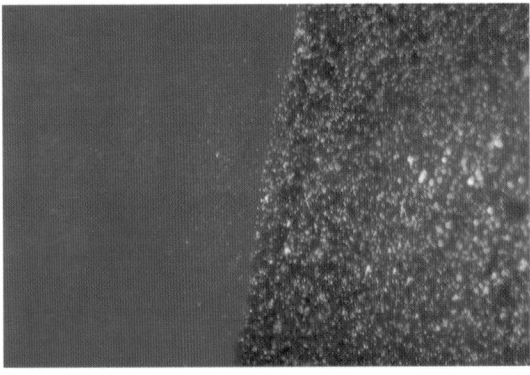

Fig. 2-12 Restoration of a Ketac-Silver cermet cement showing close adaptation to enamel walls and the burnished surface produced by flow of the silver particles (original magnification × 40).

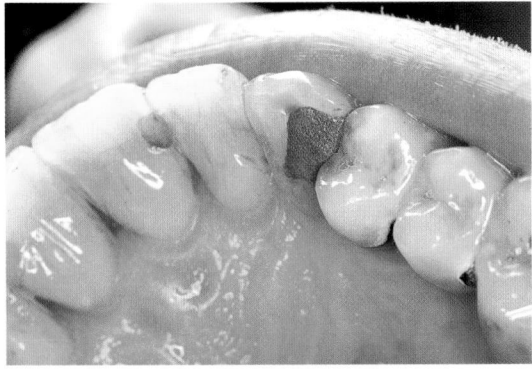

Fig. 2-13a Gold-cermet-ionomer cement on distal surface of tooth 23 showing no wear during disclusion. Note failure of the composite resin on the distal surface of tooth 21.

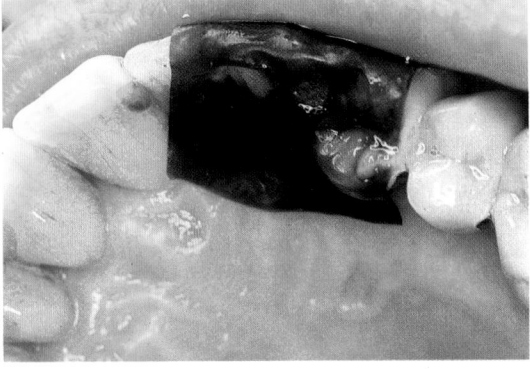

Fig. 2-13b Surface of a gold-cermet-ionomer cement on tooth 23 showing contact with the mandibular canine through the occlusal indicator wax.

(1986) considered that the silver has a lubricating effect on the surface, and McLean and Gasser (1985) suggested that the sintered metal powder was lowering the coefficient of friction. This would appear to be borne out by clinical trials. A gold-cermet restoration is shown in Fig. 2-13a, where it may be seen that after six years the cermet surface is still acting as a discluding mechanism on the canine and no load has been transferred to the adjoining enamel (Fig. 2-13b). The flexural strength of the cermet-cements is marginally better than the best glass-ionomer cements but as yet cannot be compared in strength to composite resins and amalgam alloys. They are therefore unsuitable for use in a high-stress-bearing cavity such as a large Class II lesion.

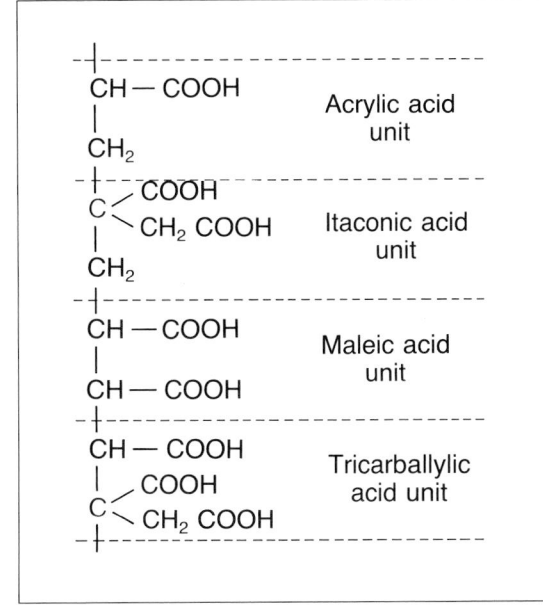

Fig. 2-14 Structure of a poly(alkenoic acid). The drawing shows various types of carboxylic acid units used in ionomer polyacids.

Polyelectrolytes

Polyelectrolytes are interesting substances, which, as their name implies, are both electrolytes and polymers. The notion that polymers are soluble in water is an unusual one, but such substances are of considerable biological importance.

The polyelectrolytes used in glass-ionomer cements can be described as poly(alkenoic acid)s; indeed, the International Organization for Standardization name for glass-ionomer cement that contains polyelectrolytes is Glass Polyalkenoate Cement. These polyacids include the homopolymers or copolymers of unsaturated mono-, di-, and tri-carboxylic acids, particularly those of acrylic acid (Crisp et al., 1980b). The more important carboxylic acids in the ionomer system include acrylic acid, maleic acid, and itaconic acid. The numbers of homopoly-

mers and copolymers that can be built from these three structural units of different configurations and molecular weights is considerable.

Examples are depicted in Fig. 2-14. The polyacid may be either in the form of a concentrated aqueous solution (40% to 50% by mass) or blended dry with the glass powder when the system is activated by mixing with either water or an aqueous solution of tartaric acid (McLean et al., 1984).

The most important of the polyacids used to date have been the poly(acrylic acid)s themselves, copolymers of acrylic and itaconic acids (Crisp et al., 1980b), and copolymers of acrylic and maleic acids (Schmitt et al., 1981b). There are differences in functionality and acid strength between these polyacids. Poly(maleic acid) contains twice as many carboxyl groups as poly(acrylic acid) and is a stronger acid. It would be ex-

Table 2-4 Composition of experimental LGC/ASPA cements

Cement	Class	Type	Powder	Liquid
ASPA I	Conventional	Filling	G-200	50% PA-1
ASPA II	Conventional	Filling	G-200	47.5% PA-1, 5% TTA
ASPA III	Conventional	Filling	G-200	45.0% PA-1, 5% TTA, 5% CH_3OH
ASPA IV	Conventional	Filling	G-200	47.5% PA-48, 5% TTA
ASPA IVa	Conventional	Luting	G-200a	47.5% PA-48, 5% TTA
ASPA V	Water-hardening	Filling	G-200: PA-2 (5:1)	10% TTA
ASPA Va	Water-hardening	Luting	G-200a: PA-2 (2.5:1)	10% TTA
ASPA X	Conventional	Filling	G-338	47.5% PA-48, 5% TTA

Key

G-200	Glass powder: maximum grain size 50 μm, composition: 29.0% SiO_2, 16.5% Al_2O_3, 7.3% AlF_3, 34.3% CaF_2, 3.0% NaF, 9.9% $AlPO_4$ (Kent et al., 1979)
G-200a	Glass powder: maximum grain size 15 μm, composition: G-200 (Wilson et al., 1977b)
TTA	(+)-tartaric acid
PA-1	Poly(acrylic acid) MW(wt. avg.) = 23,000 (Crisp et al., 1980b)
PA-2	Poly(acrylic acid) MW(wt. avg.) = 50,000 (Crisp et al., 1980b)
PA-48	Acrylic acid/itaconic acid 2:1 copolymer MW(wt. avg.) = 10,400 (Crisp et al., 1980b)

pected to be more reactive and require less reactive glasses than those used in combination with poly(acrylic acid).

The first practical glass-ionomer cement, ASPA II, used poly(acrylic acid) as the cement-forming acid (Table 2-4). However, this system was not suitable for marketing because a 50% solution of poly(acrylic acid) will gel after a period of time as the result of a slow increase in hydrogen bonding (Crisp et al., 1975). Poly(acrylic acid) chains are flexible and are constantly changing their configurations; when segments of a pair of chains approach each other, an intermolecular hydrogen bond can be formed. This is a slow but continuing process, which is, in effect, slowly cross-linking poly(acrylic acid). It ultimately reduces solubility, causing gelation.

One approach adopted by Wilson and Crisp (1974) was to add methyl alcohol to poly(acrylic acid) solutions as an agent that inhibits the ordering of structures in solution. This glass ionomer cement was known as ASPA III. Although the gelation of poly(acrylic acid) was prevented, McLean found that the cement stained in the mouth. Another approach had to be adopted.

Crisp and Wilson (1977) reasoned that copolymers of acrylic acid with other unsaturated carboxylic acids would be less regular than simple poly(acrylic acid) and so less liable to form intermolecular hydrogen bonds. They synthesized a co-

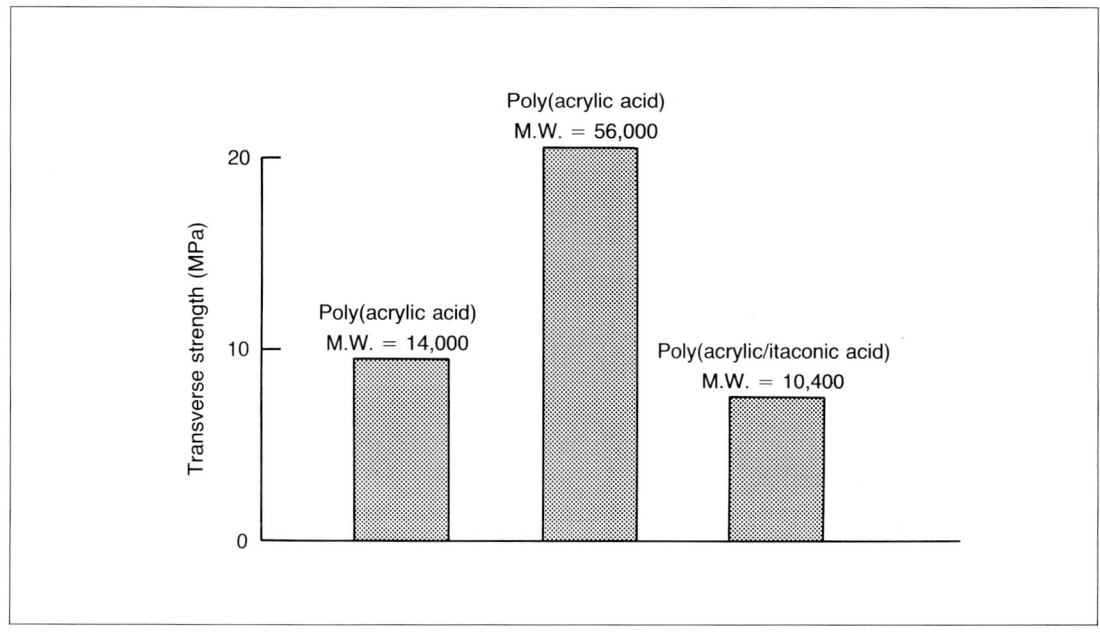

Fig. 2-15   Effect of molecular weight *(M.W.)* on the flexural strengths of glass-ionomer cements.

polymer of acrylic and itaconic acid, which proved indefinitely stable in a 50% aqueous solution. This copolymer was used in ASPA IV, which was otherwise identical to ASPA II (see Table 2-4). A commercial glass-ionomer cement was based on the ASPA IV formula.*

It would be expected that different molecular configurations would affect adhesion; recent evidence supports this hypothesis. Aboush and Jenkins (1986) have shown that cements based on poly(acrylic acid) bond more strongly to enamel and dentine than to cements based on copolymers of acrylic acid with itaconic or maleic acid. Another difference, noted by Setchell and coworkers (1985), is that cements based on copolymers of acrylic and maleic acids are apparently less resistant to acid attack than those based on poly(acrylic acid), a re-

sult confirmed by Wilson and coworkers (1986). But these cements are harder than those of poly(acrylic acid), which aids early finishing (Mount and Makinson, 1982; Matis and Philips, 1986). This can be attributed to a more highly cross-linked matrix arising from the greater number of carboxyl groups.

The molecular weight (relative molar mass) and the concentration of the polyacid affects cement strength (Fig. 2-15)—increases in either will shorten set time and increase the strength of the set cement (Wilson et al., 1977a; Prosser et al., 1986; Crisp et al., 1977).

Since strength is a welcome attribute, such modifications would appear desirable. Unfortunately, when the polyacid is present in solution, an increase in either molecular weight or concentration will increase the viscosity of the liquid, making the cement pastes progressively more difficult to manipulate. Hence, there is a trend away from using polyacid in solu-

*De Trey Aspa, Dentsply International Inc., Weybridge, England, and York, Pa. No longer marketed.

tion and toward using it in dry solid form for blending with the glass powder. The liquid for cement formation is then either plain water or an aqueous solution of tartaric acid, both of low viscosity. In this system the molecular weight and effective polyacid concentration can be increased, to some extent, without rendering the pastes unworkable. Thus, this type of glass-ionomer cement tends to be stronger than the other.

Effect of the nature of the poly(alkenoic acid) on cement properties

From the previous discussion it is apparent that the nature of the polyacid does have some effect on cement properties, although this is less marked than in the case with glass composition. The type of polyacid used is thought to affect setting time, and its molecular weight affects strength. The higher the molecular weight of the polyacid, the higher will be the strength of the cement. However, against this is the increasing viscosity of the mix, which limits the molecular weight of the polyacid employed.

Water

Water is often not considered a constituent of glass-ionomer cement, but it is, in fact, a very important one. It is the reaction medium and also plays a role in hydrating reaction products, that is, metal poly(alkenoate) salts and silica gel. Attempts to replace it even partially with another solvent, such as alcohol, gives rise to very weak cement (Hornsby, 1977).

Too much water in the system results

in weak, slow-setting cements. Some reduction in the amount of water is beneficial: cements set faster and are stronger and more durable. However, once this optimum limit is reached, there is insufficient water for the reaction and for hydration—the result is a weakening of the cement (Prosser et al., 1986).

Tartaric acid

In their early studies, Wilson and Kent (1973) found that the principal obstacle to developing a practical glass-ionomer cement was the sluggish nature of the set. Working time was minimal and hardening was slow. The future of the system appeared doubtful. However, by dint of preparing many glasses, they found that one or two glasses exceptionally high in fluoride were capable of reaching the minimal acceptable setting characteristic. Even so, these cements set sluggishly and had low translucency because of the large amounts of fluorite crystallites in the glasses. The simple two-component glass plus polyacid does not constitute an adequate system.

For this reason, a search was made for additives to control the setting reaction, and in 1976 Wilson and coworkers reported that tartaric acid was extremely effective. Depending on the nature of the glass, the working time is unaffected or even prolonged, and the setting rate is markedly increased (Wilson and Crisp, 1976; Wilson et al., 1976; Cook, 1983; Crisp and Wilson, 1976; Prosser et al., 1982). The addition of tartaric acid made the glass-ionomer cement system a practical one. It enabled the fluoride content of the glasses to be reduced, an important step in the production of clear or slightly opal glasses, which form the basis of glass-ionomer cements with en-

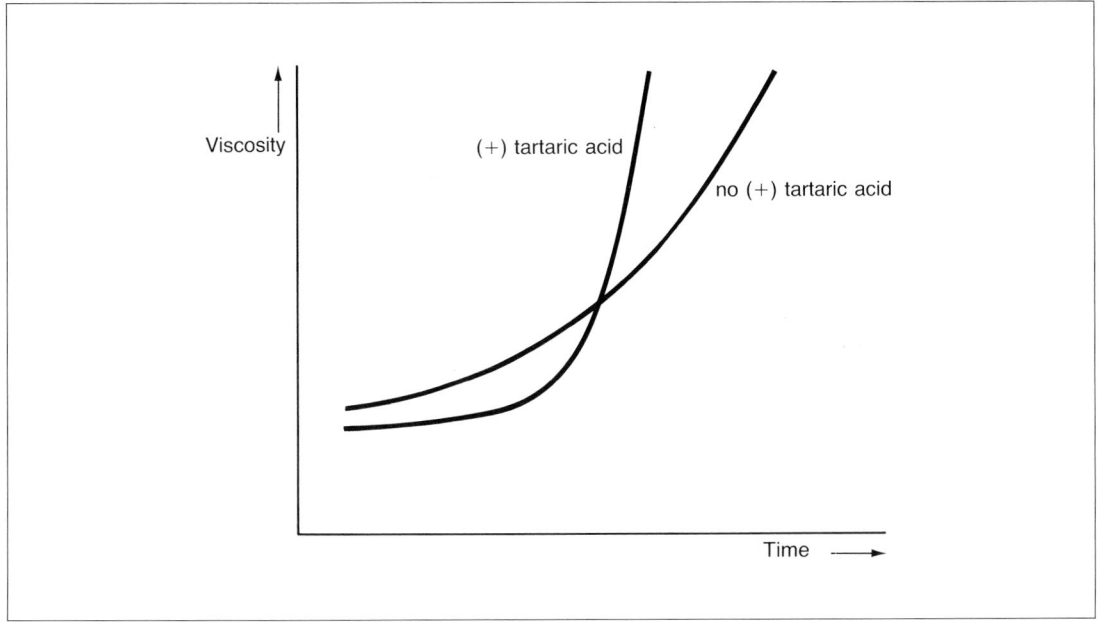

Fig. 2-16 Effect of tartaric acid concentration on the viscosity/time curve for a setting glass-ionomer cement.

hanced translucency. In addition, the number of glasses that could be used for cement formation was increased dramatically.

Rheological studies show that tartaric acid delays the onset of viscosity, and that the greater the concentration of tartaric acid, the longer the delay (Fig. 2-16) (Cook, 1983; Hill and Wilson, 1986).

The action of tartaric acid is apparently unique. Other rate-controlling additives are known, but even other hydroxycarboxylic acids do not have the unique delaying effect of tartaric acid—even meso-tartaric acid is ineffective (Crisp et al., 1979). Only the positive enantiomorph of tartaric acid produces the desired effect.

Other additives

Other additives are used to control the setting reaction of glass-ionomer ce-

ments but they either accelerate the set at the expense of working time or vice versa (Wilson et al., 1976; Tomioka et al., 1983; Crisp et al., 1980a). Polyphosphates can be used to extend working time but the set is prolonged. Certain metal salts, such as stannous fluoride, accelerate setting but reduce working time. All are useful only if used in conjunction with (+)-tartaric acid.

Packaging and dispensing

As we have seen, the modern glass-ionomer cement has four constituents: glass, polyacid, tartaric acid, and water. The material is presented to the clinician as a two-component powder/liquid pack. How are the constituents blended together to form the components of the pack?

In the older, conventional form, the powder was simply ground glass, and the liquid contained the polyacid and tartaric acid in solution. More recently a new presentation has appeared—the so-called water-hardening cements—where the polyacid is dried and mixed with the glass to form a powder blend (Prosser et al., 1984; McLean et al., 1984). The liquid is then either water (in which case dried tartaric acid is incorporated into the powder blend) or a solution of tartaric acid.

The term "anhydrous cement" has been inappropriately applied to these materials. They are water-based cements, with water playing an essential role in both the reaction and the cement structure. Zinc oxide–eugenol cements, where eugenol is the reaction medium, are the true anhydrous cements.

Types

Apart from the different packaging just described, glass-ionomer cements come in many forms. They are best distinguished by usage.

Type I: luting agents

Flow properties and minimal film thickness are essential in cements used as luting agents. Fine-grained glass powders with maximum grain sizes of 15 μm or less are employed. Some clinicians require radio-opacity, which can be obtained by replacing calcium in the glass with strontium or lanthanum. When translucency is not required, phase-separated glass, a cermet ionomer, or a glass combined with zinc oxide can be used.

Type II: aesthetic filling materials

In anterior restorations, where aesthetics is important, adequate translucency is required of a glass ionomer cement. Phase-separated glass or cermet ionomers cannot be used. Clear glasses tend to have high silica/alumina ratios, and cements formed from them tend to harden slowly.

Type II: bis-reinforced filling materials

This category covers the cermet (glass-metal) derivatives of Type II materials. These are not aesthetic but are more resistant to abrasion.

Type III: lining, base, and fissure-sealing materials

Strength and radiopacity are important when a glass-ionomer cement is to be used as a lining, base, or fissure sealant. Fine-grained glasses are often employed when translucency is not important. Some lining materials contain zinc oxide, which tends to buffer the system and render the cement radio-opaque. These are useful properties, but are obtained at the price of some loss of strength. Cermet-ionomer cements can also be used. The Type III classification could well be extended to include nonaesthetic glass-ionomer materials. Some of these materials set very quickly because they are used in the "double laminate" or "sandwich" technique.

Pit and fissure sealants

One manufacturer makes a special high-fluoride cement for use as a pit and fissure sealant. The original G-200 was, of course, a high-fluoride glass.

Type I and Type II materials have national and international specifications under the British Standards Institution (BS) and the International Standards Organization (ISO):

BS 6039:1981/Glass-Ionomer Cements
ISO 7489:1986/Glass-Polyalkenoate Cements

Type III is included in the ISO Draft Proposal for Dental Cements.

Although versions of the glass-ionomer cement are marketed specifically for pit and fissure sealing, such materials could well be included in the Type I classification.

Laboratory of the Government Chemist (LGC) materials

LGC materials have already been described. These materials are summarized in Table 2-4.

Commercial materials

Leading commercial materials that are, or have been, on the market are listed in Table 2-5. All materials are based on fluoroaluminosilicate glasses; many of them are qualitatively similar to G-200. More recent glasses, however, tend to contain more sodium and less fluoride (Table 2-6). Unlike G-200, some glasses used in Type II formulations are clear, which is one of the reasons why many modern glass-ionomer cements have improved translucency.

However, glasses used in Type I cements frequently contain fluorite crystallites (CaF_2) and are thus opal. Although this adversely affects the translucency of the cements these glasses impart favourable setting and strength qualities to the cement.

Radiopacity is found in some materials. This is attained by incorporating strontium, barium or lanthanum into the glass composition, fusing silver to the glass, or mixing in zinc oxide. Current glass-ionomer cements use a variety of polyacids—poly(acrylic acid), copolymers of acrylic acid with maleic acid—to increase reactivity, with itaconic acids for greater stability in aqueous solutions, and with tricarballylic acid. Tannic acid is found in some compositions in order to enhance bonding to dentine because tannic acid adheres to collagen. The polyacid can be present as a solution or added to the glass powder as a dry solid.

All varieties of cement contain (+)-tartaric acid to modify the setting reaction. Sometimes other additives are employed as well, for example, the polyphosphates or tetrahydrofuranetetracarboxylic acid.

Table 2-5 Major brands of glass-ionomer cement

Name	Type	Manufacturer
De Trey Aspa	II	Amalgamated Dental Co., Weybridge, England
Chembond	I	
Chem-Fil	II	
Aqua-Cem	I	
Chem-Fil II	II	Dentsply International Inc.,
Chem-Fil II	II	Weybridge, England, and York, Pa.
Chem-Fil Express	II	
Chem-Fil Junior	II	
Ketac-Fil	II	
Chelon	II	
Ketac-Cem	I	
Ketac-Cem Radio-opaque	I, Radio-opaque	ESPE GmbH, Seefeld/Oberbay, West Germany, and Valley
Ketac-Bond	III	Stream, N.Y.
Ketac-Silver	II cermet	
Chelon-Silver	II cermet	
Fuji Ionomer I	I	
Fuji Ionomer II	II	
Fuji Lining	III lining	G-C International Corp., Tokyo,
Fuji Ionomer III	Pit and fissure	and Scottsdale, Ariz.
Fuji Miracle Mix	Amalgam filled	
Glas-Ionomer Type I	I	
Glas-Ionomer Type II	II	Shofu Dental Corp., Kyoto, Japan,
Glas-Ionomer Base	III	and Menlo Park, Calif.
Shofu Lining	III	

Table 2-6 Examples of modern ionomer glasses

Species	Composition	% Mass
	A	B
SiO_2	41.9	35.2
Al_2O_3	28.6	20.1
AlF_3	1.6	2.4
CaF_2	15.7	20.1
NaF	9.3	3.6
$AlPO_4$	3.8	12.0

References

Aboush, Y.E.Y., and Jenkins, C.B.G. (1986) An evaluation of the bonding of glass-ionomer restorative to dentine and enamel. Br. Dent. J. 161:179–184.

Barry, T.I., Clinton, D.J., and Wilson, A.D. (1979) The structure of a glass-ionomer cement and its relationship to the setting process. J. Dent. Res. 58:1072–1079.

Barry, T.I., Clinton, D.J., Lay, L.A., and Miller, R.P. (1972) ASPA dental cement. Part I. Studies on microstructure in ASPA glasses. National Physical Laboratory Report. SI no. 91/0/486.

British Standards Institution (1981) British Standard for glass-ionomer cements. BS 6039.

Cook, W.D. (1983) Dental polyelectrolyte cements. III. Effect of additives on their rheology. Biomaterials 4: 85–88.

Crisp, S., and Wilson, A.D. (1976) Reaction in glass ionomer cements. V. Effect of incorporating tartaric acid in the cement forming liquid. J. Dent. Res. 55:1023–1031.

Crisp, S., and Wilson, A.D. (1977) Poly(carboxylate) cements. Br. pat. 1,484,454, August 1973.

Crisp, S., Lewis, B.G., and Wilson, A.D. (1975) Gelation of polyacrylic acid aqueous solutions and the measurement of viscosity. J. Dent. Res. 54:1173–1175.

Crisp, S., Lewis, B.G., and Wilson, A.D. (1977) Characterisation of glass-ionomer cements. 3. Effect of polyacid concentration on the physical properties. J. Dent. 5:51–56.

Crisp, S., Lewis, B.G., and Wilson, A.D. (1979) Characterisation of glass-ionomer cements. 5. The effect of tartaric acid concentration in the liquid component. J. Dent. 7:304–312.

Crisp, S., Merson, S.A., and Wilson, A.D. (1980a) Modification of ionomer cements by the addition of simple metal salts. Ind. Eng. Chem. Prod. Res. Dev. 19:403–408.

Crisp, S., Ferner, A.J., Lewis, B.G., and Wilson, A.D. (1975) Properties of improved glass ionomer cement formulations. J. Dent. 3:125–130.

Crisp, S., Kent, B.E., Lewis, B.G., Ferner, A.J., and Wilson, A.D. (1980b) Glass ionomer cement formulations. II. The synthesis of novel polycarboxylic acids. J. Dent. Res. 59:1055–1063.

Hill, R.G., and Wilson, A.D. (1986) Unpublished results.

Hornsby, P.R. (1977) The development of ionic polymer cements. Ph.D. Thesis. Brunel University.

International Standards Organization (1986) International Standard for glass polyalkenoate cements. ISO 7486.

Kent, B.E., and Wilson, A.D. (1971) Dental silicate cements. XV. Effect of particle size of the powder. J. Dent. Res. 50:1616–1620.

Kent, B.E., Lewis, B.G., and Wilson, A.D. (1973) The properties of a glass ionomer cement. Br. Dent. J. 135:322–326.

Kent, B.E., Lewis, B.G., and Wilson, A.D. (1979) Glass ionomer formulations. I. The preparation of novel fluoroaluminosilicate glasses high in fluorine. J. Dent. Res. 58:1607–1619.

McKinney, J.E., Antonucci, J.M., and Rupp, N.W. (1986) Wear and micro-hardness of a metal-filled ionomer cement. J. Dent. Res. 64(Special Issue):344 (IADR abstr. 1577).

McLean, J.W., and Gasser, O. (1985) Glass-cermet cements. Quintessence Int. 16:333–343.

McLean, J.W., Wilson, A.D., and Prosser, H.J. (1984) Development and use of water-hardening glass-ionomer luting cements. J. Prosthet. Dent. 52:175–181.

Matis, B.A., and Phillips, R.W. (1986) Glass ionomer restorative materials: Clinical evaluation of early finishing. J. Dent. Res. 65(Special Issue):193 (AADR abstr. 217).

Moore, B.K., Swartz, M.L., and Phillips, R.W. (1985) Abrasion resistance of metal reinforced glass ionomer cements. J. Dent. Res. 64:(Special Issue):371 (IADR/AADR abstr. 1766).

Mount, G.J., and Makinson, O.F. (1982) Glass-ionomer restorative cements: Clinical implications of the setting reaction. Oper. Dent. 7:134–141.

Prosser, H.J., Powis, D.R., and Wilson, A.D. (1986) Glass-ionomer cements of improved flexural strength. J. Dent. Res. 65:146–148.

Prosser, H.J., Richards, C.P., and Wilson, A.D. (1982) NMR spectroscopy of dental materials. II. The role of tartaric acid in glass-ionomer cements. J. Biomed. Mater. Res. 16:431–445.

Prosser, H.J., Powis, D.R., Brant, P., and Wilson, A.D. (1984) The characterisation of glass-ionomer cements. 7. The physical properties of current materials. J. Dent. 12:231–240.

Sced, I.R., and Wilson, A.D. (1980) Poly(carboxylic acid) hardenable compositions. Br. pat. appl. GB 2,028,855A, 1978.

Schmidt, W., Purrmann, R., Jochum, P., and Gasser, O. (1981a) Calcium aluminofluorosilicate glass powder and its use. Eur. Pat. Appl. 23,013.

Schmidt, W., Purrmann, R., Jochum, P., and Gasser, O. (1981b) Mixing compounds for glass-ionomer cements and use of a copolymer for preparing the mixing components. Eur. Pat. Appl. 24,056.

Setchell, D.J., Teo, C.K., and Kuhn, A.T. (1985) The relative solubilities of four modern glass-ionomer cements. Br. Dent. J. 158:220–222.

Simmons, J.J. (1983) The miracle mixture glass ionomer and alloy powder. Tex. Dent. J. October:6–12.

Tomioka, K., Hirota, K., Muramatsu, H., and Akahane, S. (1983) Liquid of acrylic acid copoylmer and tetrahydrofurantetracarboxylic acid for setting dental cements. U.S. Pat. 4,374,936.

Wilson, A.D. (1978) The chemistry of dental cements. Chem. Soc. Rev. 7:265–296.

Wilson, A.D., and Crisp, S. (1974) Unpublished data.

Wilson, A.D., and Crisp, S. (1976) Poly(carboxylate)-cements. Br. pat. 1,422,337, April 1972.

Wilson, A.D., and Kent, B.E. (1973) Surgical cement. Br. Pat. 1,316,129, December 1969.

Wilson, A.D., Crisp, S., and Abel, G. (1977a) Characterization of glass-ionomer cements. 4. Effect of molecular weight on physical properties. J. Dent. 5:117–120.

Wilson, A.D., Crisp, S., and Ferner, A.J. (1976) Reactions in glass-ionomer cements. IV. Effect of chelating co-monomers on setting behavior. J. Dent. Res. 55:489–495.

Wilson, A.D., Crisp, S., Lewis, B.G., and McLean, J.W. (1977b) Experimental luting agents based on the glass ionomer cements. Br. Dent. J. 142:117–122.

Wilson, A.D., Kent B.E., Clinton, D., and Miller, R.P. (1972) The formation and microstructure of dental silicate cements J. Mater. Sci. 7:220–238.

Wilson, A.D., Crisp, S., Prosser, H.J., Lewis, B.G., and Merson, S.A. (1980) Aluminosilicate glasses for polyelectrolyte cements. Ind. Eng. Chem. Prod. Res. Dev. 19:263–270.

Wilson, A.D., Groffman, D.M., Powis, D.R., and Scott, R.P. (1986) An evaluation of the significance of the impinging jet method for measuring the acid erosion of dental cements. Biomaterials 7:55–60.

Wygant, J.F. (1958) Cementitious bonding in ceramic fabrication. pp. 171–188 In W.D. Kingery (ed.) Ceramic Fabrication Processes. Cambridge, Mass.: MIT Press.

Chapter 3

The Setting Reaction and Its Clinical Consequences

The setting characteristics of the glass-ionomer cement are central to its science, and some understanding of the setting reaction—even if only in outline—is needed to appreciate the scientific technology of glass-ionomer cements and the correct clinical usage of them in dental surgery. The reader will also be able to understand the limitations of the early materials and how the working and hardening characteristics have been improved over the years.

Poor setting behaviour was the Achilles' heel of early glass-ionomer cements, because the clinical consequences of progressive setting are not confined to premature loss of workability and sluggish hardening but extend to other properties. Set cements that are not fully hardened are vulnerable to the effects of water, and slow hardening prolongs this period of sensitivity. Thus, the clinician must devote much attention to keeping the restoration protected from saliva. It is true to say that a considerable amount of research and development, both by the Laboratory of the Government Chemist and manufacturers, has been devoted to improving the setting behaviour.

The vulnerability of the freshly set cement to water can be best appreciated by considering the chemistry of the setting reaction. Fortunately, although the setting reaction is extremely complex and is imperfectly understood in detail—and it is doubtful if the reaction will ever be fully unraveled—the outline of the reaction is simple to describe and understand.

Chemistry of the setting

When the cement powder and aqueous liquid are brought together to form a paste, the glass powder, which is basic, reacts with the poly(alkenoic acid), often poly(acrylic acid), to form a salt hydrogel. This hydrogel is the binding matrix. Water is the reaction medium and is also an essential part of the hydrogel, for it is required to hydrate the metal polyalkenoate formed.

The glass-ionomer cement sets and hardens by a transfer of metal ions from the glass to the poly(acrylic acid), which causes gelation in the aqueous phase (Fig. 3-1). During the process of transfer the matrix-forming metal ions are in soluble form and vulnerable to attack by aqueous fluids (Figs. 3-1 and 3-2). Some form of limited protection during this period is essential.

There is another reason for protection. Water forms an important part of the cement structure, and loss of water of hydration disrupts the cement structure. Loss of water can occur before the cement has fully matured, for example by

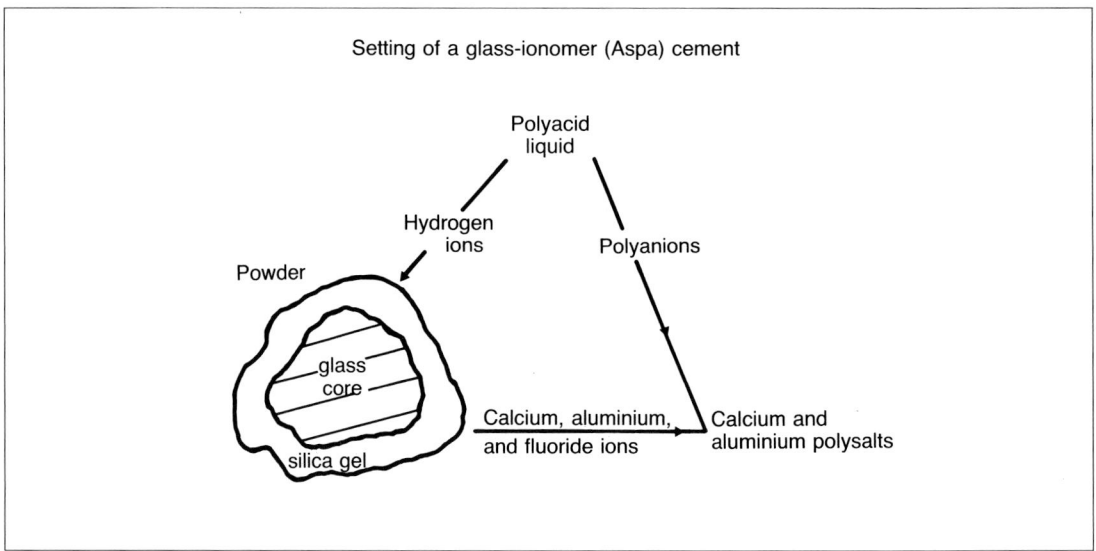

Fig. 3-1 Cement-forming reaction of glass-ionomer cements showing extraction of ions from the glass, migration into the aqueous phase, and subsequent precipitation as polyanion hydrogels.

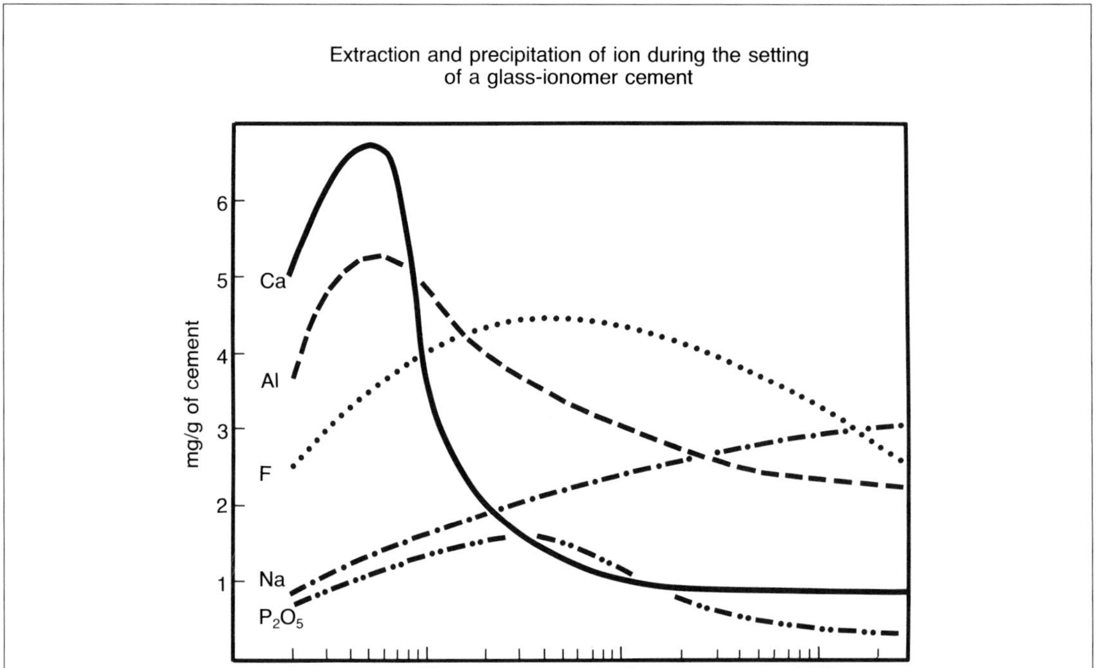

Fig. 3-2 A soluble ion/time dependant curve showing the accumulation of soluble ions in the cement, as they are extracted from the glass, and their subsequent precipitation. Reprinted with permission from Crisp and Wilson (1974b).

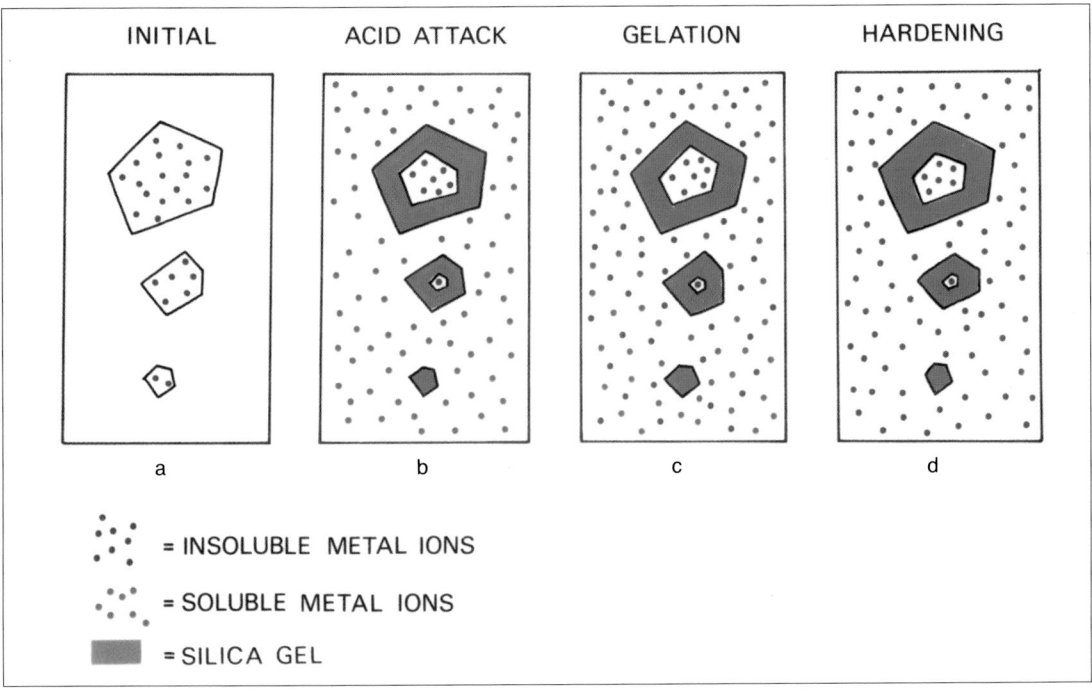

| INITIAL | ACID ATTACK | GELATION | HARDENING |
| a | b | c | d |

= INSOLUBLE METAL IONS

= SOLUBLE METAL IONS

= SILICA GEL

Fig. 3-3 Course of the cement-forming reaction from the initial state to final hardening. *(a)* Initial state. Unattacked glass particles dispersed in the polyacid liquid. Blue dots represent bound metal ions, Al^{3+} and Ca^{2+}, in the glass. *(b)* Attack on the glass particles by the acid. The outer layer of the glass particles is depleted of metal ions and degraded to a silica gel. Metal ions have migrated to the liquid phase, where they remain in soluble form *(red dots). (c)* Initial gelation. A sufficient number of metal ions have accumulated in the liquid phase to cause gelation. The insoluble gel ions are shown as blue dots. However, soluble metal ions remain, and the cement is still vulnerable to moisture. *(d)* Fully hardened glass-ionomer cement with all ions *(blue dots)* in an insoluble form. The cement is no longer vulnerable to attack by moisture.

dehydration or vigorous finishing techniques. Once the cement has fully matured—and this may take many days—this is no longer a problem.

The chemistry of the cement-forming reaction from initial mixing through the various stages of the reaction is depicted in Fig. 3-3. The initial situation is shown in Fig. 3-3a. Following are the stages in the reaction:

1. *Decomposition* of the glass and release of cement-forming metal ions (Al^{3+} and Ca^{2+}).

2. *Migration* of these metal ions into the aqueous phase of the cement (Fig. 3-3b).

3. *Gelation* of the polyacid by the metal ions leading to set (Fig. 3-3c).

4. *Post-set hardening* when metal ions become increasingly bound to the polyacid chain. Under conditions of high humidity, the cement tends to expand. The cement is vulnerable to moisture until sufficient hardness has developed. This can take up to one hour but is generally less for modern materials. Hardening continues for about 24 hours, during

which time translucency develops as the chemical reaction proceeds (Fig. 3-3d).

5. *Further slow maturation.* Even after 24 hours a further slow maturation takes place and in the first few days translucency develops further, as does resistance to desiccation and acid attack. Over a period of months the cement becomes more rigid and gathers strength. The reaction is slightly exothermic, the exotherm being less than that of any of the other water-based cements. This exotherm is reflected in a setting shrinkage, however, which can be nullified by hydroscopic expansion.

A full account of the setting reactions, as much as it is known, is given below. It is based largely on the work of Crisp and Wilson (1974a, 1974b), Crisp et al. (1974), Crisp and Wilson (1976), Wilson et al. (1976), Prosser et al. (1982b), and Cook (1983). Most of their work was carried out using the glass G-200 and poly(acrylic acid). Although now other glasses and other polyacids are also used in glass-ionomer cements, the results of these studies can generally be applied to them all.

Decomposition of the glass and migration of ions

In the early stages of the reaction, the glass powder is decomposed by the polyacid (see Fig. 2-5), a property characteristic of this type of glass (Crisp and Wilson, 1974a). In a normal cement mix where there is a considerable excess of powder over liquid, about 20% to 30% of the glass is attacked. The attack occurs at the surface of the glass, and as cations are withdrawn the glass network breaks down into silicic acid, which polymerises at the surface of the glass powder. Ions locked up in the glass network—principally Al^{3+}, Ca^{2+}, and F^-—

are released and migrate into the aqueous phase of the cement, the aluminium and fluoride as complexes (see Fig. 3-3b). Calcium ions predominate because the acid attack on the glass is not uniform, but occurs preferentially at calcium-rich sites (Barry et al., 1979).

As the reaction proceeds the concentration of these ions increases, with the preferential buildup of calcium over aluminium (Crisp and Wilson, 1974b; Crisp et al., 1974; see Fig. 3-2). The pH also increases, which reflects the conversion of the poly(acrylic acid) to polyacrylates. The viscosity of the paste also increases as the poly(acrylic acid), originally in a random coil configuration, acquires charge and unwinds under the influence of electrostatic forces of repulsion.

Gelation and vulnerability to water

At a critical pH and ionic concentration precipitation of insoluble polyacrylates begins to take place. When this process reaches a certain stage, the cement sets (see Fig. 3-3c). Even after set, in the postset hardening phase, the precipitation process continues—indeed, it is responsible for the development of hardness—until all the ions are in insoluble form (see Fig. 3-3d).

The studies of Crisp et al. (1974) and Barry et al. (1979) have shown that calcium polyacrylate is responsible for the initial set, at least in the absence of tartrate, but that the hardening process derives from the slower formation of aluminium polyacrylate, which phase ultimately predominates in the matrix.

Not all the carboxyl (COOH) groups of poly(acrylic acid) are converted to carboxylate groups (COO$^-$) during the course of the reaction, for two reasons. First, when most of the carboxylic acid groups have ionized, the negative charge on the polymer chain has increased to such an extent that the positively charged hydrogen ions become very strongly bound to the remaining un-ionized carboxylic acid groups and are not easily replaced by metal ions. Second, as the density of cross-links increases the metal ions are increasingly hindered in their movements toward carboxyl sites.

What is important for the clinician to remember is that after set, but before the cement is fully hardened, a proportion of the cement-forming aluminium, calcium, fluoride, and polyacrylate ions are in soluble form and so can be dissolved out of the cement by aqueous fluids. Once these ions are leached out they are irretrievably lost for matrix formation and the cement is permanently weakened. In particular, the surface is softened and becomes opaque as water is absorbed, causing the restoration to lose its aesthetic appeal (Mount and Makinson, 1982).

Ions released from the glass accumulate in the cement water and subsequently are removed by precipitation (see Figs. 3-1 and 3-2). Note that the concentration of soluble ions reaches a maximum as the glass is decomposed, and then declines as the insoluble matrix is formed (see Fig. 3-2). The object of a manufacturer developing the cement is to reduce this period of vulnerability to a minimum by sharpening the rate of hardening.

Although glass-ionomer cements have been improved considerably, for the best clinical results it is still advisable to adopt a strict routine to exclude water during this vulnerable stage of setting.

In this connection, calcium polyacrylate, which is more vulnerable to water than aluminium polyacrylate, is believed to predominate in freshly set cements—further reason for protecting the freshly set cement. Indeed, one manufacturer has attempted to improve his product by washing the glass powder with acid to remove calcium ions from the surface (Schmidt et al., 1981). This process delays initial set and gives excellent working and setting characteristics.

Causes of gelation

So far we have explained why calcium and aluminium ions, simple or complex, cause the polyacrylate to gel. Sodium ions do not have this effect and it is tempting to conclude that the divalent calcium and trivalent aluminium ions cross-link the polyacrylate chains ionically.

While it is easy to visualize calcium ions bridging two chains (Fig. 3-4), it is unlikely that aluminium ions could connect three chains for steric and probability reasons. The coordination of the aluminium ion has to be considered. The coordination number of aluminium is six in the presence of water; that is, there must be six ligands attached to a central aluminium ion. The ligands in the case of glass-ionomer cements would be COO^- from polyacrylate, F^- ions, OH^- ions, and water molecules. However, it is easy to see how the $[AlF \cdot 3H_2O]^{2+}$ unit can bridge just two polyacrylate chains (Fig. 3-4).

However, gelation may simply be caused by the multivalent aluminium and calcium ions displacing or partly displacing the various spheres of hydration that interpose themselves between the cation-anion ion pairs. Contact cation-polyacrylate ion pairs are formed; the cations are site-bound. Desolvation of hydration spheres renders the ionic pairs more hydrophobic and precipitation occurs. Sodium ions cannot displace the hydration sphere and are not site bound because of their low ionic charge. Consequently, they do not precipitate as polyacrylates.

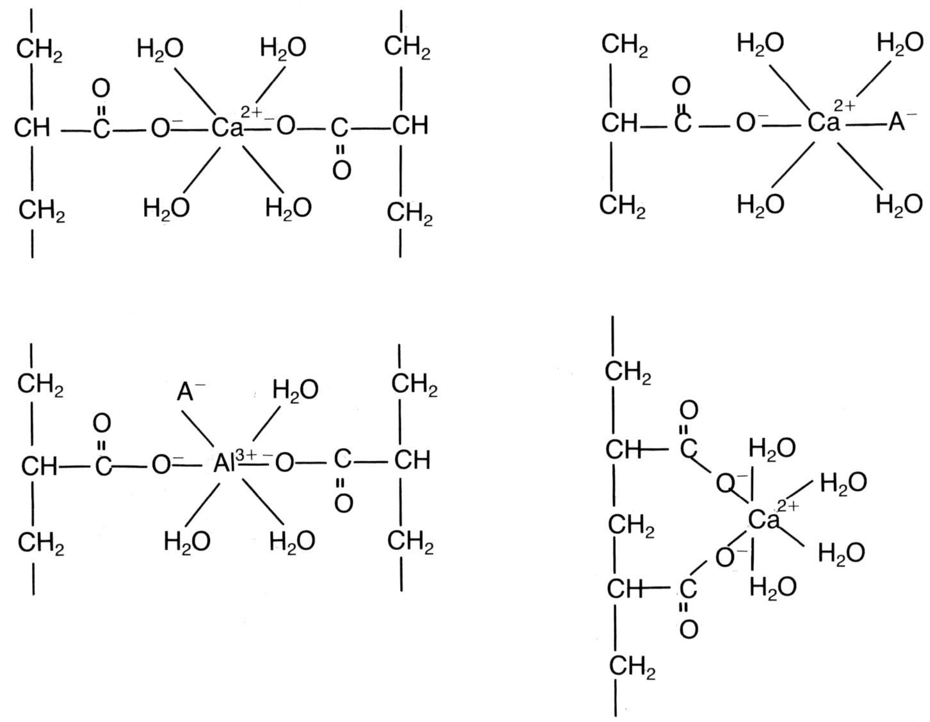

Fig. 3-4 Possible molecular structures in a set glass-ionomer cement. A^- represents either F^- or OH^- ligands. Other ligands are COO^- and H_2O. Although aluminium is trivalent, it has a coordination number of six in an aqueous environment, that is, six ligands have to be attached to it. Again, aluminium does not have to bind three polyacid chains together, which is stearically unlikely, because of the presence of negatively charged ligands. Reprinted with permission from Wilson and Crisp (1975).

In this model, cross-linking does not play a dominant role, the cohesive binding forces in the cement being attributable, in the main, to chain entanglement. Recent experimental evidence (Hill et al., 1986) indicates that chain entanglement, weak ionic cross-linking, and hydrogen bonds are all involved in matrix formation.

Hardening and slow maturation

Hardening and the precipitation process continue for about 24 hours and are ac-companied by a slight expansion under conditions of high humidity and the development of translucency. Further changes continue to take place for a considerable period—at least a year and probably more.

There are a number of indicators of these slow changes. In the first few days the translucency of the cement improves and the cement becomes resistant to desiccation. Strength continues to increase for at least a year and is apparently proportional to the logarithm of time (Fig. 3-5; Crisp et al., 1976a). The cement, which initially shows some plastic character, like the zinc polycarboxylate

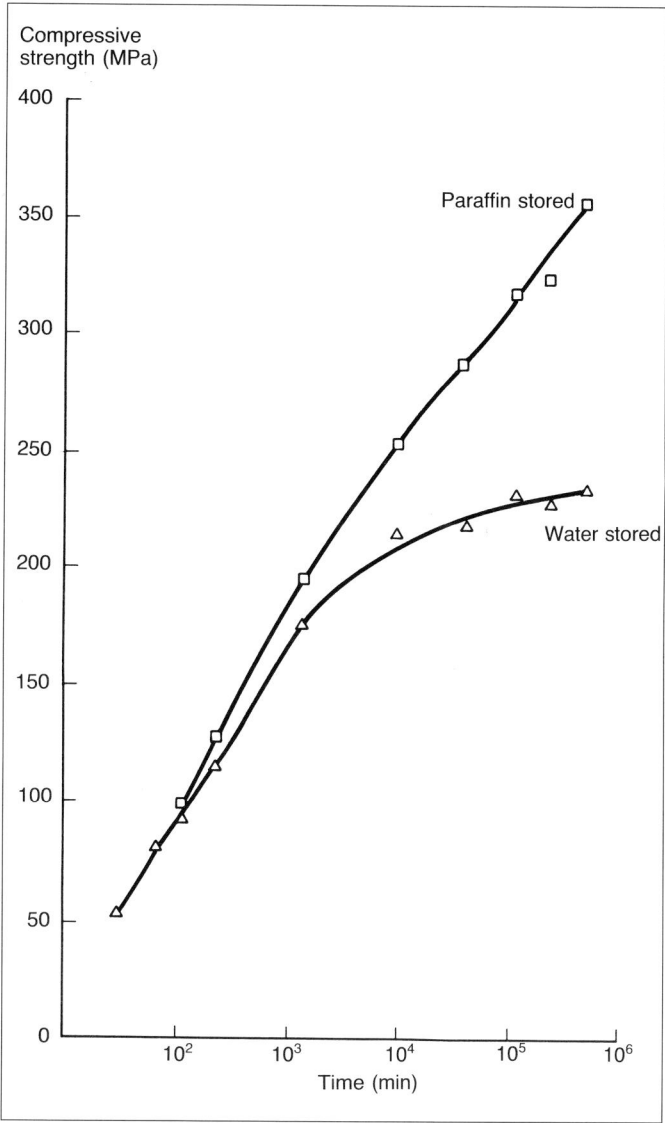

Fig. 3-5 Increase of compressive strength as a glass-ionomer cement ages. Reprinted with permission from Crisp et al. (1976a).

cement, becomes increasingly rigid as it ages until it approaches the rigidity of the phosphate-bonded cements (Paddon and Wilson, 1976). This behaviour is unique among the dental cements. Also, the ability of the cement to absorb or lose water decreases as it ages.

The underlying chemical changes causing these physical changes remain a subject for debate. But Wilson and his coworkers have shown that increases in strength are associated with increases in bound water; that is, increasing hydration of the metal-carboxylate links in a manner analogous to the hydration reactions in Portland cement (Wilson et al., 1979; Wilson et al., 1981). This progressive hydration explains the increasing stability of the cement with regard to gain or loss of water.

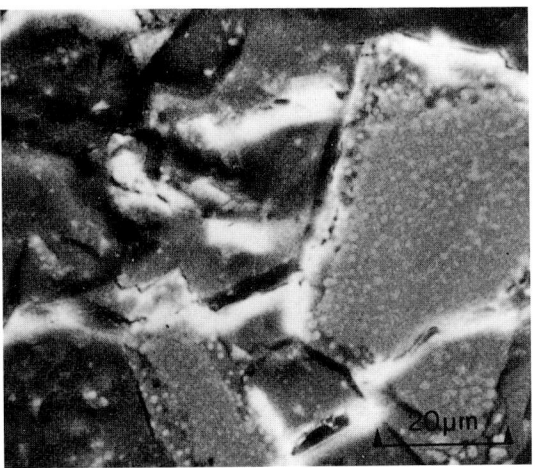

Fig. 3-6 Micrograph of a set glass-ionomer cement showing the pitted surface of the glass particles (where preferential acid attack has occurred) and the siliceous hydrogel layer. Reprinted with permission from Barry et al. (1979).

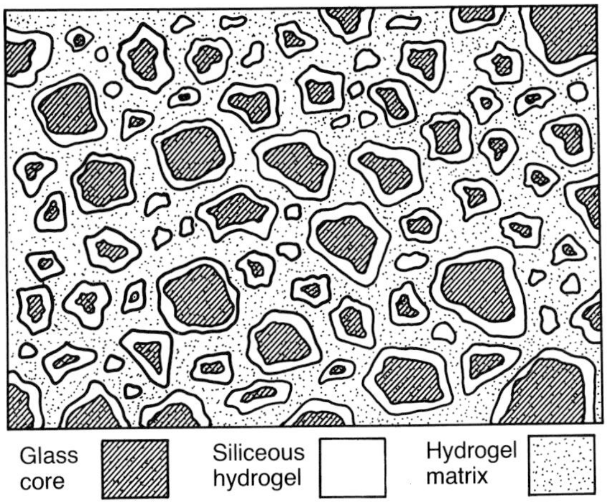

Fig. 3-7 Fully hardened glass-ionomer cement showing the matrix phase and the structure of the filler (glass core sheathed by a siliceous hydrogel). Smaller particles are completely degraded to a siliceous hydrogel. Reprinted with permission from Laboratory of the Government Chemist.

Glass core — Siliceous hydrogel — Hydrogel matrix

Increasing strength and rigidity must be associated with a slow increase in cross-linking. There is some evidence for such a time-dependent increase in cross-linking, for it has recently been observed that the glass transition temperature of the cement rises with time (Hill, 1986). Increase in cross-linking could result from the slow replacement of residue carboxyl hydrogen ions by metal ions and the increasing predominance of aluminium over calcium in the matrix.

Cement structure

Our knowledge of the structure of glass-ionomer cement comes from just two studies: Barry et al. (1979) and Brune and Smith (1982). The set cement is a highly complex composite, where a cored filler is bound together by a hydro-gel of calcium and aluminium polyacrylates that contains fluorine, probably as a fluoroaluminium polyacrylate.

The filler system is complex and is derived from the original glass powder, which is partly degraded to a siliceous hydrogel that apparently contains fluorite crystallites. The larger filler particles contain a glassy core pitted by selective etching and sheathed by a siliceous hydrogel (Fig. 3-6). Observation indicates that the bond between core and sheath is not particularly strong. The smaller filler particles are composed entirely of a siliceous hydrogel that can be presumed to be completely degraded relics of small glass particles (Fig. 3-7).

The nature of the cohesive forces binding the matrix together is a subject for speculation, but they can be presumed to be a mixture of ionic cross-links, hydrogen bridges, and chain entanglements.

The role of water

The glass-ionomer cements are water-based materials, and water plays an important role in their setting and structure. It is the reaction medium into which the cement-forming cations—calcium and aluminium—are leached and in which they are transported to react with the polyacid to form a polyacrylate matrix. Water also serves to hydrate the siliceous hydrogel and the metal polyacrylate salts formed. It is an essential part of the cement structure. If water is lost from the cement by desiccation while it is setting, the cement-forming reactions will stop.

Water present in the set cement can be classified, somewhat arbitarily, into two forms: "loosely bound" water, which is readily removed by desiccation, and "tightly bound" water, which cannot be removed (Wilson and Crisp, 1975; Crisp et al., 1976c; Elliott et al., 1975; Wilson et al., 1979; Wilson et al., 1981). Tightly bound water is associated with the hydration shell of the cation-polyacrylate bond, particularly that of aluminium, and some silica gel water.

As the cement ages, the degree of hydration, that is, the ratio of tightly bound to loosely bound water, increases. This is accompanied by an increase in strength and modulus and a decrease in plasticity (Paddon and Wilson, 1976; Wilson et al., 1981).

Water is easily lost and gained by the cement, as the loosely bound water is labile; indeed, the cement is only stable in an atmosphere of 80% relative humidity (Hornsby, 1980). In higher humidities, the cement absorbs water and the consequent hydroscopic expansion can exceed the setting shrinkage. This is a clinical advantage. The cement can lose water under drying conditions, however, leading to shrinking and crazing. The earliest clinical observations of this phenomenon were made by J. W. McLean with ASPA I in the early 1970s. Moreover, loss of water will retard cement formation, since it is the reaction medium, and will prevent strength from fully developing, since it is required for the hydration of the matrix salts.

Susceptibility to desiccation decreases as the cement ages (Saito, 1978; Hornsby, 1980). The period of vulnerability is different for different cements and has been stated to range from one to 30 days depending on the material used (Phillips and Bishop, 1985). Paradoxically, early contact with moisture is equally damaging. Glass-ionomer cements rapidly absorb water, mainly in the first day (Crisp et al., 1976c, 1980). If the cement is not sufficiently mature, this can lead to disruption of the surface by swelling or loss of substance to the oral environment, which results in surface roughness (Wilson et al., 1981; Causton, 1981; Roulet and Wälti, 1984; Phillips and Bishop, 1985). However, if glass-ionomer cements are protected for between ten and 30 minutes, depending on brand, this problem does not arise.

Thus, glass-ionomer cements must be protected against two extremes: desiccation and aqueous fluids. It is a question of water balance, and as we have seen this is achieved in an atmosphere of 80% relative humidity. Higher humidities are not harmful, for the cement will then absorb water and expand. But contact with aqueous fluids must be avoided, for these remove, irretrievably, cement-forming ions.

Protection

What are the clinical implications of this need for water balance?

A rubber dam, while useful in protecting the unset cement from moisture, can

51

have a damaging effect by allowing the cement paste to desiccate. Desiccation will retard the reaction, and can cause shrinking and crazing once the cement has set. At this stage of the clinical procedure, the clinician should work with the cement exposed to the humid condition of the mouth while at the same time ensuring that moisture droplets do not contaminate the surface of the cement.

Once set, and after the matrix has been removed, the cement should be protected by a suitable barrier. The period of protection against moisture can be quite short. Sixty minutes will usually suffice, but the exact period depends on the brand used (Mount and Makinson, 1982; Phillips and Bishop, 1985).

As yet there appears to be no ideal barrier for the purpose (Earl et al., 1985; Earl and Ibbetson, 1986), but the clinician should use a proprietary brand designed for the purpose. Copal varnish and some other varnishes are not effective, although a clear nail varnish may be used. Emollients such as petroleum jelly can be effective, but are not suitable for all clinical situations because they are easily removed by tongue movements. Perhaps the best solution is to use a light-cured bonding agent.

Factors affecting setting characteristics

There are many chemical and physical factors that affect the setting characteristics of glass-ionomer cements. Although fundamentally an acid-base reaction, the reaction is complicated by the differential release and precipitation of calcium and aluminium ions and by their chelation by fluoride and tartrate ions.

While some factors—such as temperature, powder particle size, and powder/liquid ratio—merely serve to accelerate or retard the reactions, certain chemical factors have a more profound effect and play an important role in modifying the chemical reaction itself. The two most important are fluoride and tartaric acid.

The role of fluoride

In their early studies, before the effect of tartaric acid had been discovered, Wilson and Kent had to develop a glass high in fluoride, G-200, in order to obtain any working properties at all. They observed that glasses without fluoride yielded intractable, unworkable pastes. The inference drawn was that the fluoride ion profoundly affected the nature of the cement-forming reaction. Crisp and Wilson (1974a) and Barry and coworkers (1979) demonstrated clearly that working properties were influenced by the amount of fluoride released from the glass. The action of fluoride was attributed to the formation of metal complexes that retarded the binding of cations to anionic sites on the polyelectrolyte chain, thus delaying gelation and prolonging working time. Formation of complexes also releases hydrogen ions, thus increasing the acidity of the paste and delaying pH-dependent gelation.

The effect of tartaric acid

The favourable effect of fluoride and the knowledge that this effect depended on complex formation prompted Wilson and Crisp to search for other chelating agents (Wilson and Crisp, 1975; Wilson et al., 1976; Crisp and Wilson, 1976). They quickly discovered the unique effectiveness of optically actived tartaric acid (the *meso* form does not have this effect). This was the key discovery in the development of the glass-ionomer cement as a practical dental material. So important is (+)-tartaric acid to the viability of the system, that it must be regarded as a third component.

Tartaric acid is a cement-former in its own right, but its cements are totally unstable toward water (Wilson, 1968; Crisp and Wilson, 1976). But when added in moderate amounts to glass-ionomer cement systems, tartaric acid has several favourable effects. First, it improves manipulation of the cement paste and tends to increase working time. This effect is very noticeable when glasses that do not contain fluoride are used, for the addition of tartaric acid renders workable cement pastes that otherwise would be intractable. Second, tartaric acid sharpens set by accelerating the precipitation process (Crisp and Wilson, 1976). Third, when added in moderate amounts, tartaric acid increases cement strength. More importantly, tartaric acid has vastly widened the range of glasses that can be used for cement formation. Glasses containing less fluoride can be used, laying open the way for developing cements of greater translucency and aesthetic appeal.

The mechanism of action of tartaric acid has not been entirely elucidated, despite the work of Crisp and Wilson (1976) and Prosser and coworkers (1982a, 1982b). Tartaric acid is a stronger acid than poly(acrylic acid), forming strong complexes with aluminium and so enhancing extraction of aluminium from the glass. Prosser and coworkers (1982b), using carbon-13 nuclear magnetic resonance spectroscopy, showed that the initial reaction is between the glass and tartaric acid. They found initially that tartaric acid alone complexes cations, but then as neutralization proceeds and the pH rises

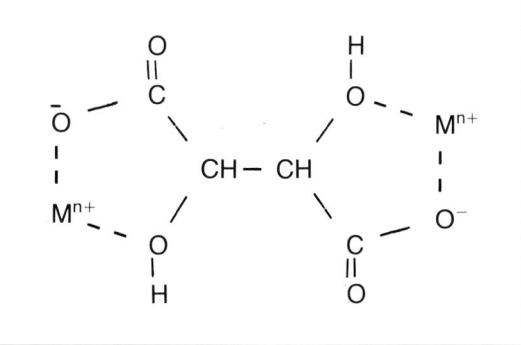

Fig. 3-8 The metal-tartrate complex bridging unit envisaged by Crisp and Wilson (1976). Reprinted with permission.

to around 3, poly(acrylic acid) becomes neutralized by metal ions until the cement sets at pH 5.0 to 5.5. In addition, the ionization of poly(acrylic acid) is suppressed and the unwinding of the poly-(acrylic acid) chain is retarded, thus reducing the viscosity of the paste and delaying gelation. However, once gelation occurs tartaric acid accelerates hardening. Tartaric acid would seem, therefore, to control the initial setting of the cement. Since tartaric acid and calcium react preferentially, the initial set is probably due to the formation of calcium tartrate.

Because glass-ionomer cements that contain tartaric acid are superior in strength to simple glass-ionomer cements, there must be some cooperative interaction between metal ions, tartaric acid, and poly(acrylic acid). Undoubtably, in the set cement tartrate is incorporated into a molecular structure together with polyacrylate and metal ions. Crisp and Wilson (1976) envisage a cross-linking unit consisting of a pair of metal ions bridged by tartrate that contains two pairs of chelating ligands (Fig. 3-8). It is also possible that fluoride ions are involved in this complex.

Figs. 3-9a to c Width of micrographs is 500 μm; original magnification ×200.

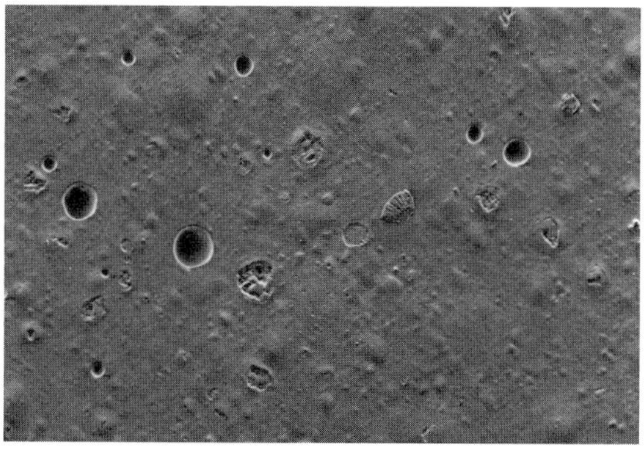

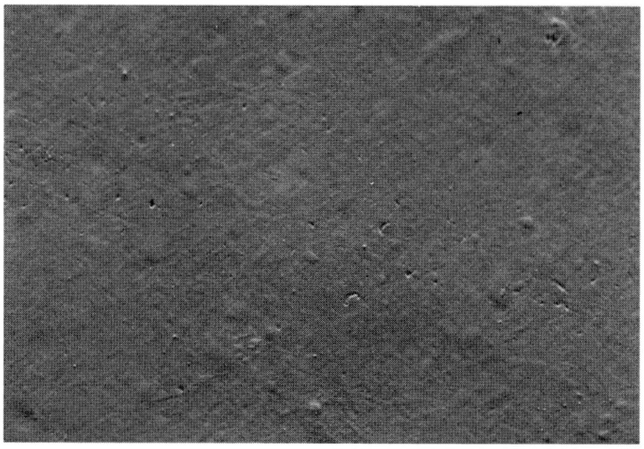

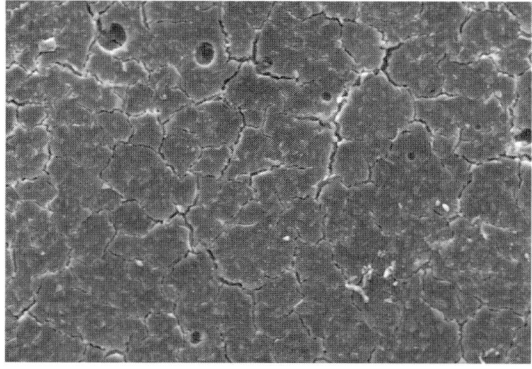

Factors affecting the rate of setting

In previous sections we have shown how certain chemical factors can affect the rate of setting. The effects of some of these—tartaric acid is a case in point—can be quite complex. Others are simple physical chemistry effects. Some are controlled in the manufacture and others lie in the hands of the clinician. A list of these factors is given below:

1. *Glass composition,* especially the alumina/silica ratio and fluoride content. Up to a limiting value, the higher the alumina/silica ratio the faster the set and the shorter the working time.
2. *Particle size* of the glass powder. The finer the powder the faster the set and the shorter the working time.
3. *Addition of tartaric acid.* Sharpens the set without shortening the working time.
4. *Relative proportions of the constituents* in the cement mix, i.e., glass/polyacid/tartaric acid/water. The greater the proportion of glass and the lower the proportion of water the faster the set and the shorter the working time (Crisp et al.; 1976b).

Fig. 3-9a *(top)* Surface of a glass-ionomer cement protected during curing. Reprinted with permission from Laboratory of the Government Chemist.

Fig. 3-9b *(middle)* Effect of early moisture contamination on the surface of a glass-ionomer cement. Reprinted with permission from Laboratory of the Government Chemist.

Fig. 3-9c *(bottom)* Effect of desiccation on the surface of a glass-ionomer cement. Reprinted with permission from Laboratory of the Government Chemist.

5. *Temperature* of mixing. The higher the temperature the faster the set and the shorter the working time.

Simple physical chemistry tells us the set will be faster when the powder is finer, the proportion of powder in the mix is greater, the amount of water in the mix is lower, and the temperature of mixing is higher. While a fast set can be an advantage, this is offset by a corresponding loss of working time.

The manufacturer has complete control over glass composition, particle size of the glass powder, and the addition of tartaric acid. The temperature of the mix is within the clinician's province and with some materials he can control the powder/liquid ratio in the mix.

McLean has, since the early 1970s, employed the technique of chilling the powder and the mixing slab. Mount and Makinson (1978) confirmed the usefulness of this technique and reported an increase in working time without loss of physical properties when slab and powder were cooled. A word of warning: if the liquid is a polyacid solution, chilling it may cause gelation. Also, if the humidity of the environment is high and the temperature of the slab is below the dew point, then moisture will condense on the cement materials and the cement will be weakened. When using this technique it is preferable to use an old-fashioned glass slab because it will have a greater thermal capacity and permit ready observation of moisture condensation when the temperature is below the dew point.

The glass/polyacid/tartaric acid/water ratio is controlled by the manufacturer when the materials are capsulated. For hand-mixed materials control is partly in the hands of the clinician, who can control the powder/liquid ratio. For filling and lining purposes the thickest mix is preferable. Setting, too, is always hastened and strength is improved by increasing the amount of glass powder in the mix. Conversely, setting is delayed and the cement is weakened if the amount of water in the mix is increased. Some of these effects are illustrated in Fig. 3-9.

References

Barry, T.I., Clinton, D.J., and Wilson, A.D. (1979) The structure of a glass-ionomer cement and its relationship to the setting process. J. Dent. Res. 58:1072–1079.

Brune, D., and Smith, D.C. (1982) Microstructure and strength properties of silicate and glass ionomer cements. Acta Odontol. Scand. 40:389–396.

Causton, B.E. (1981) The physico-mechanical consequences of exposing glass ionomer cements to water during setting. Biomaterials 2:112–115.

Cook, W.D. (1983) Degrative analysis of glass ionomer polyelectrolyte cements. J. Biomed. Mater. Res. 17:1015–1027.

Crisp, S., and Wilson, A.D. (1974a) Reactions in glass ionomer cements. I. Decomposition of the powder. J. Dent. Res. 53:1408–1413.

Crisp, S., and Wilson, A.D. (1974b) Reactions in glass ionomer cements. III. The precipitation reaction. J. Dent. Res. 53:1420–1424.

Crisp, S., and Wilson, A.D. (1976) Reactions in glass ionomer cements. V. Effect of incorporating tartaric acid in the cement liquid. J. Dent. Res. 55:1023–1031.

Crisp, S., Lewis, B.G., and Wilson, A.D. (1976a) Characterisation of glass-ionomer cements. 1. Long-term hardness and compressive strength. J. Dent. 4:162–166.

Crisp, S., Lewis, B.G., and Wilson, A.D. (1976b) Characterisation of glass-ionomer cements. 2. Effect of powder:liquid ratio on the physical properties. J. Dent. 4:287–290.

Crisp, S., Lewis, B.G., and Wilson, A.D. (1976c) Glass ionomer cements: Chemistry of erosion. J. Dent. Res. 55:1032–1041.

Crisp, S., Lewis, B.G., and Wilson, A.D. (1980) Characterisation of glass-ionomer cements. 6. A study of erosion and water absorption in both neutral and acidic media. J. Dent. 8:68–74.

Crisp, S., Pringuer, M.A., Wardleworth, D., and Wilson, A.D. (1974) Reactions in glass ionomer cements. II. An infrared spectroscopic study. J. Dent. Res. 53:1414–1419.

Earl, M.S.A., and Ibbetson, R.J. (1986) The clinical disintegration of a glass-ionomer cement. Br. Dent. J. 161:287–291.

Earl, M.S.A., Hume, W.R., and Mount, G.J. (1985) Effect of varnishes and other surface treatments on water movement across the glass-ionomer cement surface. Aust. Dent. J. 30:298–301.

Elliott, J., Holliday, L., and Hornsby, P.R. (1975) Physical and mechanical properties of glass-ionomer cements. Br. Polym. J. 7:297–306.

Hill, R.W. (1986) Unpublished data.

Hill, R.G., Warrens, C.P., and Wilson, A.D. (1986) Unpublished data.

Hornsby, P.R. (1980) Dimensional stability of glass-ionomer cements. J. Chem. Tech. Biotech. 30:595–601.

Mount, G.J., and Makinson, O.F. (1978) Clinical characteristics of a glass ionomer cement. Br. Dent. J. 145:67–71.

Mount, G.J., and Makinson, O.F. (1982) Glass-ionomer restorative cements: Clinical implications of the setting reaction. Oper. Dent. 7:134–141.

Paddon, J.M., and Wilson, A.D. (1976) Stress relaxation studies on dental materials. 1. Dental cements. J. Dent. 4:183–189.

Phillips, S., and Bishop, B.M. (1985) An in vitro study of the effect of moisture on glass ionomer cement. Quintessence Int. 16:175–177.

Prosser, H.J., Jerome, S.M., and Wilson, A.D. (1982a) The effect of additives on the setting properties of a glass-ionomer cement. J. Dent. Res. 61:1195–1198.

Prosser, H.J., Richards, C.P., and Wilson, A.D. (1982b) NMR spectroscopy of dental materials. II. The role of tartaric acid in glass-ionomer cements. J. Biomed. Mater. Res. 16:431–445.

Roulet, J.-F., and Wälti, C. (1984) Influence of oral fluids on composite resin and glass-ionomer cement. J. Prosthet. Dent. 52:182–189.

Saito, S. (1978) Characteristics of glass ionomer and its clinical application. I. Relations between hardening reactions and water. Int. J. Dent. Mater. 8:1–16.

Schmidt, W., Purrmann, R., Jochum, P., and Gasser, O. (1981) Calcium aluminofluorosilicate glass powder and its use. Eur. Pat. Appl. 23,013.

Wilson, A.D. (1968) Dental silicate cements. VII. Alternative liquid cement formers. J. Dent. Res. 47:1133–1136.

Wilson, A.D., and Crisp, S. (1975) Ionomer cements. Br. Polym. J. 7:279–296.

Wilson, A.D., Crisp, S., and Ferner, A.J. (1976) Reaction in glass-ionomer cements. IV. Effect of chelating co-monomers on setting behavior. J. Dent. Res. 55:489–495.

Wilson, A.D., Crisp, S., and Paddon J.M. (1981) The hydration of a glass-ionomer (ASPA) cement. Br. Polym. J. 13:66–70.

Wilson, A.D., Paddon, J.M., and Crisp, S. (1979) The hydration of dental cements. J. Dent. Res. 58:1065–1071.

Chapter 4

Physical Properties

Glass-ionomer cements set rapidly in the mouth, in three to eight minutes, and harden to form a body having a translucency that, at least in more recent commercial materials, matches that of tooth enamel. They are not to be regarded as completely brittle materials, for when young they behave almost like filled thermoplastic materials and deform slightly under load. However, they do lack toughness, and although high in compressive strength—200 MPa can be attained—they are comparatively weak in flexural strength (5 to 40 MPa). Of all the dental cements, they are the most resistant to erosion in the acidic stagnation regions of the mouth (Wilson et al., 1986). They are more resistant to staining and maintain their colour match better than composite resins. As with other dental cements, the powder/liquid ratio of the mix affects cement properties; thickly mixed materials have increased strength, more resistance to attack by fluids, and faster setting rates. Glass-ionomer cements slowly increase their strength as they age. A one-year-old cement is approximately twice as strong as a 24-hour-old cement and approaches 400 MPa in compressive strength.

Glass-ionomer cements are bioactive. They form permanent adhesive bonds to dentine and enamel, which enables them to help prevent the development of secondary caries by providing an almost perfect seal against the intrusion of caries-producing agents. They also have the ability to release fluoride over a prolonged period and so can arrest the progress of caries in adjacent tooth material. In these days, when more attention is being paid to biocompatibility, these are important properties. However, the hydrophilic nature of the cements also makes them susceptible to the action of aqueous fluids before they are fully set, requiring that the freshly placed restoration be protected by varnish or petroleum jelly.

The question the clinician needs to ask when approaching a restorative problem is whether it is better to have an inert resin filling material, which, while having better resistance to acid degradation, does nothing for the surrounding tooth, or to have a cement that may degrade but which releases fluoride and so protects the surrounding tooth material.

Test methods

The ultimate arbiter of the performance of a dental material, other than general experience, is the controlled clinical trial. But this is slow and expensive—not suitable for quality control of commercial products or in the early stages of formulation and development of a new material. There has to be recourse to laboratory testing to yield more rapid results.

It is useful to distinguish between the various types of in vitro tests. There are those that measure fundamental physical properties, for example, modulus. Such data cannot be questioned, although the connection between it and clinical performance may be far from obvious. Then there are the empirical tests, which seek to a greater or lesser degree to simulate clinical conditions and so predict clinical performance. If the simulation is poor then the data from such tests is worthless—or worse, for it can be misleading. Even when the simulation is good such data must be treated with the utmost caution.

The physical properties of some current glass-ionomer filling and luting cements are given in Tables 4-1 and 4-2 (Prosser et al., 1984). Many of these properties are based on specification test procedures of the International Organization for Standardization (1986) and the British Standards Institution (1981). A word of caution has to be given because they do not correspond to the clinical situation, nor are they, for the most part, fundamental material properties. Specification limits are also given in Tables 4-1 and 4-2.

Working and setting times

Both working time and setting time can be determined by indentation tests (ISO 7489:1986; BS 6039:1981). Setting in this context refers to the moment when the cement has set to an apparently rigid body; it does not represent the fully hardened state when the clinician can finish the restoration. The oscillating rheometer of Wilson (Bovis et al., 1971) gives more information and is a better measure of working time than the indentation test. Its dynamic nature is closer to the clinical situation than is the static indentation test.

Consistency and film thickness

Consistency is measured by the spread of a cement paste under a load and gives a rough idea of the mobility of the paste. Film thickness is the thickness obtained when paste mixture is pressed out under a load. It is a function of consistency and the grain size of the powder and is time dependent. The present standards insist that film thickness should not exceed 20 μm for luting agents. These tests are described in ISO 7489:1986 and BS 6039:1981.

Strength

The strength of dental cements has, in the past, always been measured as a *compressive strength.* Compressive strength is measured by applying a load to the flat ends of a cement cylinder until it fractures. This is still the specification test method, although there is a move toward the use of *flexural strength,* a more discriminating and clinically relevant test of strength (Prosser et al., 1984). Flexural strength gives a measure of tensile strength—the force required to pull two planes of atoms apart—which is a fundamental strength property. The other fundamental parameter is shear strength, which is a measure of the force required to slip two planes of atoms past each other. Failure in compression is generally by a shear mechanism, so that compressive strength is an indication of failure in shear, although other factors affect its magnitude. In the past compressive strength has been used more as a materials property than a criterion for clinical excellence. For example, phosphate-bonded cements with poor compressive strength tend to be unsatisfactory in other respects, such as durability. Chiefly, testing compressive strength has been used for quality control and is the specification test of strength. Details of the test method are given in ISO 7489:1986 and BS 6039:1981.

It is important to note that as the cement ages the compressive strength increases for at least a year, when the strength is about double what it is after only 24 hours (see Fig. 3-5; Crisp et al., 1976a).

The *diametral compressive test* (Smith, 1968) has been used to obtain figures for tensile strength. The load is applied diametrically across the cylinder. Theory demands that the material under test be absolutely brittle for the results to be meaningful measure of tensile strength, otherwise the test becomes a compression test with the load being applied diametrically. The test is probably not applicable to every dental cement, certainly not to the rather plastic zinc polycarboxylate cement. Although the glass-ionomer cement is often thought of as brittle, it, too, is somewhat plastic, especially when young.

Translucency

Translucency is a property of interest, for unless the translucency of a cement matches that of tooth enamel, a colour match can never been achieved. In practice it is measured by a property that is almost its inverse: *opacity* (Crisp et al., 1979). Opacity is a contrast ratio—the ratio of the reflectance of a specimen on a black background to its reflectance on a white background. The contrast ratio is 1.0 for an opaque body and 0.0 for a perfectly translucent one. For dental cements, opacity, or contrast ratio, is mea-sured using a 1-mm-thick disk and its value is expressed as a $C_{0.7}$ value. The 0.7 arises from the reflectivity of the white background, which is 70%. For optimum aesthetics, $C_{0.7}$ values should lie between 0.35 to 0.55. The glass-ionomer specification limits of 0.35 to 0.90 are somewhat too lenient. This topic is dealt with in more detail in chapter 5.

Solubility

Specification values for "solubility"—the term is a slight misnomer—are given for the sake of completeness (ISO 7489:1986; BS 6039:1981). However, we believe that these figures mislead rather than inform, for reasons given by Wilson in 1976.* Moreover, new harmonized specifications being developed by the International Organization for Standardization have now discarded this test in favour of an acid-erosion test. However, the "soluoility" test, when suitably modified, can be used to give an indication of early susceptibility to moisture (Prosser et al., 1984). In this modified test, a seven-minute-old cement is immersed in water and the amount of material going into solution is measured.

Acid-erosion test

A move is being made toward using Beham's impinging jet acid-erosion test to assess the durability of glass-ionomer cements and other dental cements (see Wilson et al., 1986 for a description). So far, the acid-erosion has been a good indicator of clinical durability. In the test,

---

*The test was carried out on immature specimens, for too brief a period (24 hours), using test solutions that were not representative of oral fluids, particularly acidic conditions, and without any element of erosion.

Table 4-1 Properties of filling materials*

Property	Test method	Limits	Conventional			
			ASPA X[†]	De Trey Aspa[‡]	Fuji Ionomer II[§]	Shofu Hy-Bond Restorative[¶]
Powder/liquid ratio (g/ml)	—	—	2.0	3.0	2.75	3.2
Consistency disc diam. (mm)	ISO 7489/BS 6039	—	29	33	34	26
Rheometer working time, 23°C (min)	Wilson et al. (1976)	—	2.4	2.7	3.8	1.3
Indentation working time, 23°C (min)	ISO 7489/BS 6039	1.75 min.	2.25	5.0	5.0	2.75
Setting time, 37°C (min)	ISO 7489/BS 6039	5.0 max.	3.5	4.25	3.75	3.8
Compressive strength, 24 h (MPa)	ISO 7489/BS 6039	125 min.	141	140	174	195
Diametral tensile strength, 24 h (MPa)	Smith (1968)	—	9.0	14.0	13.5	12.7
Flexural strength (MPa)	Prosser et al. (1984)	—	30.0	9.8	8.9	12.7
Creep, 24 h (%)	Wilson & Lewis (1980)	—	0.33	0.25	0.32	0.17
Water-leachable material, 7 min (%)	Prosser et al. (1984)	—	1.04	2.10	1.90	0.76
Water-leachable material, 1 h (%)	ISO 7489/BS 6039	0.7 max.	0.32	0.30	0.70	0.13
Opacity, $C_{0.7}$	ISO 7489/BS 6039	0.35–0.90	0.44	0.85	0.69	0.74

*Based on Prosser et al. (1984).
[†]Laboratory of the Government Chemist, London.
[‡]Amalgamated Dental Co., Weybridge, England.
[§]G-C International Corp., Tokyo, and Scottsdale, Ariz.
[¶]Shofu Dental Corp., Kyoto, Japan, and Menlo Park, Calif.

Table 4-1 (continued)

Property	Test method	Limits	Water-hardening			
			Ketac-Fil[#]	ASPA V[†]	Chem-Fil[**]	Chelon[#]
Powder/liquid ratio (g/ml)	—	—	—	7.2	6.8	6.7
Consistency disc diam. (mm)	ISO 7489/BS 6039	—	29	28	18	36
Rheometer working time, 23°C (min)	Wilson et al. (1976)	—	1.7	3.0	1.5	2.7
Indentation working time, 23°C (min)	ISO 7489/BS 6039	1.75 min.	2.75	5.75	2.0	3.5
Setting time, 37°C (min)	ISO 7489/BS 6039	5.0 max.	3.0	4.7	2.75	3.75
Compressive strength, 24 h (MPa)	ISO 7489/BS 6039	125 min.	185	147	161	178
Diametral tensile strength, 24 h (MPa)	Smith (1968)	—	19.3	12.8	17.4	16.0
Flexural strength (MPa)	Prosser et al. (1984)	—	30.3	25.7	19.5	13.5
Creep, 24 h (%)	Wilson & Lewis (1980)	—	0.21	0.22	0.19	0.23
Water-leachable material, 7 min (%)	Prosser et al. (1984)	—	0.29	2.12	0.90	0.36
Water-leachable material, 1 h (%)	ISO 7489/BS 6039	0.7 max.	0.13	0.55	0.28	0.16
Opacity, $C_{0.7}$	ISO 7489/BS 6039	0.35–0.90	0.61	0.84	0.70	0.75

[†]Laboratory of the Government Chemist, London.
[#]ESPE GmbH, Seefeld/Oberbay, West Germany, and Valley Stream, N.Y.
[**]Dentsply International Inc., Weybridge, England, and York, Pa.

Table 4-2 Properties of luting agents

Property	Test method	Limits	Conventional				Water-hardening		
			ASPA IVa†	Chembond‡	Fuji Ionomer I§	Shofu Hy-Bond Luting¶	ASPA Va†	Ketac-Cem#	Aqua-Cem‡
Powder/liquid ratio (g/ml)	—	—	1.67	1.86	1.75	1.83	3.6	3.4	3.3
Consistency disc diam (mm)	—	—	29	30	31	26	31	38	21
Maximum particle size (µm)	Prosser et al. (1984)	—	20	28	40	37	—	—	20
Film thickness (µm)	ISO 7489/BS 6039	25 max.	24	28	40	40	22	20	20
Rheometer working time, 23°C (min)	Wilson et al. (1978)	—	—	3.1	3.0	2.3	4.0	5.75	3.15
Indentation working time, 23°C (min)	ISO 7489/BS 6039	2.0 min.	2.5	4.5	5.0	4.25	4.3	5.75	3.5
Setting time, 37°C (min)	ISO 7489/BS 6039	7.5 max.	4.5	6.25	4.75	5.2	5.0	4.5	4.5
Compressive strength, 24 h (MPa)	ISO 7489/BS 6039	65 min.	128	118	139	162	124	105	82
Diametral tensile strength, 24 h (MPa)	Smith (1968)	—	—	6.4	7.5	10.9	7.8	5.3	7.6
Flexural strength, 24 h (MPa)	Prosser et al. (1984)	—	—	6.6	5.8	6.6	15.5	4.1	15.2
Creep, 24 h (%)	Wilson & Lewis (1980)	—	—	0.52	0.51	0.32	0.7	0.63	1.37
Water-leachable material, 7 min (%)	Prosser et al. (1984)	—	—	1.9	2.0	3.2	1.8	1.0	0.9
Water-leachable material, 1 h (%)	ISO 7489/BS 6039	1.0 max.	0.9	1.0	1.2	0.3	0.7	0.4	0.46
Opacity, $C_{0.7}$	Crisp et al. (1979)	—	—	0.77	0.67	0.83	0.76	0.87	0.88

*Based on Prosser et al. (1984).
†Laboratory of the Government Chemist, London.
‡Dentsply International Inc., Weybridge, England, and York, Pa.
§G-C International Corp., Tokyo, and Scottsdale, Ariz.
¶Shofu Dental Corp., Kyoto, Japan, and Menlo Park, Calif.
#ESPE GmbH, Seefeld/Oberbay, West Germany, and Valley Stream, N.Y.

cement specimens are subjected to an impinging jet of dilute lactic acid, and erosion is measured after a number of hours. Test results indicate that the glass-ionomer cements are the most durable of dental cements. The results are discussed more fully in chapter 7.

Dimensional stability

There has been some misunderstanding about the setting shrinkage of glass-ionomer cements. It is, in fact, difficult to disentangle setting shrinkage from other factors affecting the dimensional stability, such as humidity. Therefore, statements in the literature about setting shrinkage are to be taken with some reserve. The exotherm of glass-ionomer cement on setting indicates that there will be a setting shrinkage, but this will be low and obscured by gain or loss of water. The glass-ionomer cement is in equilibrium with an environment of 80% to 85% relative humidity. At greater humidities or in the presence of water the cement will absorb water, which tends to make the cement expand (Hornsby, 1980). In general, the extent of this expansion is sufficient to exceed the setting shrinkage, so that in practice, there is a net expansion of the cement. However, if the cement is allowed to desiccate it will shrink, for once the relative humidity drops below 80% to 85% the cement loses water.

Adhesion

Adhesion to enamel and dentine is discussed at length in chapter 6.

Restorative cements

Our discussion on the properties of glass-ionomer filling materials is based on the work of Prosser et al. (1984), who examined a number of commercial and experimental cements. Prosser and his coworkers found a clear difference between the mixing qualities of water-hardening and conventional cements; water-hardening cements were much easier to mix because of the low viscosities of the aqueous solutions used in them, compared with the thick polyacid solutions used in conventional materials. However, Chem-Fil,* a water-hardening cement, proved to be noticeably thicker when mixed than all the other cements tested, as shown by the smallness of its consistency spread.

Each of the glass-ionomer cements tested passed specification limits for working time (measured by indentation test) and setting times. However, some cements, particularly Fuji Ionomer II,† had more favourable working time (measured by rheometer)/setting time ratios than others. (The rheometer test values are quoted here because this test is a more realistic simulation of clinical conditions than the indentation test.)

More important and clinically relevant than either compressive or diametral tensile strength is flexural strength. The flexural strength of glass-ionomer cements is quite low and varies considerably between the different cements studied (8.9 to 30.3 MPa). The variation was proportionately much greater than that found for compressive strength, which suggests there is still considerable scope for improving this property.

*Dentsply International Inc., Weybridge, England, and York, Pa.
†G-C International Corp., Tokyo, and Scottsdale, Ariz.

The compressive strength of glass-ionomer cements is quite high; in all cases it exceeded 140 MPa for 24-hour-old cements, and in some cases it approached 200 MPa. Note that the relative differences between cements were not great. All brands exceeded the specification limit, which is set rather low at 125 MPa. However, the clinical significance of this property is limited.

The diametral compressive (tensile) strength values are given in Table 4-1, but will not be discussed because the validity of the test is uncertain.

Material water-leached from seven-minute-old cements is an inverse measure of early resistance to moisture. Of the older materials based on the original ionomer glass, G-200, De Trey Aspa* (the first commercial cement) and ASPA V (the first water-hardening material derived from ASPA IV) had the least early resistance to water. Ketac-Fil,† a more recent material, stood out in having the most early resistance to water.

Opacity ($C_{0.7}$) values were all within the specification limits of 0.35 to 0.90. However, it must be admitted that the upper specification limit in glass-ionomer cement specifications ISO 7489 and BS 6039 was set very high to accommodate early glass-ionomer materials that were deficient in translucency. A more clinically relevant upper limit is 0.55, the upper limit in the dental silicate cement specifications ISO 1565 (1978) and BS 3365/1 (1980). Only one glass-ionomer cement met this requirement—ASPA X, based on an improved glass, G-338, from the Laboratory of the Government Chemist. Of the other cements, only Ketac-Fil has satisfactory translucency. However, there has been a marked improvement in this property over the years. The early glass-ionomer cements De Trey Aspa and ASPA IV had much higher $C_{0.7}$ values (0.85) than those of more recent cements, such as ASPA X ($C_{0.7} = 0.44$) and Ketac-Fil ($C_{0.7} = 0.61$). More improvements are needed in the translucency of glass-ionomer cements. The topic is discussed more fully in chapter 5.

Overall, it must be noted that the capsulated material, Ketac-Fil, has the most favourable combination of properties. It is the least affected by early contamination with water, and is one of the strongest (judged by flexural strength). The indication is that it is the hardest, probably because the use of a acrylic acid/maleic acid copolymer yields a more highly cross-linked matrix. In addition, it has the greatest translucency apart from the experimental ASPA X. Working time is limited, although there is some gain in actual manipulation time because of the rapid mixing in the mechanical mixer used in this system. However, it is probably less resistant to acid erosion and less adhesive than cements based on poly(acrylic acid) (Setchell et al., 1985; Wilson et al., 1986; Thornton et al., 1986).

Luting cements

Not all examples of glass-ionomer luting cements are satisfactory as judged by the ISO specifications (see Table 4-2). The property that most commonly causes failure is film thickness. All conventional commercial luting agents, that is, those supplied with the polyacid present as a solution, have inadequate film thickness. Indeed, the Laboratory of the Government Chemist's experimental material ASPA IVa is the only luting agent of this type that passes the specification requirement. By contrast, all water-harden-

*Amalgamated Dental Co., Weybridge, England.
†ESPE GmbH, Seefeld/Oberbay, West Germany, and Valley Stream, N.Y.

ing cements meet the film thickness requirement.

All the luting cements meet the specification requirements for working and setting time, but there are, however, considerable differences among them. Ketac-Cem* has particularly favourable setting properties, combining the shortest setting time with the longest working time (as measured by rheometer). These favourable properties probably arise from an acid-wash treatment of the glass powder and are well illustrated by the rheograms presented in Fig. 4-1. Both Ketac-Cem and Chembond have a sharp set (judged by the shape of the envelope of the rheogram to the setting point). However, Ketac-Cem shows a much extended working time and flows more readily than other cements. Indeed, the consistency spread is very high (38 mm in diameter) compared with other cements. This cement can be painted on substrates with a fine brush (McLean et al., 1984).

The compressive strength of glass-ionomer cement is high when compared with other luting agents, and far exceeds those of the zinc phosphate and polycarboxylate cements. In all cases they are well above the specification limit, which is set low at 65 MPa. One cement, Shofu Hy-bond† has a particuarly high compressive strength of 162 MPa. This value even exceeds the compressive strengths of some glass-ionomer filling materials. The effect of the low powder/liquid ratio is offset by the finer grain size of the glass powder.

Flexural strengths of luting materials, taken as a group, are significantly lower than the best of the filling materials.

*ESPE GmbH, Seefeld/Oberbay, West Germany, and Valley Stream, N.Y.
†Shofu Dental Corp., Kyoto, Japan, and Menlo Park, Calif.

The creep value of one of the water-hardening luting cements is significantly higher than that of the conventional luting cements. This difference is not apparent with filling materials. However, it may be an indication that the setting of water-hardening cements is different from that of the conventional cements. Conductance and permittivity values (Prosser et al., 1984; Tay and Braden, 1984) confirm this supposition. It would seem that, for some reason, water-hardening cements contain more unbound water than their conventional equivalents, at least for several hours. Unbound water will tend to act as a plasticizer.

Luting glass-ionomer cements are much more affected by early contamination by water than are the filling materials, because of the low powder/liquid ratio employed.

Comparison of cement types

Glass-ionomer cements are universal materials and have a wide range of applications: aesthetics, luting restorations, luting crowns and inlays, lining cavities, constructing cores, and sealing pits and fissures. The tendency has been for manufacturers to develop a range of glass-ionomer cements with properties appropriate for each application: a material for pit and fissure sealing is high in fluoride, for example. It is interesting to note that the Laboratory of the Government Chemist used a glass high in fluoride, G-200, in the original glass-ionomer cements ASPA II and ASPA IV—which was successful as a pit and fissure sealant.

The remaining applications for the various types of glass-ionomer cements are well illustrated by one manufacturer's

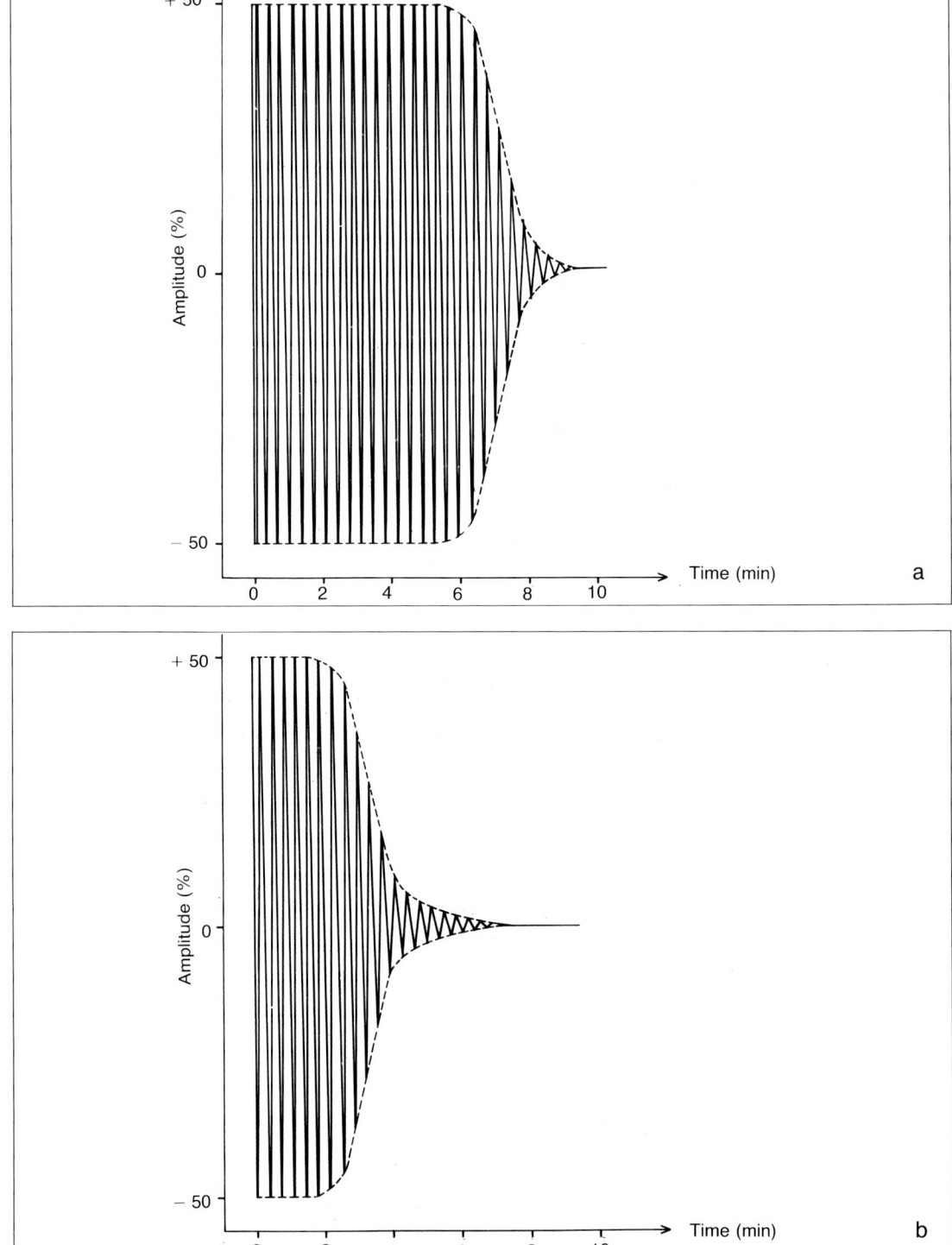

Fig. 4-1 Wilson rheometer trace for *(a)* Ketac-Cem and *(b)* Chembond.

range of materials, listed in Table 4-3. These show interesting variations in properties and demonstrate how the glass-ionomer cement can be easily tailored to specific applications.

The Type I luting agent Ketac-Cem has an extended working time and sharp set in comparison with Types II and III cements. It is a comparatively weak material; seemingly this price has been paid for its excellent setting characteristic. There is a radio-opaque version of this luting agent, in which some of the calcium in the glass is replaced by lanthanum.

The Type II aesthetic filling materials (Ketac-Fil and Chelon) are stronger than the Type I luting agents. However, the glasses for these materials have to be clear in order to achieve good aesthetics. This means that the SiO_2/Al_2O_3 ratio must be kept high with the consequence that hardening is sluggish. Despite this, the Type II filling materials are the strongest in the range.

The Type III materials, used for lining, are fast setting. They need to harden rapidly because they are often acid-etched.

Factors affecting cement properties

In chapter 2 we noted that cement properties are affected by the composition of the cement. The temperature of cement preparation affects working time, which is prolonged as the temperature of preparation is reduced. Advantage is taken of this when the mixing slab is cooled in order to prolong working time.

Powder/liquid ratio affects several properties. The thicker the mix, the faster the cement sets and the stronger and more durable it becomes (Crisp et al., 1976b).

Conclusions

Glass-ionomer cements show a wide range of properties and are clearly very diverse materials. The filling materials are broadly satisfactory apart from translucency, although even here there are one or two materials that are satisfactory. Of the luting cements, all of the water-hardening types are satisfactory, while all of the conventional commercial types have inadequate film thickness. Over the years, marked improvements have been made in working and setting properties, early resistance to moisture, and translucency. But clearly there is still much room for further development.

Table 4-3 Comparative properties of various types of glass-ionomer cement*

Property	Type 1		Type II				Type III	
	Ketac-Cem	Ketac-Cem Radio-opaque	Ketac-Fil	Chelon	Ketac-Silver	Chelon-Silver	Ketac-Bond	
P:L, by mass	3.4	3.8	caps	3.2	2.0	3.8	3.4	4.2
Working time (min)	3.5	3.5	2.0	3.0	2.0	4.0	2.0	2.0
Final setting time (min)	7.0	7.0	15.0	15.0	5.0	7.0	4.0	3.5
Compressive strength (MPa)	120	120	170	170	190	150	120	170
Diametral tensile strength (MPa)	9	9	15	15	14	13	6	13
Flexural strength (MPa)	12	—	18	18	32	32	13	16
Surface hardness (MPa)	160	160	200	300	240	—	120	235
Film thickness (μm)	20	20	—	—	—	—	—	—
Dentine adhesion (MPa)	5	—	5	—	—	—	4	4
Enamel adhesion (MPa)	5	—	5	—	—	—	—	—
Coeff. thermal expansion, K^{-1}	—	—	13×10^{-6}	—	15×10^{-6}	—	8×10^{-6}	8×10^{-6}
Solubility (%)	0.1	0.1	0.1	0.1	—	0.1	0.2	0.1

*All products of ESPE GmbH, Seefeld/Oberbay, West Germany, and Valley Stream, N.Y. Data supplied by ESPE GmbH.

Appendix: Test methods for glass-ionomer cements

We consider it useful to give an outline of the test procedures used to evaluate glass-ionomer cements in order to familiarize the reader with this aspect of materials science. It would be inappropriate for us to go into more detail in a book of this nature. Those interested in the fine details of testing should go to the original papers or specifications where they are described in detail.

Preparation of cements

For hand-mixed cements, pastes for specimens are prepared by spatulating together, as quickly as possible, measured portions of the powder and liquid into a smooth paste. Mixing time must not exceed one minute. Atmospheric conditions are carefully controlled at 23°C and 50% relative humidity (ISO 7489:1986 and BS 6039:1981).

Capsulated materials are also available and these are prepared by mechanical mixing.

Consistency

A cylinder of cement paste, 0.5 cm^3 in volume, is placed between two horizontal glass plates two minutes after start of mix and a vertical load is applied to it. The diameter of the disk so formed is measured and taken as an indication of the consistency of the cement paste. The load applied is 220 g for Type I luting cements and 2.5 kg for Type II filling cements. The test is carried out at 23°C and 50% relative humidity (ISO 7489:1986 and BS 6039:1981).

Film thickness (for Type I luting cements only)

A small quantity of cement paste is placed between two horizontal glass plates, and a vertical load of 15 kg is applied to it two minutes after start of mix. After the cement has set the thickness of the film formed is measured. The test is carried out at 23°C and 50% relative humidity (ISO 7489:1986 and BS 6039:1981).

Working time

The cement paste is tested with an indentor, mass 28 g and diameter 2 mm. Working time is taken as the time when the needle fails to indent the surface measured from the start of mix. The test is carried out at 23°C and 50% relative humidity (ISO 7489:1986 and BS 6039:1981).

Setting time

The cement paste is tested with an indentor, mass 400 g and diameter 1 mm. Setting time is taken as the time when the needle fails to indent the surface measured from the time of mix. The test is carried out in a humidifier at 37°C (ISO 7489:1986 and BS 6039:1981).

Oscillating rheometry

The reader is referred to original publications for details. The test can be run at 23°C and 37°C. The cement paste is placed between the platens of an oscillating rheometer and the trace of the amplitude of the oscillations is recorded.

The amplitude decreases as the cement paste thickens. Working time is taken when the amplitude of the oscillations decreases to 95% of the original value. This test is carried out at 23°C. Setting time is taken as the point when the amplitude of the trace reaches a constant value. This test is carried out at 37°C (Bovis et al., 1971).

Compressive strength

A cement cylinder, either 12 mm × 6 mm in diameter or 6 mm × 4 mm in diameter (for capsulated materials), is aged in a humidifier for 24 hours at 37°C. It is then placed upright on the horizontal platen of a mechanical testing machine. A progressively increasing compressive load is applied to the flat ends of the specimen. The load at fracture is recorded and the compressive strength is calculated from the following formula:

$$\text{Compressive strength} = P/\pi r^2$$

where P is the load at fracture and r is the radius of the cylinder (ISO 7489:1986 and BS 6039:1981).

Diametral tensile strength

A cement cylinder, 4 mm × 8 mm in diameter, is aged in a humidifier for 24 hours at 37°C. It is then placed on its side on the horizontal platen of a mechanical testing machine. A progressively increasing compressive load is applied to the flat ends of the specimen. The load at fracture is recorded and the tensile strength calculated from the following formula:

$$\text{diametral tensile strength} = P/2\pi rh$$

where P is the load at fracture, r is the radius of the cylinder, and h is the height of the cylinder (ISO 7489:1986 and BS 6039:1981).

Flexural strength

A cement beam 25 × 3 × 3 mm is aged in a humidifier for 24 hours at 37°C. It is then laid between two horizontal parallel rollers placed 20 mm apart. A progressively increasing load (applied by a knife edge to the middle of the specimen) is applied to the flat ends of the specimen. The load at fracture is recorded and the flexural strength is calculated from the following formula:

$$\text{Flexural strength} = 3Pl/2bd^2$$

where P is the load at fracture, l is the distance between the two rollers, b is the breadth of the specimen, and d is the depth of the specimen (Prosser et al., 1986).

Opacity

Opacity is determined using a disk 1.0 mm thick after it has aged in a humidifier for 24 hours at 37°C. The cement disk, contained in a small shallow trough of water, is placed within a reflectometer on a black background. It is then illuminated with diffuse light and the light reflected from it is measured (R_0). The cement disk is then placed on a white background of 70% reflectivity and the measurement is repeated to give another reflectivity value ($R_{0.7}$). The contrast ratio $R_0/R_{0.7}$ is the $C_{0.7}$ opacity (Crisp et al., 1979).

Water-soluble materials—one hour

Two cement disks (20 mm in diameter × 1.5 mm thick), after being aged in a humidifier for one hour at 37°C, are placed in 50 cm^3 water. After 24 hours the disks are removed and the amount of material going into the solution is measured by evaporation to dryness and weighing (ISO 7489:1986 and BS 6039:1981).

Water-soluble materials—seven minutes

This test is identical to the one above except that the cement is only aged for seven minutes at 37°C before being immersed in water. It is used as a measure of early resistance to moisture (Prosser et al., 1984).

Acid-erosion

The method employed is the impinging jet method of Beham. The description given here of this complex test method is necessarily brief, and recourse must be made to the reference for full details. In this method a row of cylindrical holes (4 mm in diameter × 7 mm deep) in a rack are filled with cement paste. The cements are cured for 24 hours before an impinging jet of lactic acid (pH = 2.7) is directed on the flat surface of the cement for between one and seven hours. The depth of the erosion is measured (Wilson et al., 1986).

References

Bovis, S.C., Harrington, E., and Wilson, H.J. (1971) Setting characteristics of composite filling materials. Br. Dent. J. 131:352–356.

British Standards Institution (1981) British Standard for glass-ionomer cements. BS 6039.

Crisp, S., Abel, G., and Wilson, A.D. (1979) The quantitative measurement of the opacity of aesthetic dental filling materials. J. Dent. Res. 58:1585–1596.

Crisp, S., Lewis, B.G., and Wilson, A.D. (1976a) Characterisation of glass-ionomer cements. 1. Long-term hardness and compressive strength. J. Dent. 4:162–166.

Crisp, S., Lewis, B.G., and Wilson, A.D. (1976b) Characterisation of glass-ionomer cements. 2. Effect of powder:liquid ratio on the physical properties. J. Dent. 4:287–290.

Hornsby, P.R. (1980) Dimensional stability of glass-ionomer cements. J. Chem. Tech. Biotech. 30:595–601.

International Organization for Standardization (1986) International Standard for glass polyalkenoate cements. ISO 7486.

McLean, J.W., Wilson, A.D., and Prosser, H.J. (1984) The clinical development of water-hardening glass-ionomer luting cements. J. Prosthet. Dent. 52:175–181.

Prosser, H.J., Powis, D.R., and Wilson, A.D. (1986) Glass-ionomer cements of improved flexural strength. J. Dent. Res. 65:146–148.

Prosser, H.J., Powis, D.R., Brant, P., and Wilson, A.D. (1984) Characterisation of glass-ionomer cements. 7. The physical properties of current materials. J. Dent. 12:231–240.

Setchell, D.J., Teo, C.K., and Kuhn, A.T. (1985) The relative solubilities of four modern glass-ionomer cements. Br. Dent. J. 158:220–222.

Smith, D.C. (1968) A new dental cement. Br. Dent. J. 125:381–384.

Tay, W.M., and Braden, M. (1984) Dielectric properties of glass ionomer cements—further studies. J. Dent. Res. 63:74–75.

Thornton, J.B., Retief, D.H., and Bradley, E.L. (1986) Fluoride release from and tensile bond strength of Ketac-Fil and Ketac-Silver to enamel and dentin. Dent. Mater. 2:241–245.

Wilson, A.D. (1976) Specification test for the solubility and disintegration of dental cement: A critical evaluation of its meaning. J. Dent. Res. 55:721–729.

Wilson, A.D., and Lewis, B.G. (1980) The flow properties of dental cements. J. Biomed. Mater. Res. 14:383–391.

Wilson, A.D., Crisp, S., Lewis, B.G., and McLean, J.W. (1977) Experimental luting agents based on the glass-ionomer cements. Br. Dent. J. 142:117–122.

Wilson, A.D., Groffman, D.M., Powis, D.R., and Scott, R.P. (1986) An evaluation of the significance of the impinging jet method for measuring the acid erosion of dental cements. Biomaterials 7:55–60.

Chapter 5

Aesthetics

A dental material used to restore a cavity on the labial side of an anterior tooth must match the appearance of the enamel if it is to be aesthetically satisfactory. This is not just a question of matching colour. For two surfaces to match they must be alike in colour, translucency, and texture. Enamel is a glossy and translucent material with a pearl-like appearance. Light falling on it is reflected by scattering after it has entered the translucent enamel. Because there is dentine of a less translucent material underlying enamel, the situation is complex. Be that as it may, a restorative material can only be matched to tooth enamel if it has a similar degree of translucency and gloss. Translucency gives a sense of depth to a dental restorative material that would otherwise appear dull and lifeless against tooth enamel. It is for this reason that dental porcelain enamels are so lifelike.

Translucency

The glass-ionomer cement is an aesthetic filling material because it has a degree of translucency. Its translucency arises because its filler is a glass and not an opaque substance, like zinc oxide. The translucency of the glass-ionomer cement depends on its formulation, and much attention has been paid to optimizing this property.

Early examples of glass-ionomer cements, both experimental and commercial, were insufficiently translucent and could not, therefore, be exactly colour matched to tooth enamel (Crisp et al., 1979). Clinical results were disappointing. However, these research workers reported an experimental glass-ionomer cement—ASPA X—which was as translucent as tooth material (Fig. 5-1). Since then there has been a notable improvement in the translucency of some commercial materials, although none have yet matched ASPA X. In the future, the clinician will have fully aesthetic glass-ionomer cements for the restoration of anterior teeth.

It is important to note that, because of slow hydration reactions, glass-ionomer cements take at least 24 hours to fully mature and to develop full translucency; only after this waiting period can a glass-ionomer cement completely match tooth enamel. Unless the patient is recalled a day or two later, the clinician will fail to observe this, which can perhaps account for clinical reports of colour mismatch and some apparent disappointments. However, if this characteristic of the glass-ionomer cement is accepted, it will prove to have long-term aesthetic advantages because, unlike composite resins which stain and lose their colour

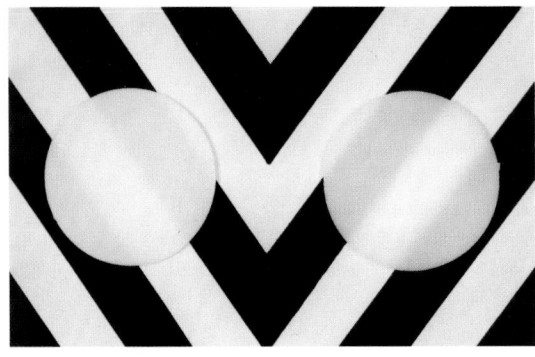

Fig. 5-1 Examples of glass-ionomer cements of varying degrees of translucency. *(left)* An early example of a glass-ionomer cement showing poor translucency; *(right)* a modern glass-ionomer cement with improved translucency. Reprinted with permission from Laboratory of the Government Chemist.

Table 5-1 Opacity ($C_{0.7}$) values for glass-ionomer cements*

Filling materials		Luting agents		Composite resins	
ASPA I‡	0.76	ASPA IVa‡	0.77	Concise‡‡	0.75
ASPA II‡	0.73	ASPA Va‡	0.84	Sevriton§	0.40
ASPA IV‡	0.73	Chembond†§	0.77		
ASPA X‡	0.52	Aqua-Cem#	0.88		
De Trey Aspa†§	0.84	Fuji Type I**	0.67		
Chem-Fil#	0.70	Ketac-Cem¶	0.87		
Fuji Type II**	0.69	Shofu Hy-Bond	0.83		
Ketac-Fil¶	0.61	Luting(†)††			
Chelon¶	0.75				
Shofu Hy-Bond Filling(†)††	0.74				

*Modified from Crisp et al. (1979) and Prosser et al. (1984).
†Superseded materials.
‡Experimental materials, Laboratory of the Government Chemist, London.
§Amalgamated Dental Co., Weybridge, England.
#Dentsply International Inc., Weybridge, England, and York, Pa.
¶ESPE GmbH, Seefeld/Oberbay, West Germany, and Valley Stream, N.Y.
**G-C International Corp., Tokyo, and Scottsdale, Ariz.
††Shofu Dental Corp., Kyoto, Japan, and Menlo Park, Calif.
‡‡3M Dental Products, St. Paul, Minn.

match in the mouth, the colour of glass-ionomer cements remains unaffected by oral fluids. P. J. Knibbs and coworkers (1986), in a three-year study of Class III glass-ionomer cement restorations, found that none were in need of replacement as the result of a poor colour match.

The translucency of dark shades is less than that of the light shades (Crisp et al., 1979; Asmussen, 1983). Also, early contamination of the cement surface with moisture adversely affects translucency (Asmussen, 1983). Thus, it is in the hands of the clinician to maximize translucency by adopting careful clinical techniques.

Opacity

What are the fundamental factors that control translucency? In discussing this it is easier to talk about its inverse, *opacity,* which is the property generally measured in the laboratory.

Materials like the zinc oxide cements are almost 100% opaque because their filler is opaque. Glass-ionomer cements have a degree of translucency because the filler is clear or opalescent. However, opacity can arise even if both filler and matrix are clear, when the refractive indices of the glass filler and the matrix are not identical. This mismatch gives rise to light scattering—the greater the mismatch of refractive indices the greater will be the scattering of light and the greater the opacity. The particle size of the glass particles also has an effect, and particles of the same dimensions as the wavelength of light will absorb that light, becoming, in effect, opaque. Opacity is also increased if the glass particles are themselves not clear, as is often the case with glass-ionomer cements. Clear or slightly opalescent glasses need to be used to minimize opacity. Heavily phase-separated glasses or glass-ceramics are to be avoided.

So far we have discussed aesthetics, translucency, and opacity in purely qualitative terms. In order to discuss the topic in more detail, it is necessary to define these parameters quantitatively. This is best done in terms of opacity.

Opacity is not a material property since, as will be shown, it depends on other parameters. Opacity can also be termed *contrast ratio* (C_r), for it is defined quantitatively as the ratio of the light reflected from a laminar of the material placed on a black background (R_0) to that when it is placed on a white background (R_r):

$$C_r = R_0/R_r,$$

where r is the reflectivity of the white surface. In the specification for dental cements the value chosen for r is 0.70, i.e., the reflectivity of the white surface is 70% of that of a "pure" white surface of magnesium oxide (Paffenbarger, 1937; Judd, 1937; Paffenbarger et al., 1938). Thus, we speak of $C_{0.7}$ values as a measure of opacity for a laminar 1.0 mm thick. Obviously, $C_{0.7}$ will increase with the thickness of the disc.

If a material is opaque, $C_r = 1$, and if perfectly translucent, $C_r = 0$.

Opacity values ($C_{0.7}$) for a number of current, experimental, and past glass-ionomer cements are given in Table 5-1. The $C_{0.7}$ value of a cement should not exceed 0.55 if it is to match the translucency of tooth enamel. This value is the upper limit specified in the dental silicate cement standards ISO 1565 (1978) and BS 3365/I (1980). As yet, only Chem-Fil II and ASPA X (now eight years old) meet this requirement. Of course, all glass-ionomer cements meet the opacity requirement of the glass-ionomer cement standards ($C_{0.7} < 0.9$), but these are far too lenient for an aesthetic filling material.

As mentioned previously, translucency

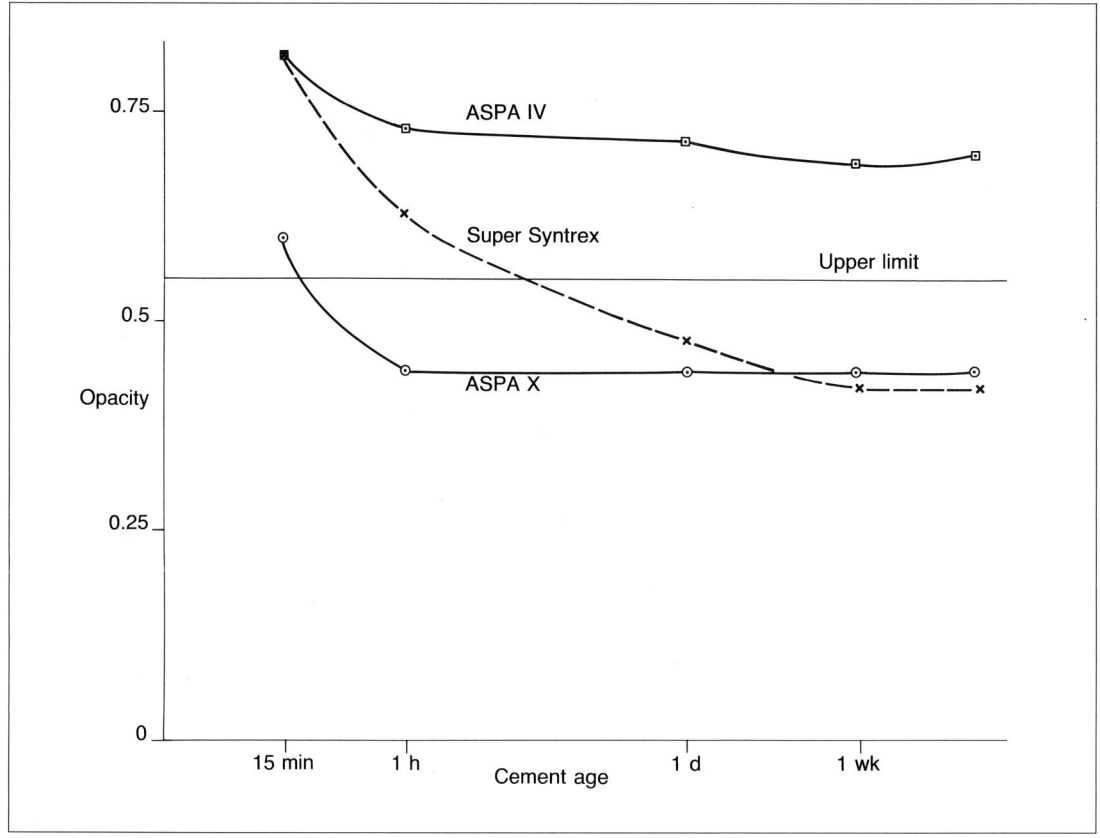

Fig. 5-2 Changes in the opacity of glass-ionomer cements as they age. Reproduced with permission from Crisp et al. (1979).

of glass-ionomer cements increases as they age, and is reflected by a decrease in their opacity (Fig. 5-2). This change is rapid during the first hour of maturation, but thereafter changes are slow. In the case of ASPA X, opacity attains a minimum value in 24 hours. But ASPA IV shows further decreases, although very slight, in $C_{0.7}$ values over a few days. The practical implication is that the clinician needs to wait for at least an hour before he can judge colour match. The clinician could be aided if manufacturers developed a shade guide of paired hues: those obtained immediately after the cement has set and those of the fully matured cement.

Scattering power and reflectance

As we have noted previously, opacity is not a material property but depends on other, more fundamental, properties: the scattering coefficient, S, the light reflectance from an infinite depth of material, R_∞, and the thickness of the specimen, θ. Scattering power is $S\theta$. If no light is absorbed by a translucent body, $R_\infty = 1.0$. If the light is totally absorbed, $R_\infty = 0$. For a perfectly translucent body, $S\theta = 0$, and for one which is totally opaque, $S\theta = \infty$. In practice, if $S\theta$ attains a reasonable value, say 3.0, the body is, for all practical purposes, opaque.

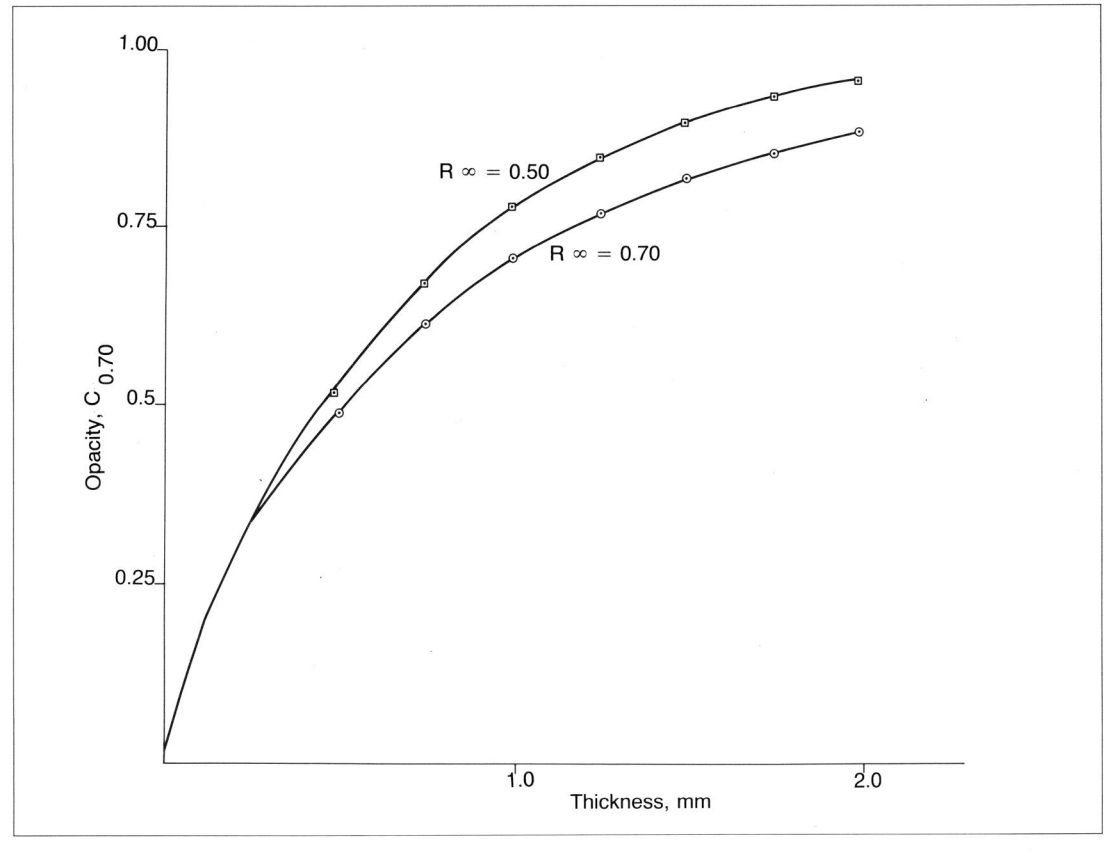

Fig. 5-3   Effect of pigmentation and cement thickness on the opacity of a glass-ionomer cement.

Opacity or contrast ratio, R_0/R_r, is a function of S, R, and θ, since R_0 and R_r are functions of those basic parameters. It is also dependent on r, the reflectance of the white background used in its determination. Equations relating R_0 and R_r, and, hence, C_R, to S, R_∞, θ, and r were developed more than 50 years ago by Kubelka and Munk (1931) and are given in the appendix to chapter 5. Suffice it to say at if R_0, R_r, and θ are measured, then S and R_∞ can be calculated using nonograms developed by Judd (1934, 1937).

The implication of these relationships is that opacity is affected by *(1)* pigmentation, because pigments absorb light

(rather than increase S) and so reduce R_∞, and *(2)* cement thickness, θ, since scattering power, $S\theta$, increases with θ. Thus, as Fig. 5-3 and Table 5-1 show, opacity increases with θ and its pigmentation; see curves in Fig. 5-3 for the unpigmented ASPA IV cement and the cement pigmented dark yellow with sienna. The effect of pigmentation is shown in more detail in Table 5-2. Note that S is not affected by pigmentation, but that R_∞ is reduced because of the light absorbed by the pigment; consequently, $C_{0.7}$ is reduced. The relationship between opacity and reflectivity is shown in Fig. 5-4.

Both Crisp et al. (1979) and Asmussen (1983) have, in fact, noted that dark

Table 5-2 Effect of pigmentation on opacity ($C_{0.7}$), scattering coefficient (S), and reflectance value (R_∞) of ASPA IV*

Pigmentation (%)	$C_{0.7}$ (1 mm)	S (mm^{-1})	R_∞
None	0.75	1.2	0.65
Yellow ochre			
0.05	0.75	1.2	0.65
0.075	0.77	1.3	0.64
0.1	0.73	1.1	0.65
0.2	0.78	1.3	0.62
0.5	0.83	1.2	0.47
Sienna			
0.05	0.79	1.1	0.50
0.075	0.81	1.2	0.49
0.1	0.84	1.2	0.44
0.2	0.91	1.2	0.33
0.5	0.95	1.0	0.21
Carbon black			
0.01	0.81	1.1	0.45
0.1	0.91	1.0	0.28

*Modified from Crisp et al. (1979).

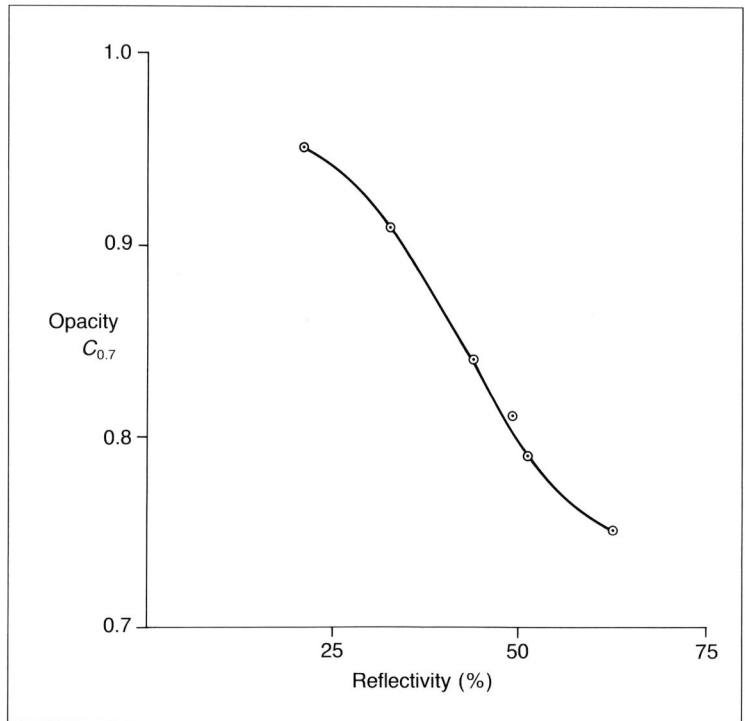

Fig. 5-4 The relationship between opacity ($C_{0.7}$) and reflectivity (R_∞) for a cement pigmented to different degrees.

Table 5-3 Opacity ($C_{0.7}$) scattering coefficient *(S),* and reflectance value (R_∞) for various filling materials*

Filling material	$C_{0.7}$	S (mm^{-1})	R_∞
Glass-ionomer cements			
ASPA I‡	0.76	1.25	0.75
ASPA II‡	0.73	1.23	0.78
ASPA IV‡	0.73	1.19	0.72
ASPA X‡	0.52	0.61	0.70
De Trey Aspa†§	0.84	1.85	0.77
Fuji Type II¶	0.64	0.78	0.55
Silicate cements			
Biotrey#	0.56	0.65	0.50
Achatit**	0.49	0.51	0.56
Restorative resins			
Concise††	0.75	1.09	0.56
Sevriton§	0.40	0.36	0.45

*Modified from Crisp et al. (1979).
†Superseded materials.
‡Experimental materials, Laboratory of the Government Chemist, London.
§Amalgamated Dental Co. Weybridge, England. (Now Dentsply International, Inc., Weybridge, England and York, Pa.)
¶G-C International Corp., Tokyo, and Scottsdale, Ariz.
#Dentsply International Inc., Weybridge, England, and York, Pa.
**Vivadent Inc., Tonawanda, N.Y.
††3M Dental Products, St. Paul, Minn.

shades increase opacity. But, as stated above, this is merely a consequence of fundamental relationships and may have little clinical significance because the stained enamel to which these are matched will also have reduced translucency.

Values for $C_{0.7}$, S, and R_∞ are given in Table 5-3 for several light-coloured glass-ionomer cements and other filling materials. It can be seen that satisfactory materials have an S value of not more than 0.65. The $C_{0.7}$ values of a number of glass-ionomer cements are no greater than that of the composite resin Con-

cise,* although all are greater than the simple filling resin Sevriton.† Only the most translucent glass-ionomer cement, ASPA X, has $C_{0.7}$ and S values comparable with those of the dental silicate cements Biotrey‡ and Achatit.§ In practice, despite the complexities of the equation relating $C_{0.7}$ to S, both parameters increase together.

*3M Dental Products, St. Paul, Minn.
†Amalgamated Dental Co., Weybridge, England.
‡Dentsply International Inc., Weybridge, England, and York, Pa.
§Vivadent Inc., Tonawanda, N.Y.

Colour match

Apart from the question of translucency, colour does not seem to have been too much of a problem, principally because the glass-ionomer, unlike composite resins, is chemically stable.

Stains penetrate into the glass-ionomer cement to a much lesser extent than is the case with composite resins (Lingard et al., 1978). However, resistance to stain is largely dependent on obtaining a good surface finish.

Clinical observations

Knibbs and coworkers (1986) have reported on opacity and colour match of a new glass-ionomer cement after two years in service.* They found 61% of the restorations had good opacity match and 37% had slight mismatch. Fifty-seven percent had good colour match and 40% had slight mismatch. In addition, 92% had no surface staining and 72% had no marginal staining. The inference from this study is that the modern glass-ionomer cement is aesthetically satisfactory.

*Chem-Fil, Dentsply International Inc., Weybridge, England, and York, Pa.

Appendix: Kubelka-Munk equation

The Kubelka-Munk equation relates fundamental opacity parameters to measured quantities. The fundamental opacity parameters are:

S the scattering coefficient
$S\theta$ the scattering power
R_∞ the light reflectance (the reflectance of a laminar of infinite thickness)

The measured quantities are:

R_r and R_0, the light reflectances of a laminar, thickness θ, of a translucent body placed respectively on a white background reflectance, r, and a black background R_0/R_r is the contrast ratio, C_r

The Kubelka-Munk equations are:

$$R_0 = R_\infty(\exp\phi - 1)/(\exp\phi - R^2_\infty)$$
$$\text{and}$$
$$R_r = \frac{R_\infty(1 - rR_\infty)\exp\phi + (r - R_\infty)}{(1 - rR_\infty)\exp\phi + R_\infty(r - R_\infty)}$$
$$\text{where } \phi = S\theta(1/R_\infty - R_\infty)$$

These equations cannot be solved algebraically for S and Rr and recourse has to be made to charts constructed by Judd (1937) or modern computer programmes.

References

Asmussen, E. (1983) Opacity of glass-ionomer cements. Acta Odontol. Scand. 41:155–157.

Crisp, S., Abel, G., and Wilson, A.D. (1979) The quantitative measurement of the opacity of aesthetic dental filling materials. J. Dent. Res. 58:1585–1596.

Judd, D.B. (1934) Opacity standards. RP 706 J. Res. Nat. Bur. Stands. 13:281–291.

Judd, D.B. (1937) Optical specification of light-scattering materials. RP 1026 J. Res. Nat. Bur. Stands. 19:287–317.

Knibbs, P.J., Plant, C.G., and Pearson, G.J. (1986) A clinical assessment of an anhydrous glass-ionomer cement. Br. Dent. J. 161:99–103.

Kubelka, P., and Munk, F. (1931) Ein Beitrag zur Optik der Farbanstriche. Z. Tech. Phys. 12:539–601.

Lingard, G.L., Davies, E.H., and von Fraunhofer, J.A. (1978) An in vitro study of the staining of anterior restorative materials. J. Dent. 6:247–258.

Paffenbarger, G.C. (1937) Dental silicate cements. In D.B. Judd Optical specifications of light scattering materials. RP 1026 J. Res. Nat. Bur. Stands. 19:314–316.

Paffenbarger, G.C., Schoonover, I.C., and Souder, W. (1938) Dental silicate cements: Physical and chemical properties and a specification. J. Am. Dent. Assoc. 25:52–87.

Prosser, H.J., Powis, D.R., Brant, P., and Wilson, A.D. (1984) The characterisation of glass-ionomer cements. 7. The physical properties of current materials. J. Dent. 12:231–240.

Chapter 6

Adhesion

Glass-ionomer cements, as many research workers have shown, have the important property of permanently adhering to untreated enamel and dentine under the moist conditions of the mouth (Tables 6-1 and 6-2). They share this property with the zinc polycarboxylate cements. Whether the cement penetrates the acquired pellicle on enamel or bonds to it is uncertain, but it does react with the smear layer on cut dentine. This is an important attribute for a filling material and, to a lesser degree, for a luting agent. Glass-ionomer cements also bond to other reactive polar substrates, such as the base metals (Fig. 6-1).

Acid etching or other surface-roughening procedures are deprecated, for the bonding is of a chemical rather than a micromechanical nature. About 80% of maximum bond strength is developed in 15 minutes (Aboush and Jenkins, 1986), but strength slowly increases for several days after that (Powis et al., 1982).

Table 6-1 Tensile bond strengths (MPa) of glass-ionomer cements to untreated enamel and dentine

Material	Enamel	Dentine
ASPA IV*	2.6[a], 3.2[j]	1.5[a], 3.1[j]
De Trey Aspa†	3.6[b], 4.8[c], 4.5[h]	1.8[b] 2.4[c] 1.1[d] 4.0[g]
	4.5[k], 5.2[m]	2.4[h] 2.4[k], 3.3[m]
Chem-Fil‡	9.6[m]	4.1[m]
Chembond‡	4.8[e]	1.3[d], 2.3[e]
Fuji Ionomer II§	4.5[e], 4.5[l], 4.2[m]	2.5[e], 4.5[k], 2.2[l], 3.1[m]
Ketac-Cem¶	4.2[f]	2.2[f]
Ketac-Fil¶	6.4[m]	3.3[m]

[a]Hötz et al. (1977), [b]Prodger and Symonds (1977), [c]Levine et al. (1977), [d]Öilo (1981), [e]Peddey (1981), [f]Shalabi et al., (1981), [g]Coury et al. (1981), [h]Negm et al. (1982), [i]Powis et al. (1982), [k]Vougiouklakis et al. (1982), [l]Beech et al., (1985), [m]Aboush and Jenkins (1986).
*Laboratory of the Government Chemist, London.
†Amalgamated Dental Co., Weybridge, England.
‡Dentsply International Inc., Weybridge, England, and York, Pa.
§G-C International Corp., Tokyo, and Scottsdale, Ariz.
¶ESPE GmbH, Seefeld/Oberbay, West Germany, and Valley Stream, N.Y.

Table 6-2 Shear bond strengths (MPa) of glass-ionomer cements to untreated enamel and dentine

Material	Enamel	Dentine
De Trey Aspa*	1.6[a]	6.8[c], 4.0[d], 4.0[e] 0.7[a]
Fuji Ionomer II†	4.2[b]	2.4[f], 3.3[b]

[a]Negm et al. (1982), [b]Lacefield et al. (1985), [c]Hood et al. (1977), [d]Causton and Johnson (1979), [e]Causton and Johnson (1982), [f]Nation et al. (1980).
*Amalgamated Dental Co., Weybridge, England.
†G-C International Corp, Tokyo, and Scottsdale, Ariz.

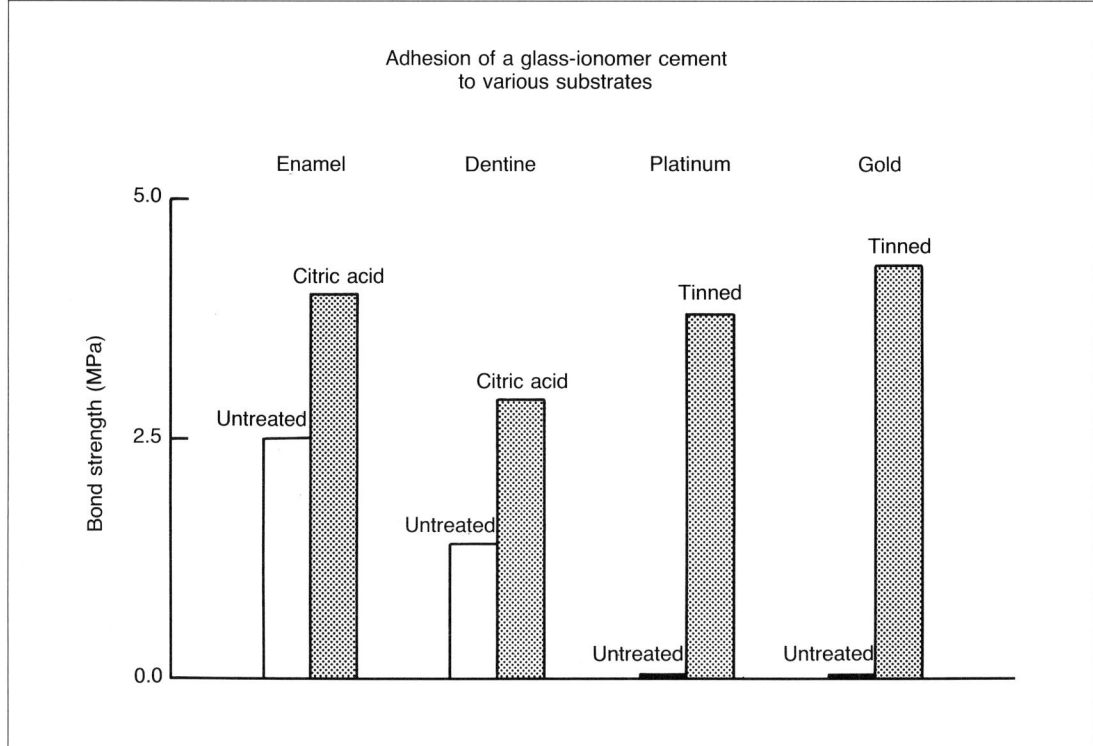

Fig. 6-1 The bonding of glass-ionomer cements to various substrates, both untreated and conditioned with citric acid. Based on Hötz et al. (1977).

Adhesion is the most important property of the glass-ionomer cement. It allows a conservative approach to restoration, because undercutting to provide mechanical keying is unnecessary in low-stress-bearing areas. This is of particular advantage in restoring cervical erosion lesions and in sealing pits and fissures (McLean and Wilson, 1974, 1977a, 1977b).

Adhesion to dentine and enamel enables the glass-ionomer cement to provide a perfect seal. Bearing in mind that the percolation of bacteria along the cavity wall/restoration interface has been cited as the cause of pulpal inflammation (Brännström, 1981) it follows that adhesion has important implications for biocompatibility.

Another barrier to adhesion is the dynamic nature of tooth material. Because enamel is an ion exchanger and dentine is a living material subject to change, one is trying to bond to shifting sand rather than to solid rock. Under such conditions the adhesive bond must have a dynamic character too. It will be broken as the substrate changes, and must be capable of being re-formed. Once broken, covalent chemical bonds cannot be re-formed. Dentine adhesives may fail because of this very point. By contrast, the ionic and polar bonds that attach the glass-ionomer cement to the substrate can be re-established, which, together with the multiplicity of the adhesive bonds, may account for this cement's unique property of being permanently adhesive under oral conditions.

Barriers to adhesion

The principal barrier to effective adhesion to dental tissue is water. Dentine is permeated by aqueous fluids transported from the pulp, and there is both loosely and tightly bound water in the surface of enamel. In the oral situation, organic adhesives are either insufficiently polar to compete with water for the surface of dental tissue, or, if highly polar, the bond they form is hydrolytically unstable. By contrast, the hydrophilic, highly ionic glass-ionomer cement competes successfully with water because of its multiplicity of carboxyl groups that form hydrogen bonds with the substrate. Water is displaced or even incorporated into the cement. Adhesion is permanent, because of the multiplicity of hydrogen and ionic bonds that attach the glass-ionomer cement to the substrate in an octopuslike fashion, making temporary scission of one such bond inconsequential.

Mechanism of adhesion to enamel and dentine

The precise mechanism of adhesion of polyelectrolyte cements has yet to be fully elucidated. Several hypotheses have been advanced. It is certain that the adhesive bond is a chemical one, affected by chemical and not mechanical factors.

Chemically, tooth material consists of apatite, which makes up over 98% of enamel and 70% of dentine by weight, and collagen, which is found in dentine alone (McLean, 1980). The bond of glass-ionomer cement to enamel is better than to dentine—evidence that bonding to apatite is the principal mode of adhesion. If the cement bonds mainly to the apatite constituent of dentine with little or no bonding to collagen, then the bond strength will be lowered but there will be no adhesive failure at the apatite sites.

This may explain the general observation that the failure of bonds to dentine, like those to enamel, is adhesive rather than cohesive.

Smith (1968) speculated that chelation of calcium, contained in apatite, was involved in adhesion, but Beech (1973) considered this mechanism was unlikely as it would involve the formation of an eight-membered ring. Instead he proposed, on the basis of an infrared spectroscopic study, that the interaction between apatite and poly(acrylic acid) produced polyacrylate ions which then formed strong ionic bonds with the surface calcium ions of apatite in enamel and dentine.

Wilson (1974) looked at the mechanism of adhesion more broadly. He suggested that initially, when the cement paste is applied to tooth material and is fluid, wetting and initial adhesion is by hydrogen bonding provided by free carboxyl groups present in the fresh paste. As the cement ages, hydrogen bonds are progressively replaced by ionic bonds, the cations coming either from the cement or the hydroxyapatite. Wilson stressed the important role of the polyelectrolyte moiety, for the older phosphate-bonded cements, unlike the polyelectrolyte cements, do not adhere to tooth substances. It follows that the polymeric polar chains of polyacid are essential for the achievement of adhesion. Their role must be one of bridging the interface between the cement and the substrate, a role that isolated orthophosphate ions cannot assume.

More recently, Wilson, Prosser, and Powis (1983), on the basis of adsorption and infrared spectroscopic studies, postulated that, during adsorption, polyacrylate entered the molecular surface of hydroxyapatite, displacing and replacing surface phosphate (Fig. 6-2). Calcium ions are displaced from hydroxyapatite along with phosphate as part of a complex series of ionic exchanges. These workers inferred that, as a consequence of these interactions, an intermediate layer of calcium and aluminium phosphates and polyacrylates would form at the interface between the cement and apatite (Fig. 6-3). Interestingly, much earlier, McLean and Wilson (1977a) had partly anticipated this model when they hypothesized on the presence of an intermediate interfacing layer between cement and tooth surface.

Chain length must also be an important factor in adhesion. The dental silicate cement does not bond to tooth tissue, although nearly all arguments applied to glass-ionomer adhesion apply to the silicate also. The difference is that whereas the dental silicate cement is an assembly of discrete cations and phosphate anions, the glass-ionomer cement is based on a polymer chain that is capable of bridging gaps between the cement body and the substrate.

While there is general agreement that bonding to enamel, which is almost entirely apatite, results from ionic and polar forces, there is no consensus of opinion on bonding to dentine, which contains a large proportion of the organic constituent collagen. Beech (1973) maintained that bonding is to the apatite constituent of dentine only, citing the weaker adhesion of the glass-ionomer cement to dentine and the nonexistence of adhesion to decalcified dentine. Wilson (1974) considered the possibility of polyacrylates bonding to collagen also. Collagen contains both amino and carboxylic acid groups, so there could be adhesion by hydrogen bonding or cationic bridges. Recent adsorption studies at the Laboratory of the Government Chemist, however, indicate that poly(acrylic acid) and polyacrylate are not absorbed on collagen (Jackson, 1986). The probability is that glass-ionomer cements do not bond to collagen.

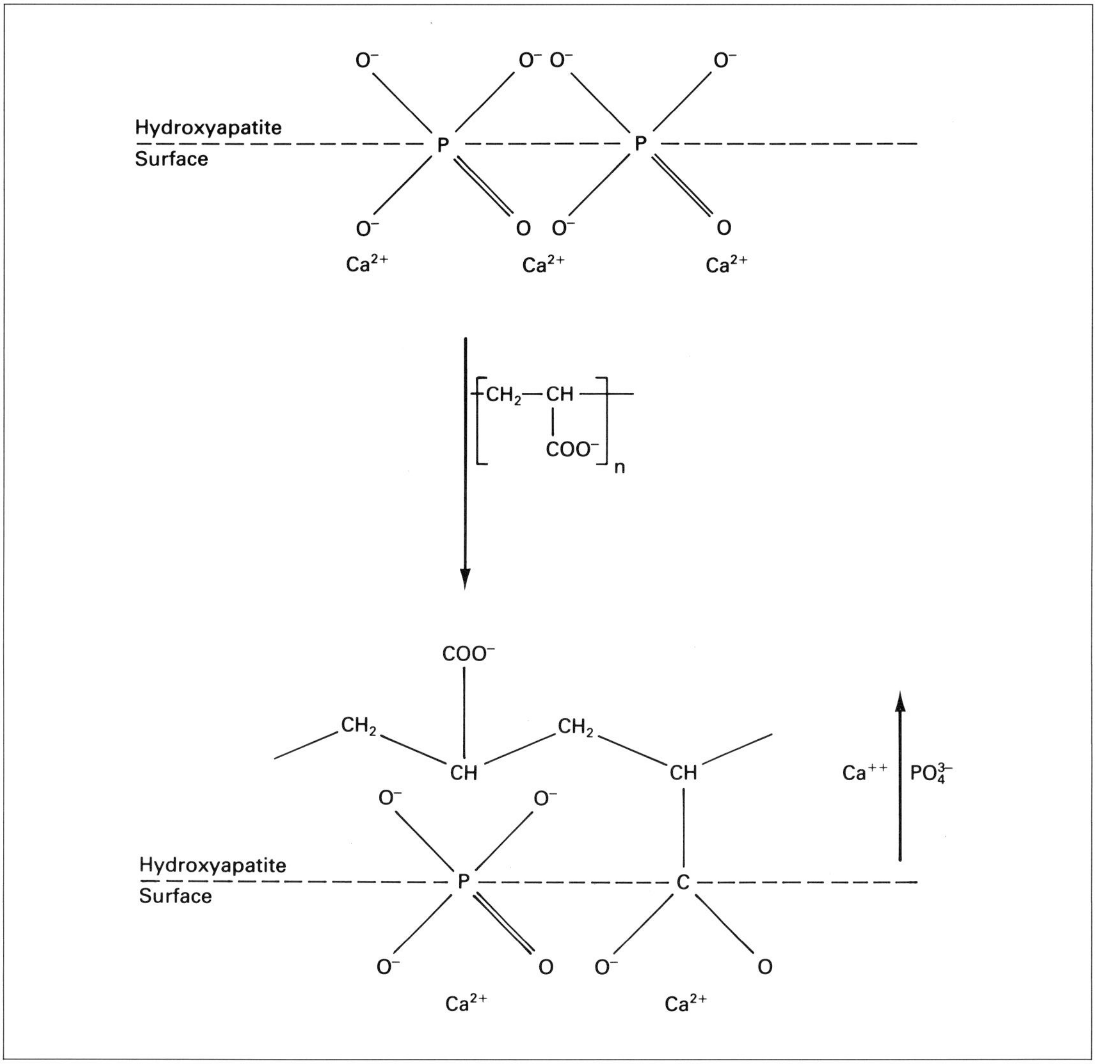

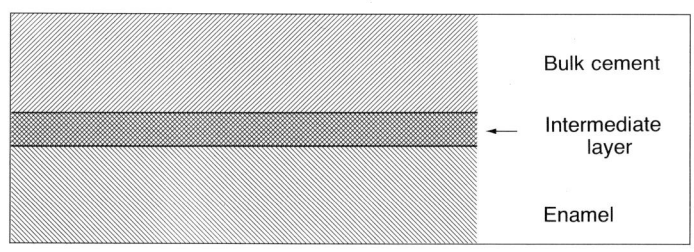

Fig. 6-2 A postulated mechanism for the adsorption of polyacrylate onto hydroxyapatite showing the displacement of phosphate and calcium by polyacrylate. Reprinted with permission from Wilson et al. (1983).

Fig. 6-3 Structure of the adhesive bond between glass-ionomer cement and enamel showing the presence of an intermediate layer. Reprinted with permission from Wilson et al. (1983).

87

Evidence is accumulating that bond strength to tooth substances depends on the nature of the polyacid used. Cements based on poly(acrylic acid) appear to bond more strongly than those based on copolymers of acrylic acid with itaconic or maleic acids (Aboush and Jenkins, 1986). If this proves to be so then the molecular configuration of the polyacid would be an important factor in controlling adhesion.

Only one study on the adhesion of cermet cements has been reported (Thornton et al., 1986). Research workers found that the adhesion of a cermet cement to enamel and dentine was inferior to that of a conventional glass-ionomer cement, a result that was attributed to poorer flow properties. They suggested that mechanical keying may be necessary. Powis (1986) recommended the pretreatment of enamel and dentine with poly(acrylic acid), which is not subsequently washed off, so that a bonding intermediary is formed.

Improving adhesion

When the cement tooth bond fractures it is by cohesive failure within the cement rather than adhesive failure at the interface. Thus, the strength of the bond is limited by the cohesive strength of the cement used.

The tensile bond strength to enamel is greater than that to dentine; the bond strength to enamel varies from 2.6 to 9.6 MPa, depending on the material, and from 1.1 to 4.5 MPa to cut but untreated dentine (see Table 6-1). Interestingly, bonding is achieved to both enamel and dentine without any sort of surface treatment, although a smear layer is present on the surface of cut enamel and dentine. Indeed, this layer may be beneficial if it is consolidated. However, Prodger and Symonds (1977) reported that salivary contamination of a freshly prepared dentine surface reduced bond strength, but whether this was because of its water content or contamination of the dentine surface is uncertain.

Surface conditioning

A number of research workers have sought to improve adhesion. One way that is common to nearly all adhesive technologies is by pretreatment of the surface (Fig. 6-4). McLean and Wilson (1977b) first used the term *surface conditioning* for this treatment in order to differentiate it from *acid etching*. Surface conditioning is needed in order to eliminate the wide variation found in the structures of tooth surfaces following cutting. The case for surface treatment, however, is still one of controversy. The issue is unlikely to be finally resolved until stronger glass-ionomer cements are available to make distinctions clearer. However, on one point all agree: rough tooth surfaces are contraindicated. In general, the smoother the surface the stronger the bond, and this is not a marginal effect (Powis et al., 1982; Aboush and Jenkins, 1986). Indeed, the smoothing of the cut dentine and enamel surfaces may be the mechanism whereby surface conditioners improve adhesion, for the most effective surface conditioners, as will be shown, while having different actions on tooth surfaces, all tend to smooth it. Good interfacial contact is important for adhesion. The smoothing of surface irregularities may be necessary to prevent air entrapment and to minimize sites where stress concentration could occur.

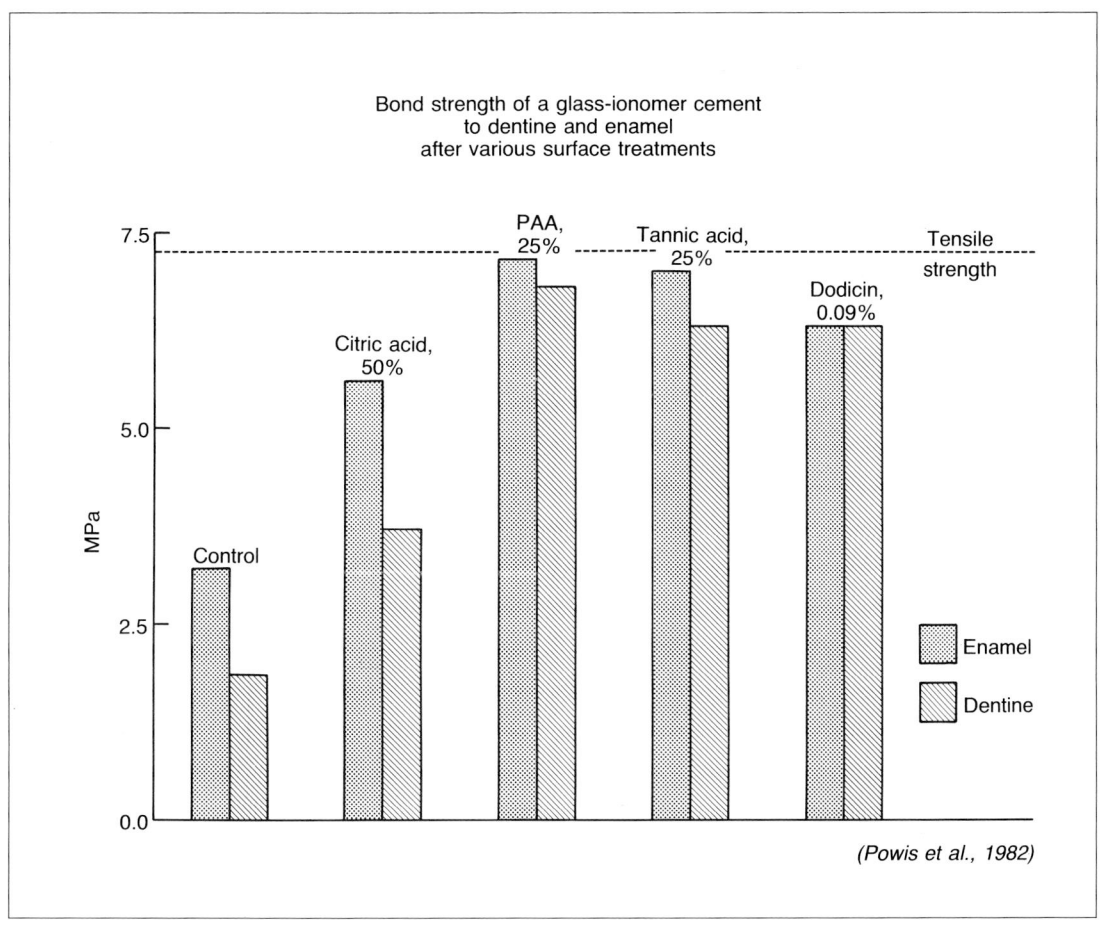

Bond strength of a glass-ionomer cement
to dentine and enamel
after various surface treatments

(Powis et al., 1982)

Fig. 6-4 Effect of various surface conditioners on bond strength of a glass-ionomer cement to dentine and enamel.

The majority of investigators find that surface conditioners improve bond strength, especially to dentine (see Tables 6-3 and 6-4 for results and references); a few maintain that there is no effect (Prodger and Symonds, 1977; Beech et al., 1985). Rarely is a reduction in bond strength reported. In the nature of things one would expect both positive and negative effects from surface treatments. If the whole body of evidence is accepted, then the very fact that there are differences between research workers, who use a variety of techniques and operate on teeth of varying natures, indicates that the condition of the surface is important. It would appear logical that if a surface treatment is proven never to be deleterious then it should be used in all cases, for the condition of teeth and the techniques of operators will vary widely. The perfect surface treatment would be one that eliminated all these variables.

Again, these surface treatments are conditioning treatments and are to be distinguished from the etching techniques used for bonding composite resins to enamel. Surface demineralization,

Table 6-3 Effect of various surface conditioners on the bond strengths (MPa) of ASPA IV to enamel and dentine*

Surface treatment	Time of application (seconds)	Enamel	Dentine
None	—	3.2	3.1
Citric acid, 50% aq	30	5.6	3.7
Citric acid, 2% aq/alc	30	5.6	3.7
Poly(acrylic acid), 25% aq	30	7.1	6.8
Tannic acid, 25% aq	60	7.0	6.3
Surface-active solution†	60	7.5	6.6
Dodicin, 0.9% aq	60	6.3	6.3
Na₂ EDTA, 2% aq	30	5.0	2.1
Na₄ EDTA, 15% aq	30	5.3	1.9
Sodium fluoride, 3% aq	30	4.7	4.8
Ferric chloride, 2% aq/alc	30	4.5	5.4

*Data obtained by Powis et al. (1982). The test employed was a tensile one.
†Chlorhexidine gluconate, 0.1%; docidin, 0.08%; sodium fluoride, 3%. The formulation of the original Tubulicid (Dental Therapeutics, AB, Nacka, Sweden; this formulation has been superseded).

Table 6-4 Effect of various surface conditioners on the bond strengths (MPa) of glass-ionomer cements to dentine

Surface conditioner	Cement	Conditioned	No treatment	Investigators*
Poly(acrylic acid)	ASPA IV†	6.8	3.1	Powis et al. (1982)t
Poly(acrylic acid)	Fuji Ionomer II‡	2.7	2.2	Beech et al. (1985)t
Ferric chloride	ASPA IV	5.4	3.1	Powis et al. (1982)t
Ferric chloride	De Trey Aspa§	4.7	2.2	Shalabi et al. (1981)t
ITS	De Trey Aspa	6.0	4.0	Causton & Johnson (1982)s
ITS	Fuji Ionomer II	3.3	2.2	Beech et al. (1985)t
Mineralizing solution	De Trey Aspa	4.8	2.4	Levine et al. (1979)t

*s = shear test; t = tensile test.
†Laboratory of the Government Chemist, London.
‡G-C International Corp., Tokyo, and Scottsdale, Ariz.
§Amalgamated Dental Co., Weybridge, England.

associated with etching techniques, is undesirable and deprecated for the bonding of glass-ionomer cements to dentine and enamel (Powis et al., 1982). Decalcifying freshly cut dentine opens up and widens dentinal tubules, allowing ingress of bacteria, and so causing inflammation (Brännström, 1981).

Citric acid

The earliest surface conditioner for the bonding of glass-ionomer cements to tooth substrates, proposed by McLean and Wilson (1977a, 1977b), was citric acid (50%), which was chosen because of its compatibility with the cement—citric acid is a cement-former. It has had its advocates (Hötz et al., 1977; Vliestra et al., 1978; Prodger and Symonds, 1977) and its detractors (Cotton and Siegal, 1978; Negm, Beech, and Grant, 1982; Vougiouklakis et al., 1982; Hood et al., 1977). Its use has fallen into some disfavour but it is still commonly employed in adhesive studies for comparative purposes. It generally increases bond strength or has no effect (Tables 6-5 and 6-6). On these grounds its use cannot be deprecated, although there are now better surface conditioners available.

There has also been controversy over the effectiveness of citric acid on the bonding of the glass-ionomer cement to dentine. However, this controversy has now been resolved and again illustrates the danger of generalising on the basis of limited experiments. The nature of the bonding to dentine is now known to depend on the particular glass-ionomer cement used (Vougiouklakis et al., 1982). Glass-ionomer cements adhere to citric acid–treated dentine by two mechanisms: chemical bonding and micromechanical attachment to the opened-up tubules. In the case of De Trey Aspa* (based on a copolymer of itaconic and acrylic acid) the gain of bonding by micromechanical attachment exceeded the loss brought about by partial decalcification of dentine. The reverse was found to be true for poly(acrylic acid)-based Fuji Ionomer II.† Thus, the appropriateness of the surface treatment depends on the material used.

Although not a strong acid, citric acid can be extremely erosive because of its ability to chelate metal ions. Powis et al. (1982) found that the effect of citric acid was drastic, with the surfaces of both dentine and enamel being attacked. The enamel surface was heavily etched, as comparison of Fig. 6-5.1a to Fig. 6-5.2a shows. The smear layer was removed from dentine and the dentinal tubules were opened up with loss of perihedral dentine (compare Fig. 6-5.1b to Fig. 6-5.2b). Optimum adhesion was not achieved with this severe treatment. Removal of the smear layer and the opening of tubules can lead to demineralization and hence decrease the chemical interaction of the cement with the tooth. For this reason Brännström (1981) advocates a treatment time of only five seconds.

Other surface conditioners

The most extensive study of surface conditioners was made by Powis et al. (1982), who examined a range of surface treatments, including simple cleansers and chelating polyfunctional carboxylic and phenolic acids, using adhesion tests and scanning electron microscopy. Their

---

*Amalgamated Dental Co., Weybridge, England.
†G-C International Corp., Tokyo, and Scottsdale, Ariz.

Table 6-5 Bond strengths (MPa) of glass-ionomer cements to untreated and citric-acid-conditioned enamel*

Investigators	Cement	No treatment	Citric acid
Hötz et al. (1977)	ASPA IV†	2.9	4.1
Powis et al. (1982)	ASPA IV	3.2	5.6
Prodger & Symonds (1977)	De Trey Aspa‡	3.6	3.2
Lacefield et al. (1982)	Fuji Ionomer II§	4.5	5.0
Aboush & Jenkins (1986)	De Trey Aspa	5.2	5.9
Aboush & Jenkins (1986)	Chem-Fil¶	9.6	9.9
Aboush & Jenkins (1986)	Ketac-Fil#	6.4	6.1
Aboush & Jenkins (1986)	Fuji Ionomer II	4.2	4.8

*All are tensile tests.
†Laboratory of the Government Chemist, London.
‡Amalgamated Dental Co., Weybridge, England.
§G-C International Corp., Tokyo, and Scottsdale, Ariz.
¶Dentsply International Inc., Weybridge, England, and York, Pa.
#ESPE GmbH, Seefeld/Oberbay, West Germany, and Valley Stream, N.Y.

Table 6-6 Bond strengths (MPa) of glass-ionomer cements to untreated and citric-acid-conditioned dentine

Investigators*	Cement	No treatment	Citric acid
Hötz et al. (1977)t	ASPA IV†	1.5	2.9
Powis et al. (1982)t	ASPA IV	3.1	3.7
Prodger & Symonds (1977)t	De Trey Aspa‡	1.8	1.7
Hood et al., (1977)s	De Trey Aspa	6.8	4.1
Shalabi et al. (1983)t	De Trey Aspa	2.2	1.9
Negm et al., (1982)t	De Trey Aspa	2.4	1.6
Lacefield et al. (1982)t	Fuji Ionomer II§	3.3	2.5
Aboush & Jenkins (1986)t	De Trey Aspa	1.8	3.3
Aboush & Jenkins (1986)t	Chem-Fil¶	2.3	4.1
Aboush & Jenkins (1986)t	Ketac-Fil#	1.6	3.3
Aboush & Jenkins (1986)t	Fuji Ionomer II	2.6	3.1

*s = shear test; t = tensile test.
†Laboratory of the Government Chemist, London, England.
‡Amalgamated Dental Co., Weybridge, England.
§G-C International Corp., Tokyo, and Scottsdale, Ariz.
¶Dentsply International, Inc., Weybridge, England, and York, Pa.
#ESPE GmbH, Seefeld/Oberbay, West Germany, and Valley Stream, N.Y.

results are shown in Table 6-3 and are supplemented by results from other research workers in Table 6-4.

Powis et al. (1982) found other treatments to be more effective than citric acid. The best agents for improving adhesion to enamel and dentine proved to be 25% poly(acrylic acid), 25% tannic acid, and a surface-active detergent, 0.9% dodicin, which contains fluoride (see Table 6-3). These treatments had different effects on the surfaces of dentine and enamel, but all were equally as effective as and less disruptive than citric acid.

Mount (1984) has suggested that surface conditioners should, ideally, meet the following requirements:

1. Be isotonic to minimise osmotic effects
2. Have a pH ranging from 5.5 to 8.0, that is, be broadly neutral
3. Be nontoxic to dentine, pulp, and gingival tissues
4. Be compatible with the chemistry of the cement
5. Have water solubility and be easily removed
6. Not deplete enamel and dentine chemically
7. Enhance the surface chemically in preparation for bonding

Of course, not all of these criteria can be met, and it is not certain whether they always need to be fully met. This useful advice may be extended and amended. Acidic solutions are not the only chemical substances to decalcify enamel and dentine—neutral complexing agents can have a similar effect. However, when these acid and complexing agents form insoluble cementitious substances, their adverse effect is negated.

Surface-active microbicidal solutions

Powis et al. (1982) examined the use of the old-style Tubulicid* formulations (0.1% chlorhexidine gluconate; 0.08% dodicin; 3% sodium fluoride), both with and without fluoride, as surface conditioners. These are approximately neutral solutions and a 60-second treatment produces no adverse effects. Results are given in Table 6-3. The fluoride containing version produces the best results on both enamel and dentine. This surface conditioner appears to be as effective an adhesion promoter as poly(acrylic acid) and tannic acid (see Table 6-3).

The active conditioning agents appear to be dodicin, a surface-active agent, and fluoride. (It should be emphasized that currently available Tubulicid is of a different composition and its effectiveness is unknown.) When applied to enamel it smoothes out the ragged edges of grooves and removes debris produced by polishing (Fig. 6-5.3a). On dentine it smoothes out polishing grooves and, although dentinal tubules can be seen beneath a reduced smear layer, the tubules are not opened up (Fig. 6-5.3b). The solution is not chemically compatible with the cement system but is readily washed off.

Dodicin

The surface-active agent dodicin by itself produces effects on dentine and enamel similar to the surface-active microbicidal solutions (Powis et al., 1982). Remarks in the previous section apply here.

*Dental Therapeutics, AB, Nacka, Sweden (no longer available).

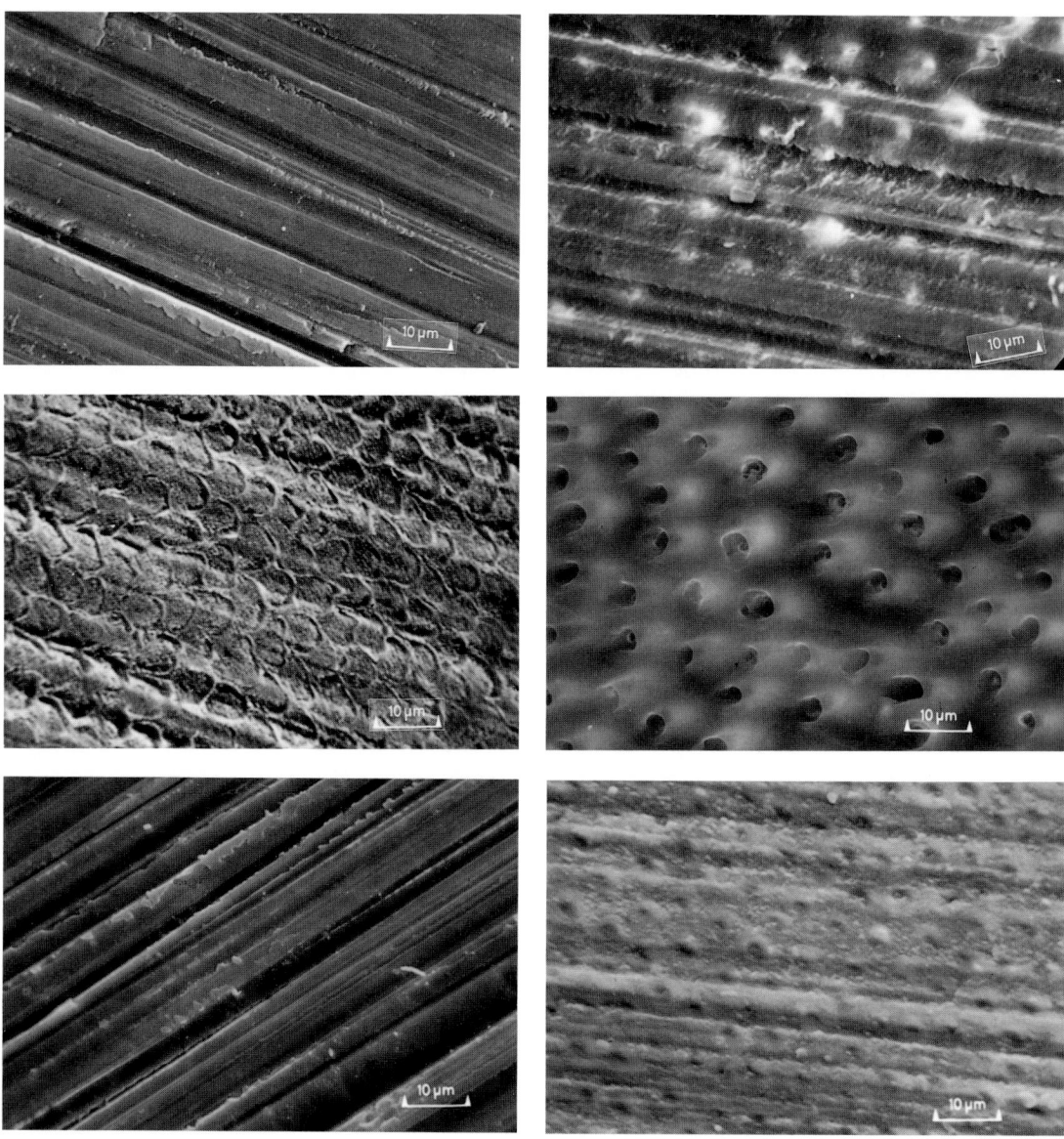

Figs. 6-5.1a to 6-5.6b SEMs of enamel and dentine surfaces after various surface treatments. Reprinted with permission from Powis et al. (1982).

Fig. 6-5.1a SEM of enamel without treatment.

Fig. 6-5.2a SEM of enamel after treatment with citric acid showing the etching of the enamel and revealing its prismatic structure.

Fig. 6-5.3a SEM of enamel after treatment with surface-active solution showing removal of debris and smoothing of the edges of polishing grooves.

Fig. 6-5.1b SEM of dentine without treatment. Note smear layer and cutting debris.

Fig. 6-5.2b SEM of dentine after treatment with citric acid showing the opening up of the dentinal tubules and removal of perihedral dentine.

Fig. 6-5.3b SEM of dentine after treatment with surface-active solution showing smoothing out of polishing grooves. Dentinal tubules can be seen beneath a reduced smear layer.

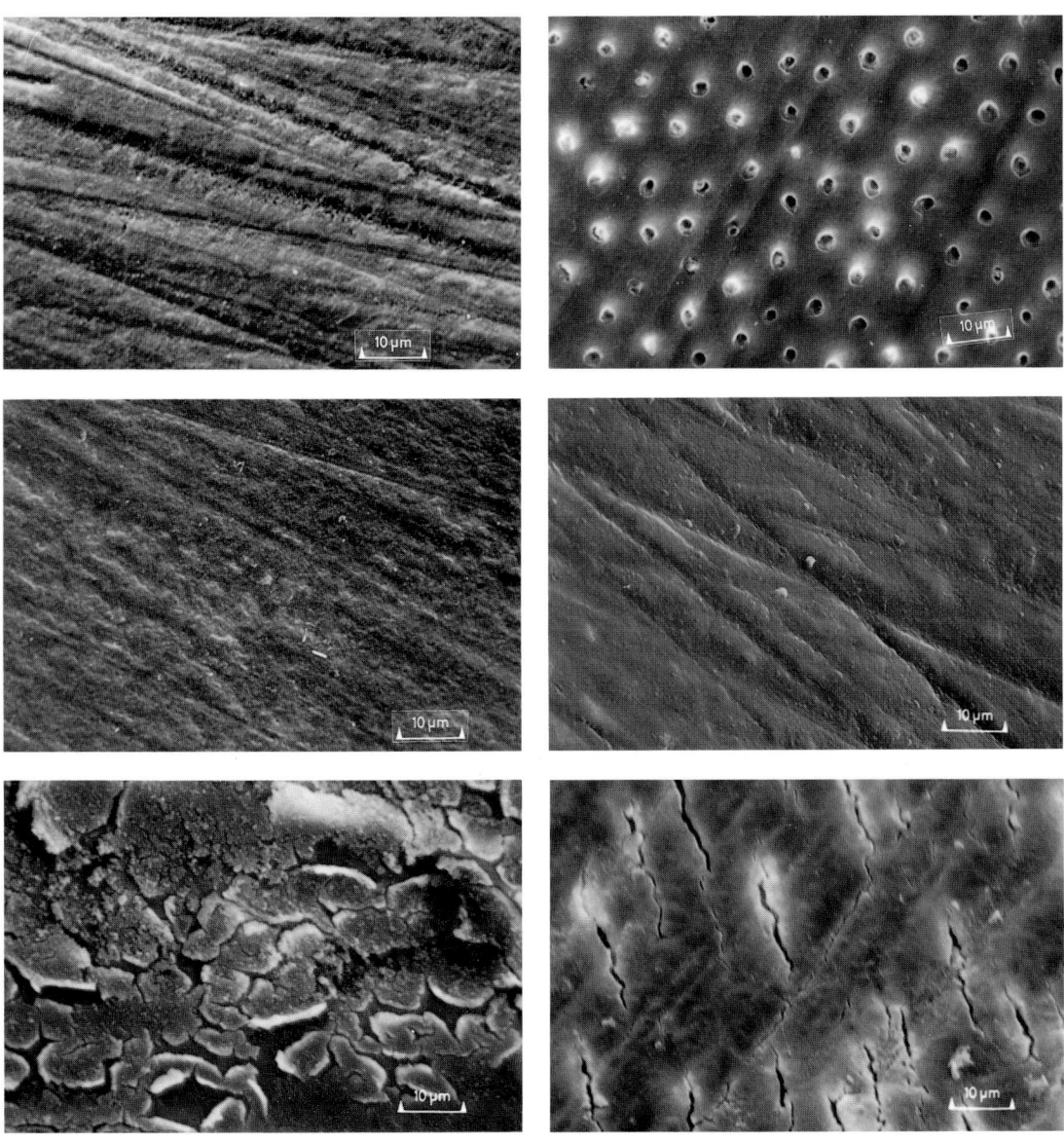

Fig. 6-5.4a SEM of enamel after treatment with poly(acrylic acid) showing slight etching of enamel and removal of polishing marks.

Fig. 6-5.4b SEM of dentine after treatment with poly(acrylic acid) showing removal of debris and smoothing out of surface irregularities with some opening of dentinal tubules.

Fig. 6-5.5a SEM of enamel after treatment with tannic acid showing the formation of a smooth featureless reaction layer.

Fig. 6-5.5b SEM of dentine after treatment with tannic acid showing formation of a smooth featureless reaction layer. Dentinal tubules as blisters.

Fig. 6-5.6a SEM of enamel after treatment with ferric chloride showing an extensively fissured surface.

Fig. 6-5.6b SEM of dentine after treatment with ferric chloride solution showing virtual elimination of polishing grooves. The surface is fissured and there is no sign of dentinal tubules.

Poly(acrylic acid)

Poly(acrylic acid) in 25% aqueous solution was recommended as an effective surface conditioner by Powis et al. (1982) (see Tables 6-3 and 6-4). Because poly(acrylic acid) complexes metal ions and is also acidic, its solutions have a decalcifying action. For this reason, Mount (1984) recommends a short application time of 10 seconds. Its action is less drastic than that of citric acid, but it does etch enamel slightly while removing polishing marks (Fig. 6-5.4a). On cut dentine, its general effect is to remove surface debris and smooth out surface irregularities, although it does open up dentinal tubules (Fig. 6-5.4b).

We are tempted to say that poly(acrylic acid) is the conditioner of choice because it is part of the cement-forming system. Indeed, it must be used for the bonding of cermet cements, because the formation of an intermediate bonding layer between the restoration and the cavity wall is essential. However, there must be some reservation about its use on dentine, since, like citric acid, it opens the tubules. There is the possibility that this could lead to sensitivity, especially with luting agents. Although poly(acrylic acid) will not penetrate tubules because of its high molecular weight, opened tubules may offer a route for the movement of water.

Long et al. (1986) found that the optimum concentration for poly(acrylic acid) lies between 30% to 35%, and cited results which show a bond strength of 3.9 MPa with 35% poly(acrylic acid) against 3.0 MPa obtained with a 25% concentration.

Tannic acid

Tannic acid, as its name implies, is an organic tanning agent. It reacts with collagen. Since it is also known to form cements with aluminosilicate glasses (Wilson, 1968), it would appear to have potential to couple the cement to collagen and so have advantages as a surface conditioner, at least for dentine. Powis et al. (1982) have found that tannic acid in 25% aqueous solution is at least as effective a surface conditioner as poly(acrylic acid) (see Table 6-3).

Tannic acid has an acidic reaction (pH = 2.5) and is not isotonic. Powis et al. (1982) recommend a 30-second period for treatment. When applied to enamel it forms a smooth featureless surface without etching or decalcification (Fig. 6-5.5a). On dentine it also forms a smooth featureless layer and tubules are not opened but appear as blisters (Fig. 6-5.5b). Tannic acid probably undergoes a tanning reaction with collagen and so serves to consolidate the smear layer (Vaidyanthan et al., 1984).

Tannic acid could well be considered the material of choice for treating dentine because it forms a protective layer and dose not open up tubules. It could prove to be the answer to the problem of sensitivity sometimes found when the glass-ionomer cement is used as a luting agent, but this has yet to be proved. In effect it would be acting as a lining agent.

Ferric chloride

The use of ferric chloride as a surface conditioner has been investigated by Powis et al. (1982), who used a 2% aqueous/alcoholic solution, and Shalabi et al. (1981). Ferric chloride is an inorganic tanning agent and a mordant and is probably capable of being incorporated into both apatite and glass-ionomer cement. It has potential to provide metal linkages between collagen and glass-ionomer cement. It is also very acidic;

ferric chloride hydrolyzes to give free hydrochloric acid, an acid stronger than phosphoric acid. Thus, its effect on enamel is dramatic, producing a surface with extensive fissuring, although whether this surface is the enamel or a reaction product is uncertain (Fig. 6-5.6a).

When ferric chloride is applied to dentine a unique surface is formed (Fig. 6-5.6b). Polishing grooves are almost obliterated but dentinal tubules are not exposed. Fissures are apparent in the surface but these are probably in a deposited coating rather than in the dentine itself. Although bond strengths (see Tables 6-5 and 6-6) are high, its use cannot be recommended in light of our present knowledge and its highly acidic nature. There could be a future in the treatment if an iron-containing complex is prepared that has a tanning action without the acidity of ferric chloride.

Sodium fluoride

Somewhat surprisingly, Powis and co-workers (1982) found that sodium fluoride strengthened the adhesive bond both to enamel and dentine (see Table 6-3). Hydrogen bonds to fluoride are known to be the strongest hydrogen bonds and so this result, namely that fluoride enhances adhesion, supports the view that hydrogen bonding is of importance in adhesion.

Mineralizing solutions

Mineralizing solutions have been developed by both Causton and Johnson (1979, 1982)—the ITS solution—and Levine et al. (1977), although Beech and coworkers (1985) consider these treatments ineffective. These solutions are approximately neutral and are isotonic. Details of preparation are given below.

Levine et al. solution

This solution is prepared by mixing two stable solutions, A and B. *Solution A* is a 0.5 mol/l solution of potassium dihydrogen phosphate (pH = 4.5) saturated with brushite (calcium hydrogen phosphate dihydrate). *Solution B* is a 0.5 mol/l solution of disodium hydrogen phosphate (pH = 9) containing 2,000 ppm fluoride.

ITS solution

Composition of the ITS solution is in g/L; application time is two minutes and shelf life is 18 months (refrigerated).

$CaCl_2 = 0.2$
$KCl = 0.2$
$MgCl_2 \cdot 6H_2O = 0.5$
$NaCl = 8.0$
$NaHCO_3 = 1.0$
$NaH_2PO_4 \cdot H_2O = 0.05$
$Glucose = 1.0$

The object of these treatments is to promote mineralization of the dentine and increase the concentrations of calcium and phosphate ions within the smear layer. The time of application is two to three minutes, a relatively long one.

These workers found mineralizing treatments more effective for the zinc polycarboxylate cements than for the glass-ionomer cements. The relative ineffectiveness of these treatments on glass-ionomer cement is probably related to calcium and phosphate in the cement and the formation of a calcium- and phosphate-rich layer between the cement and the tooth surface (Wilson et al., 1983). Obviously, further work is needed on these systems, but the same result might be achieved with modifications in the cement formulation.

EDTA

Ethylenediaminetetracetic acid (EDTA) is an extremely powerful complexing agent for metal ions—more so than citric acid. It is a weak acid, almost insoluble in water, and so is used in the form of soluble sodium salts: the Na_2EDTA half-salt is approximately neutral, and the Na_4EDTA salt is alkaline in solution. Both are strong decalcifying agents because of the strong, soluble chelates they form with calcium. The effect of solutions of EDTA on dentine and enamel surfaces is broadly similar to that of citric acid. This decalcifying effect is reflected in the observation that they reduce the bond strength of glass-ionomer cement to dentine. Their use on dentine and enamel is, therefore, deprecated. Moreover, solutions of Na_4EDTA will attack the matrix of the glass-ionomer cement itself and so are incompatible with it. Therefore, their use as surface conditioners is to be deprecated.

Marginal leakage

In recent years following the increasing interest in biocompatibility, attention has been focused on attaining an efficient marginal seal. A gap at the margin between a restoration and the cavity wall can result in the percolation of harmful microorganisms and chemicals that can give rise to secondary caries beneath the restoration. Adhesion of glass-ionomer cement to enamel and dentine led to the expectation that this cement would act as an efficient seal.

The expectation has been borne out by a number of workers using different in vitro methods of assessment (Hembree and Andrews, 1978; Kidd, 1978; Maldonado et al., 1978; Powis et al., 1985; Gordon et al., 1986). Powis et al., (1985)

found that glass-ionomer cements effected a permanent seal against the diffusion of sucrose (radiolabeled) for at least a year. No other restorative material was as effective, and all, including the etched composite resins, allowed leakage to some extent.

In addition, carious lesions in adjacent enamel have been shown to be reduced; Kidd (1978) attributed this result to fluoride released by the cement being taken up by the enamel.

Conclusions

Good interfacial contact is important for adhesion. The smoothing of surface irregularities may be necessary to prevent air entrapment and to minimize sites where stress concentration could occur. Clearly, the most effective conditioners are those capable of forming hydrogen bonds with the tooth surface, so aiding wetting. They may also serve to consolidate the smear layer. Currently we recommend a ten-second application of a 25% solution of poly(acrylic acid) for the surface conditioning of cavities and a 30-second application of 25% percent tannic acid where large areas of dentine are involved, as in crown preparation.

The idea that surface smoothness is important comes from the recent work of Aboush and Jenkins (1986), who showed that bond strength decreased as surface roughness increased. The smoothest surface attainable, that obtained by using a jet of water and cleaning powder (Prophy-Jet*), gave the highest bond strength, while the roughest surface gave the weakest.

The strongest bonds that have been reported in the literature are for the cement Chem-Fil* and are 9.9 MPa

*Dentsply International Inc., Weybridge, England, and York, Pa.

to enamel (citric acid) and 7.2 MPa to dentine (Prophy-Jet treatment). The next highest are for ASPA IV: 7.5 MPa to enamel (fluoride-containing surface cleaner) and 6.8 MPa to dentine (25% poly(acrylic acid) treatment).

Bonding composite resins to glass-ionomer cements

The use of glass-ionomer cements for replacement of carious dentine prior to attachment of composite resins to acid-etched enamel was first described by McLean and Wilson (1977a). This work has resulted in the widespread use of glass-ionomer cements in the so-called "sandwich" or "double-laminated" technique, in which both cement and enamel are etched prior to attachment of a light-cured composite resin (Fig. 6-6). This technique improves the bonding between the glass-ionomer cement and the composite resin. Overall, the laminate restoration has reduced microleakage compared with the simple composite resin restoration. These conclusions are supported by the findings of numerous research workers (McLean et al., 1985; Sneed and Looper, 1985; Welsh and Hembree, 1985; Gordon et al., 1985, 1986; Hinoura et al., 1987; Hembree, 1987; Merlo et al., 1987; Nara and Dogon, 1987).

Clinical applications of the sandwich technique have been reported by an increasing number of workers (Bitter, 1986; Garcia-Godoy and Malone, 1986). In the sandwich technique a glass-ionomer cement is packed into the bottom of a cavity, in effect to replace the lost dentine, and allowed to set and harden. When it has hardened it is acid etched (for up to

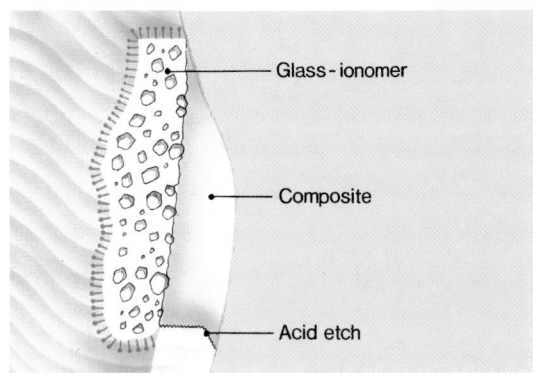

Fig. 6-6a The glass-ionomer/composite resin laminate.

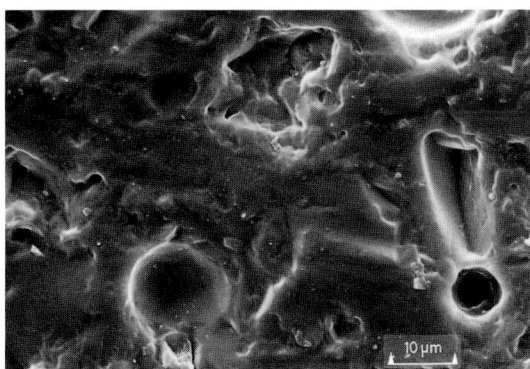

Fig. 6-6b Surface of a glass-ionomer cement prior to acid etching.

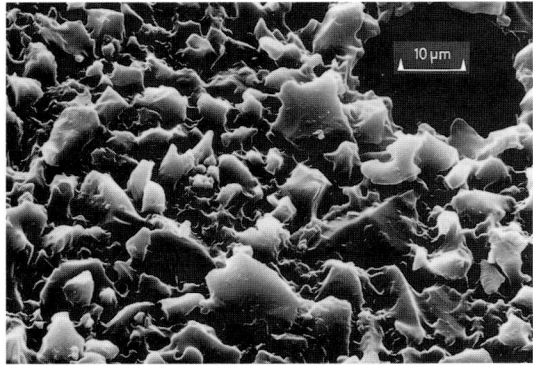

Fig. 6-6c Surface of a glass-ionomer cement after acid etching. Note that the glass particles now stand proud of the matrix, giving a surface suitable for mechanical keying.

Table 6-7 Effect of surface treatment of glass-ionomer cement on bond strength (MPa) to composite resins*

Laminate combination	Surface treatment		
	Smooth	Etched	Ground
Fuji Ionomer Type II† Silux‡ Scotchbond‡	5.2	5.2	4.9
Ketac-Bond§ Visio-Dispers§ Visio-Bond§	0.3	3.4	2.7
Ketac-Silver§ Silux‡ Scotchbond‡	4.6	6.0	4.7

*Based on data obtained from Hinoura et al. (1987).
†G-C International Corp., Tokyo, and Scottsdale, Ariz.
‡3M Dental Products, St. Paul, Minn.
§ESPE GmbH, Seefeld/Oberbay, West Germany, and Valley Stream, N.Y.

Table 6-8 Bond strengths (MPa) between various combinations of composite resins and etched glass-ionomer cements*

Cements	Cement tensile strength	Composite resin bonding agent		
		Microrest AP† G-C Bond†	Visio-Dispers†/ Visio-Bond‡	Silux§/ Scotchbond§
G-C Lining Cement‡	1.8	1.8	2.9	2.9
Fuji Ionomer I‡	3.5	0.8	4.7	4.9
Fuji Ionomer II‡	4.7	1.0	5.1	5.2
Miracle Mix‡	4.5	4.9	4.1	5.7
Ketac-Bond§	2.8	1.2	3.4	2.7
Ketac-Silver§	4.7	4.5	4.9	6.0

*Based on data obtained from Hinoura et al. (1987).
†G-C International Corp., Tokyo, and Scottsdale, Ariz.
‡ESPE GmbH, Seefeld/Oberbay, West Germany, and Valley Stream, N.Y.
§3M Dental Products, St. Paul, Minn.

one minute) using phosphoric acid solutions (37% aqueous). This treatment results in a rough surface in which glass particles stand proud of the matrix (Fig. 6-6c), suitable for mechanical keying. A thin liquid dimethacrylate resin is then applied that penetrates into the interstices between the proud particles. The composite resin is subsequently packed into the cavity.

The feasibility of bonding a composite resin, Visio-Dispers,* to glass-ionomer cements was examined by McLean et al. (1985), using Visio-Bond* as the liquid bonding resin and Ketac-Fil* as the glass-ionomer cement. Chemical analysis and scanning electron micrographs showed that phosphoric acid etches the cement by dissolving the matrix. This treatment effectively roughens the surface, increases the area available for attachment, and allows the resin to penetrate into the irregularities, where it hardens and forms retentive tags. Mechanical testing of the strength of the adhesive bond between the two materials, using flexural, shear, and tensile strength tests, revealed that the bond strength between resin and cement appeared to be greater than the cohesive strength of the cement (Table 6-7) (McLean et al., 1985; Sneed and Looper, 1985; Hinoura et al., 1987). Thus, bond strength is limited by the cohesive strength of the cement. Further, the results of Hinoura and coworkers (1987) show that bond strength can vary widely (from 0.3 to 6.0 MPa tensile strength), depending on the combination of glass-ionomer cement, composite resin, and surface treatment used (Tables 6-7 and 6-8). Consideration of the role of glass-ionomer cements in the sandwich technique has revealed that there are a number of parameters to be considered (Mount, 1987; Hinoura et al.,

1987; Hassan and Nathanson, 1987). These include length of acid-etch period, strength of the glass-ionomer cement and its rate of set, thickness of cement, radio-opacity and translucency, viscosity and wettability of the bonding resin, and shrinkage of the composite resin. Importantly, citric acid is not an effective etchant for this technique (Causton et al., 1987).

Acid etching

In general, acid etching markedly improves bond strength; see, for example, the results for the combination of Ketac-Bond, Visio-Dispers, and Visio-Bond (see Table 6-7). Grinding the cement surface is less effective than acid etching. However, in one case, surface treatment had no effect, which led Hinoura and coworkers (1987) to presume that a chemical bond would occur between certain composite resins and glass-ionomer cements. A more likely explanation is that the bonding resin itself is acidic.

Time factor

Attachment of composite resins to a glass-ionomer cement is best achieved when acid etching removes just enough matrix material to leave the unreacted glass particles proud on the surface. The question therefore arises: how much matrix material should be removed? In the early stages of set, glass-ionomer cements are particularly prone to moisture contamination because the matrix containing the calcium and aluminium ions for salt formation is comparatively weak. For this reason, etching should be restricted to the minimum period required to remove enough matrix material to provide a surface that is mechanically retentive while preserving the strength of the

*ESPE GmbH, Seefeld/Oberbay, West Germany, and Valley Stream, N.Y.

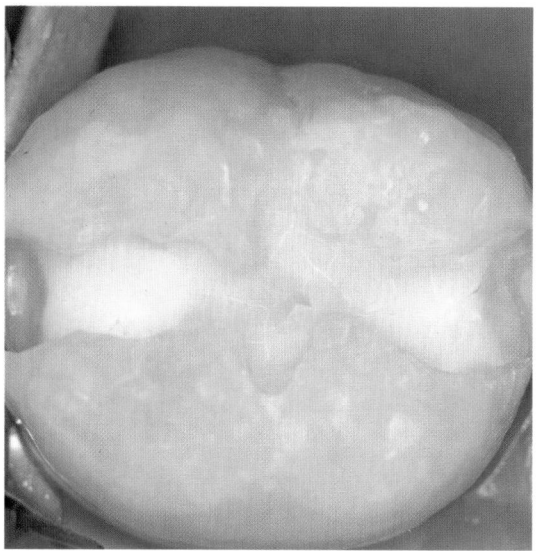

Fig. 6-7 Crazing of a glass-ionomer cement.

the highest bond strengths, followed by the Type II restorative materials (see Table 6-8). However, rate of set also will influence the result. A slower setting Type II glass-ionomer cement will be considerably weakened if etched prematurely because excess water will remove calcium and aluminium ions required for salt formation.

For the above-stated reasons, the ideal glass-ionomer cement for use with the sandwich technique is very difficult to produce. Fast-setting cements that can be etched after two to five minutes require higher alumina content in the glass and are often, therefore, more opaque (see chapter 2). In addition, these materials are generally made for hand-mixing at low powder/liquid ratios and are weaker in flexural strength. The more translucent materials, such as the Type II restoratives, are slower-setting due to lower alumina/silica ratio, and therefore require a setting period of at least eight minutes prior to acid etching.

underlying cement. Etching with a solution of 37% phosphoric acid for 20 to 30 seconds is generally recognised as the optimum time to achieve good bonding (McLean et al., 1985; Garcia-Godoy and Malone, 1986). This topic is the subject of much current research (Hassan and Nathanson, 1987; Joynt et al., 1987; Quiroz and Lentz, 1987; Smith and Soderholm, 1987).

Influence of cement strength and rate of set on bond strength

The strength of glass-ionomer cement will influence bond strength both at the dentine interface and the glass-ionomer/composite resin interface. It is now well established that the higher the strength of the cement, the better the clinical result will be providing low-contact-angle bonding resins are used (Hinoura et al., 1987; Mount, 1987). Hinoura and co-workers (1987) found that metal-reinforced glass-ionomer cements provided

Effect of cement thickness on bond strength

Obviously, the thinner the cement lining, the more likely damage will occur during acid etching. Not only will dehydration during drying remove the water needed for the cement to set and hydrate, but after air drying, excess water from the acid will penetrate the weakened polysalt matrix and invade any craze areas (Fig. 6-7). A thin lining of glass-ionomer cement may bond to the composite resin, but stress at the interface can soon cause a cohesive failure in the weakened cement or an adhesive failure at the dentine bond. Penetration of acid through the cement into the dentine will not occur if the cement thickness is greater than 0.5 mm (Walker et al., 1986).

The original concept by McLean and

Wilson (1977a) is, therefore, still valid. Glass-ionomer cement should be used as a *dentine replacement,* not as a thin wash lining. Then the cement will be stronger, provide a better surface for acid etching, and will not be subject to high stress from the shrinking composite. By increasing the bulk of glass-ionomer cement and reducing the bulk of composite resin, stable bonds can be more easily achieved. A cement thickness greater than 0.5 mm is recommended.

Radio-opacity and translucency

Radio-opacity in a lining cement is of particular value in detecting subsequent microleakage and secondary caries under the restoration. The metal-reinforced cements are therefore of considerable value under posterior composite resins and materials such as Ketac-Silver* provide strong bonding both to the dentine and the composite resin (Hinoura et al., 1987; McCullock and Smith, 1986). Where aesthetics is of major importance, the fast-setting lining cements that are also radio-opaque may be used, providing they can be covered by at least 1 mm of composite resin in thin areas. Where thickness is critical the more translucent Type II restorative materials are preferred, even though there is an increased time factor to be considered.

Viscosity and wettability of the bonding resins

Good penetration of the acid-etched surface of glass-ionomer cement by the bonding resin is highly dependent upon

*ESPE GmbH, Seefeld/Oberbay, West Germany, and Valley Stream, N.Y.

wettability. Mount (1987) observed that when using certain composite resins and their prescribed bonding resins, the failure under tensile stress was adhesive at the union rather than cohesive in the cement. He attributed this to the higher viscosity of the bonding resins used and suggested that bonding resins with low contact angles were preferred because of their increased wettability. However, Hinoura and coworkers (1987) have postulated that bond strengths could be influenced by chemical reaction between the resin bonding agent and the cement.

Setting contraction

As previously explained, the glass-ionomer cements have minimal shrinkage providing they are in a humid environment. Composite resins by their nature suffer a polymerization shrinkage from 1.67 to 5.68 vol% (Goldman, 1983). This setting contraction has been shown to produce quite severe contraction stresses of 2.8 to 3.9 MPa (Davidson and de Gee, 1984), to the point where cusps can be distorted (Causton et al., 1985). The sandwich or double-laminate technique is therefore of particular value in reducing the effects of composite resin shrinkage, since the glass-ionomer base reduces the volume of composite material used. In addition, the glass-ionomer base provides a better seal against dentine than resin-bonding agents. In general, the microfilled composite resins will shrink more than heavily filled hybrid or small-particle-size resins, so that in the posterior region the lower shrinkage materials should be used. In the anterior region the volume of the composite resin veneer is generally less, so that the more translucent and aesthetic microfilled resins can be used with safety.

Clinical recommendations

The parameters involved in glass-ionomer cement/composite resin bonding are now becoming clearer and certain recommendations can be made:

1. Condition the dentine with 25% poly-(acrylic acid) for ten seconds prior to applying the glass-ionomer base. In cases where extensive areas of dentine are involved, a 25% tannic acid solution applied for 30 seconds is preferred.

2. Never use a thin wash of cement that, during drying, can be easily dehydrated and then hydrated by the acid.

3. Wherever high stresses are involved, use stronger cements such as cermets or Type II restoratives (see Table 6-8).

4. Where radiopacity is required, use a cermet cement for the posterior restorations and a radio-opaque fast-setting lining cement for the anterior restorations. Cermet cements should be allowed to set for a minimum of five minutes prior to etching, and the fast-setting lining cements for a minimum of three to four minutes. However, the cement should be tested clinically and be hard to the touch prior to acid etching.

5. Where optimum aesthetics is required and there is limited space for the composite veneer, use a Type II restorative glass-ionomer material. Allow a minimum setting period of eight minutes prior to acid etching. Reduce the etch time to ten to 15 seconds for the slower-setting materials.

6. Wherever possible, use a minimum cement base thickness of 0.5 mm and completely line out the dentine.

7. Do not over-instrument the surface of the cement if removal of excess material is required from cavity edges. Glass-ionomer bases are preferably allowed to set undisturbed prior to acid etching.

8. Never exceed a 30-second etch period for both cement and enamel, even with the fast-setting glass-ionomers cements.

9. After acid etching the cement base, the surface must be thoroughly washed and dried to provide a high-energy surface for wetting with the bonding resin. Apply the bonding resin immediately after drying to prevent surface contamination.

10. Use a low-viscosity light-cured bonding resin for best results. This may be easily checked by viewing contact angles of the bonding resins when applied to a specimen disc of acid-etched cement. The easier they spread over the surface the better the wetting. When applying the bonding resin, avoid pooling by removing excess with a gentle stream of clean, dry compressed air.

11. Light cure the bonding resin for at least 20 seconds prior to bulk packing the composite veneer. This can prevent lifting of the higher-viscosity pastes during packing.

12. When a cermet-ionomer cement lining is used in the posterior region, it may be extended 2 mm from the cervical aspect to provide a cariostatic seal and reduce the volume of bulk composite approximally.

Causes of failure

The two main causes of failure when using the glass-ionomer/composite resin laminate technique are, first, using thin wash linings and, second, acid etching the cement before it has reached a proper state of hardening. The cement-forming ions should be locked in the matrix and the surface hard to the touch.

References

Aboush, Y.E.Y., and Jenkins, C.B.G. (1986) An evaluation of the bonding of glass-ionomer restoratives to dentine and enamel. Br. Dent. J. 161:179–184.

Beech, D.R. (1973) Improvement in the adhesion of polyacrylate cements to human dentine. Br. Dent. J. 135:442–445.

Beech, D.R., Solomon, A., and Bernier, R. (1985) Bond strength of polycarboxylic acid cements to treated dentine. Dent. Mater. 1:154–157.

Bitter, N.C. (1986) Glass ionomer-microfil technique for restoring cervical lesions. J. Prosthet. Dent. 55:661–662.

Brännström, M. (1981) Pretreatment before the placing of restorations. p. 93 In Dentine and Pulp in Restorative Dentistry. Nacka, Sweden: Dental Therapeutics AB.

Causton, B.E., and Johnson, N.W. (1979) The role of diffusible ionic species in the bonding of polycarboxylate cements to dentin. An in vitro study. J. Dent. Res. 58:1383–1393.

Causton, B.E., and Johnson, N.W. (1982) Improvement of polycarboxylate adhesion to dentine by use of a new calcifying solution. Br. Dent. J. 152:9–11.

Causton, B.E., Miller, B., and Sefton, J. (1985) The deformation of cusps by bonded posterior composite resins: An in vitro study. Br. Dent. J. 159:397–403.

Causton, B.E., Sefton, J., and Williams, A. (1987) Bonding Class II composite to etched glass ionomer cement. Br. Dent. J. 163:321–324.

Cotton, W.R., and Siegal, R.L. (1978) Human pulpal response to citric acid cavity cleanser. J. Am. Dent. Assoc. 96:639–644.

Coury, M.L., Miranda, F.J., Willer, R.D., and Probst, R.T. (1981) Adhesiveness of glass ionomer cement to enamel and dentin: A laboratory study. Oper. Dent. 7:2–5.

Davidson, C.L., and de Gee, A.J. (1984) Relaxation of polymerization contraction stresses by flow in dental composites. J. Dent. Res. 63:146–148.

Garcia-Godoy, F., and Malone, W.F.P. (1986) The effect of acid etching on two glass ionomer lining cements. Quintessence. Int. 17:621–623.

Goldman, M. (1983) Polymerisation shrinkage of resin-based restorative materials. Aust. Dent. J. 28:156–161.

Gordon, M., Plasschaert, A.J.M., Soelberg, K.G., and Bogdon, M.S. (1985) Microleakage for composite resin over a glass-ionomer cement base in Class V restorations. Quintessence Int. 16:817–820.

Gordon, M., Plasschaert, A.J.M., and Stark, M.M. (1986) Microleakage of several tooth colored restorative materials in cervical cavities: A comparative study in vitro. Dent. Mater. 2:228–231.

Hassan, F., and Nathanson, D. (1987) Shear bond strengths of composite to etched glass ionomer cement. J. Dent. Res. 66(Special Issue):132 (abstr. 203).

Hembree, J.H. (1987) Marginal leakage of Class II composite resin using a glass ionomer cement as liner. J. Dent. Res. 66(Special Issue):293 (abstr. 1493).

Hembree, J.H., and Andrews, J.T. (1978) Microleakage of several class V anterior restorative materials: A laboratory study. J. Am. Dent. Assoc. 97:179–183.

Hinoura, K., Moore, B.K, and Phillips, R.W. (1987) Tensile bond strength between glass ionomer cement and composite resins. J. Am. Dent. Assoc. 114:167–172.

Hood, J.A.A., Childs, W.A., and Evans, D.F. (1977) Bond strengths of glass-ionomer and polycarboxylate cements to dentine. N.Z. Dent. J. 77:141–144.

Hötz, P., McLean, J.W., Sced, I., and Wilson, A.D. (1977) The bonding of glass ionomer cements to metal and tooth substrates. Br. Dent. J. 142:41–47.

Jackson, A. (1986) Personal communication.

Joynt, R.B., Williams, D., Davis, E.L., and Wieczkowski, G. (1987) Effects of etching time on surface morphology and adhesion of resin to glass ionomer. J. Dent. Res. 66(Special Issue):131 (abstr. 198).

Kidd, E.A.M. (1978) Cavity sealing ability of composite resin and glass ionomer restorations: An assessment in vitro. Br. Dent. J. 144:139–142.

Lacefield, W.R., Reindl, M.C., and Retief, D.H. (1985) Tensile bond strength of a glass-ionomer. J. Prosthet. Dent. 53:194–198.

Levine, R.S., Beech, D.R., & Garton, B. (1977) Improving bond strength of polyacrylate cements to dentine. Br. Dent. J. 143:275–277.

Long, T.E., Duke, E.S., and Norling, B.K. (1986) Polyacrylic acid cleaning of dentin and glass ionomer bond strengths. J. Dent. Res. 65(Special Issue):345 (abstr. 1583).

McCullock, A.L., and Smith, B.G.N. (1986) In vitro studies of cusp reinforcement with adhesive restorative material. Br. Dent. J. 161:450–452.

McLean, J.W. (1980) Aesthetics in restorative dentistry: The challenge for the future. Br. Dent. J. 149:368–373.

McLean, J.W., and Wilson, A.D. (1974) Fissure sealing and filling with an adhesive glass-ionomer cement. Br. Dent. J. 136:269–276.

McLean, J.W., and Wilson, A.D. (1977a) The clinical development of the glass-ionomer cement. II. Some clinical applications. Aust. Dent. J. 22:120–127.

McLean, J.W., and Wilson, A.D. (1977b) The clinical development of the glass-ionomer cement. III. The erosion lesion. Aust. Dent. J. 22:190–195.

McLean, J.W., Powis, D.R., Prosser, H.J., and Wilson, A.D. (1985) The use of glass-ionomer cements in bonding composite resins to dentine. Br. Dent. J. 158:410–414.

Maldonado, A., Swartz, M.L., and Phillips, R.W. (1978). An in vitro study of certain properties of a glass ionomer cement. J. Am. Dent. Assoc. 96:785–791.

Merlo, B.J., Cooley, R.O., Fan, P.L., Cannon, M., and Fippinger, T. (1987) Microleakage with glass ionomer and dentin adhesives in composite restorations. J. Dent. Res. 66 (Special Issue):293 (abstr. 1492).

Mount, G.J. (1984) Glass ionomer cements: Clinical considerations. Chapt. 20A In J.W. Clark (ed.) Clinical Dentistry. Philadelphia: Harper & Row.

Mount, G.J. (1987) Unpublished data.

Nara, Y., and Dogon, I.L. (1987) Bonding of light cured posterior composite to glass ionomer cement. J. Dent. Res. 66(Special Issue):131 (abstr. 200).

Nation, W., Jedrychowski, J.R., and Caputo A.A. (1980) Effect of surface treatments on the retention of restorative materials to dentin J. Prosth. Dent. 44:638–641.

Negm, M.M., Beech, D.R., and Grant, A.A. (1982) An evaluation of mechanical and adhesive properties of polycarboxylate and glass ionomer cements. J. Oral. Rehabil 9:161–167.

Öilo, G. (1981) Bond strength of new ionomer cements to dentin. Scand. J. Dent. Res. 89:344–347.

Peddy, M. (1981) The bond strength of polycarboxylic acid cements to dentine: Effect of surface modification and time after extraction. Aust. Dent. J. 26:178–180.

Powis, D.R. (1986) Personal communication.

Powis, D.R., Folleras, T., Merson, S.A., and Wilson, A.D. (1982) Improved adhesion of a glass ionomer cement to dentin and enamel. J. Dent. Res. 61:1416–1422.

Powis, D.R. Prosser, H.J., and Wilson, A.D. (1985) Marginal leakage of dental restorative materials. Unpublished report. London: Laboratory of the Government Chemist.

Prodger, T.E., and Symonds, M. (1977) ASPA adhesion study. Br. Dent. J. 143:266–270.

Quiroz, L., and Lentz, D.L. (1987) Laboratory evaluation of etching time on three different glass ionomers. J. Dent. Res. 66(Special Issue):131 (abstr. 197).

Shalabi, H.S., Asmussen, E., and Jörgensen, K.D. (1981) Increased bonding of a glass-ionomer cement to dentin by means of $FeCl_3$. Scand. J. Dent. Res. 89:348–353.

Smith, D.C. (1968) A new dental cement. Br. Dent. J. 125:381–384.

Smith, G.E., and Soderholm, K.J.M. (1987) Etching time effects upon glass ionomer-resin shear bond strengths. J. Dent. Res. 66(Special Issue):131 (abstr. 199).

Sneed, W.D., and Looper, S.W. (1985) Shear bond strength of a composite resin to an etched glass ionomer. Dent. Mater. 1:127–128.

Thornton, J.B., Retief, D.H., and Bradley, E.L. (1986) Fluoride release from and tensile bond strength of Ketac-Fil and Ketac-Silver to enamel and dentin. Dent. Mater. 2:241–245.

Vaidyanthan, J., Vaidyanthan, T.K., and Schulman, A. (1984) Demineralization and ion binding action of a polycarboxylate cement liquid on human dental enamel. J. Biomed. Mater. Res. 18:871–880.

Vliestra, J.R., Plant, C.G., Shovelton, D.S., and Bradnock, G. (1978) The use of glass ionomer cement in deciduous teeth. Br. Dent. J. 145:164–166.

Vougiouklakis, G., Smith, D.C., and Lipton, S. (1982) Evaluation of the bonding of cervical restorative materials. J. Oral Rehabil. 9:231–251.

Walker, T.M., Jensen, M.E., and Chan, D.C.N. (1986) Acid penetration through glass-ionomer base. J. Dent. Res 65:344 (abstr. 1580).

Welsh, E.L., and Hembree, J.H. (1985) Microleakage of the gingival wall with four Class V anterior restorative materials. J. Prosthet. Dent. 54:370–372.

Wilson, A.D. (1968) Dental silicate cements. VII. Alternative liquid cement formers. J. Dent. Res. 47:1133–1136.

Wilson, A.D. (1974) Alumino-silicate polyacrylic acid and related cements. Br. Polym. J. 6:165–179.

Wilson, A.D., Prosser, H.J., and Powis, D.R. (1983) Mechanism of adhesion of polyelectrolyte cements to hydroxyapatite. J. Dent. Res. 62:590–592.

Chapter 7

Erosion and Longevity

For many years the longevity of a restoration was judged solely by its ability to withstand erosion and wear. However, a restoration is only as good as the condition of the tooth tissues that surround it. If these are carious, the mechanical condition of the restorative material is immaterial—it has failed in its main task of protecting the tooth from further decay. Mjör has correctly directed our attention away from creep and corrosion toward the major cause of amalgam failure: the development of secondary caries under the restoration (Mjör, 1985; Mjör and Leinfelder, 1985). This aspect is particularly relevant in the case of the glass-ionomer cement because it is not just an inert mechanical plug but also an adhesive bioactive material with therapeutic action. One interesting contrast is that while an amalgam can fail even when it remains physically intact, because of the development of secondary caries, the cariostatic effect of the glass-ionomer cement persists even when the restoration is lost.

Another aspect of longevity, which became apparent when the composite resin replaced the dental silicate, is staining, both at the surface and at the margins. Staining at the surface is an indication of breakdown at the filler/matrix interface, and staining at the margins reveals microleakage. Surprisingly, the anterior composite resin is no more durable than a good, well-prepared, and well-placed silicate cement. Only the mode of failure differs.

In discussing the longevity of the glass-ionomer cement, durability, caries development, and colour stability all have to be considered. In addition, since an adhesive material is often placed in cavities that have not been undercut, there is an additional mode of failure: loss of adhesion.

Dissolution and erosion

There are two aspects to be considered: the leaching of soluble constituents from the cement and actual erosion. The loss of soluble species from the cement can lead to disintegration if they are matrix formers, but if they are not, then this will have no effect on durability. Indeed, the release of certain chemical species can be beneficial, as is the case with fluoride release, and the matrix can act as a reservoir for soluble material.

Erosion proper is the result of chemical attack and mechanical wear, and there are short-term and long-term aspects. Damage arises from deficiencies of technique in preparing and placing glass-ionomer cement restorations. This damage is of two kinds: damage by moisture before the cement has hardened and desiccation before the cement has fully

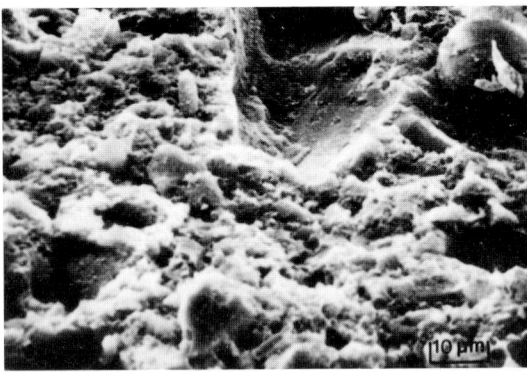

Fig. 7-1a Effect of acid on the surface of dental silicate cement. Reprinted with permission from Kent et al. (1973).

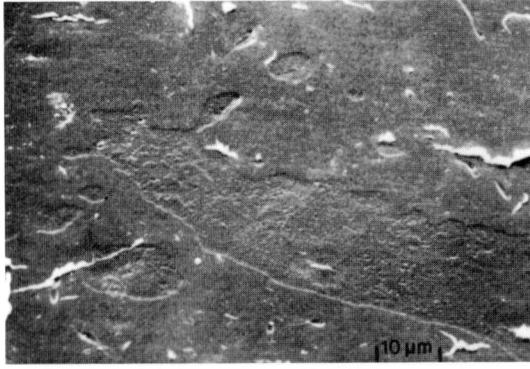

Fig. 7-1b Effect of acid on the surface of glass-ionomer cement. Reprinted with permission from Kent et al. (1973).

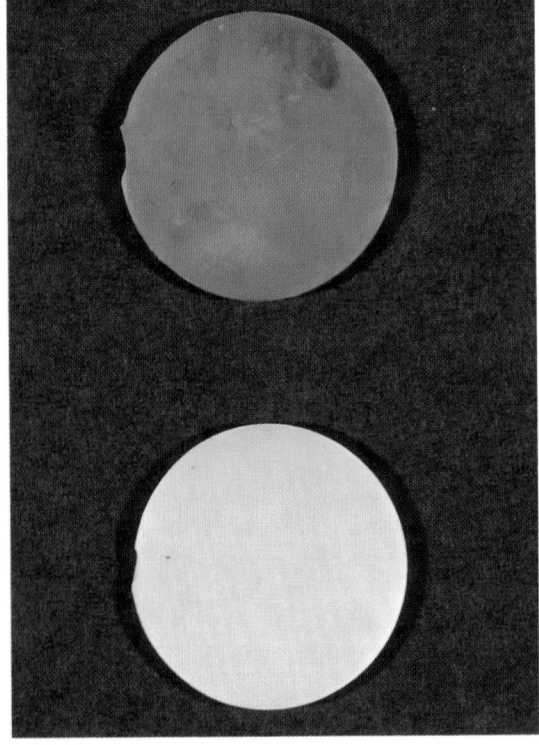

Fig. 7-2a Effect of staining on dental silicate cement. Reprinted with permission from Kent et al. (1973).

Fig. 7-2b Effect of staining on glass-ionomer cement. Reprinted with permission from Kent et al. (1973).

matured. In the long term there is the question of the cement's resistance to a combination of chemical and mechanical action. Chemical erosion is now known to be determined by acids generated by dental plaque or contained in food and beverages, and not by salivary parameters (Pluim and Arends, 1987; Henschel, 1949; Wilson and Batchelor, 1968).

In an early paper on glass-ionomer cements, Kent and coworkers (1973) demonstrated that the surface of a glass-ionomer cement was much less disrupted by acid attack and stained to a much lesser degree than the surface of a dental silicate cement (Figs. 7-1 and 7-2). This was a promising finding; the authors concluded that glass-ionomer cements should prove to be much more durable in the mouth than other dental cements. Such a finding is in accord with the chemical structures of the various dental cements. The matrix of a traditional phosphate cement is an aggregate of discrete cations and phosphate anions held together solely by ionic bonds. Acid attack easily disrupts ionic bonds. Purely ionic aggregates will then decompose into discrete phosphate ions and cations (Fig. 7-3a). The situation is quite different in the case of glass-ionomer cement, for the anion is a polymer where the active carboxylate groups are connected by covalent linkages impervious to acid attack. Only the cross-links are ionic, and many of these would have to be broken before the matrix would decompose (Fig. 7-3b).

These early findings and speculations have been confirmed. Clinical evidence is that once properly set the glass-ionomer cement is the most durable of all dental cements. The chief problem is the vulnerability of the cement to moisture before it has fully hardened.

Although in vitro studies on the solubility of dental cements have been a favourite, if often clinically irrelevant, topic for research, the number of clinical trials on the in vivo solubility of cements, including glass-ionomer cements, have been few. Fortunately, this situation is being remedied. Clinical trials that have been made indicate that the glass-ionomer cement is the most durable of all the dental cements and has but a fraction of the in vivo solubility of zinc phosphate and polycarboxylate cements (Mitchem and Gronas, 1978, 1981; Sidler and Strube, 1983; Mesu and Reedijk, 1983; Theuniers, 1984; Pluim et al., 1984; Pluim and Arends, 1987). These clinical findings are summarized in Tables 7-1 and 7-2. Further confirmation comes from studies on the in vitro acid-erosion of dental cements using Beham's impinging jet method (Wilson et al., 1986). This test is now generally believed to give a reasonable representation of the clinical situation, unlike the old specification test carried out in static distilled water on immature specimens (Wilson, 1976). Wilson and coworkers (1986) found that the acid-erosion of the various types of water-based dental cements increased in this order:

glass ionomer < silicate < zinc phosphate < polycarboxylate (Fig. 7-4)

These findings have been generally confirmed by other research workers (Crisp et al., 1980; Beech and Bandyopadhyay, 1983; Setchell et al., 1985; Matsuya et al., 1984; Walls et al., 1985). They also agree with the results from the clinical studies cited above. Setchell and coworkers (1985) also make the point, confirmed by Wilson and coworkers (1986), that glass-ionomer cements based on maleic acid copolymers are less resistant to acid attack than those based on poly(acrylic acid). This result has been observed even when the same glass has been used to prepare both types of cement (Billington, 1986).

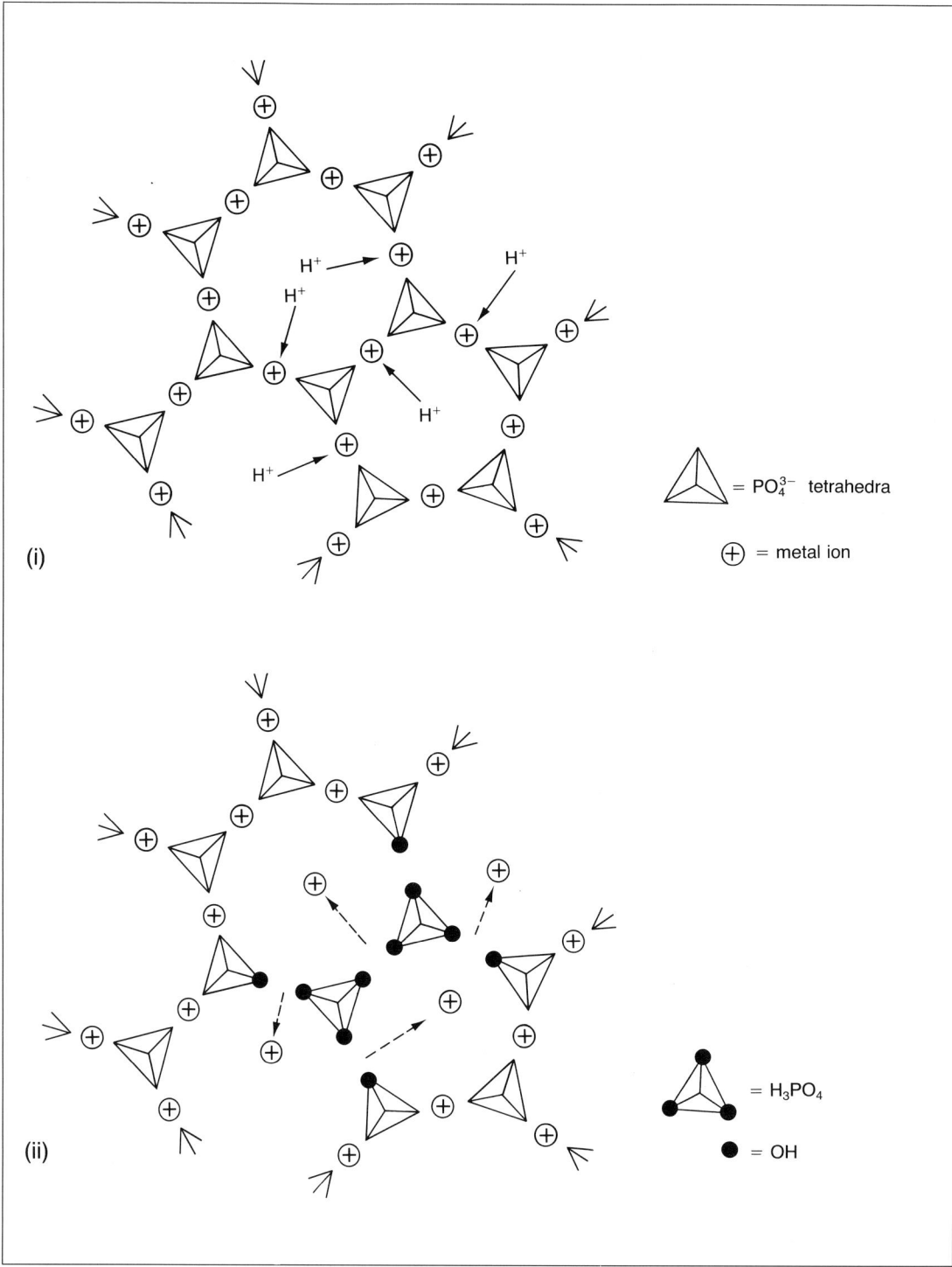

Fig. 7-3a *(i)* Initial stage of acid attack by hydrogen ions (H⁺) on the matrix of a dental silicate cement. *(ii)* Dissolution of the ionically bound phosphate-bonded matrix into isolated phosphoric acid units as the metal ions are removed, leading to the complete disruption of the cement.

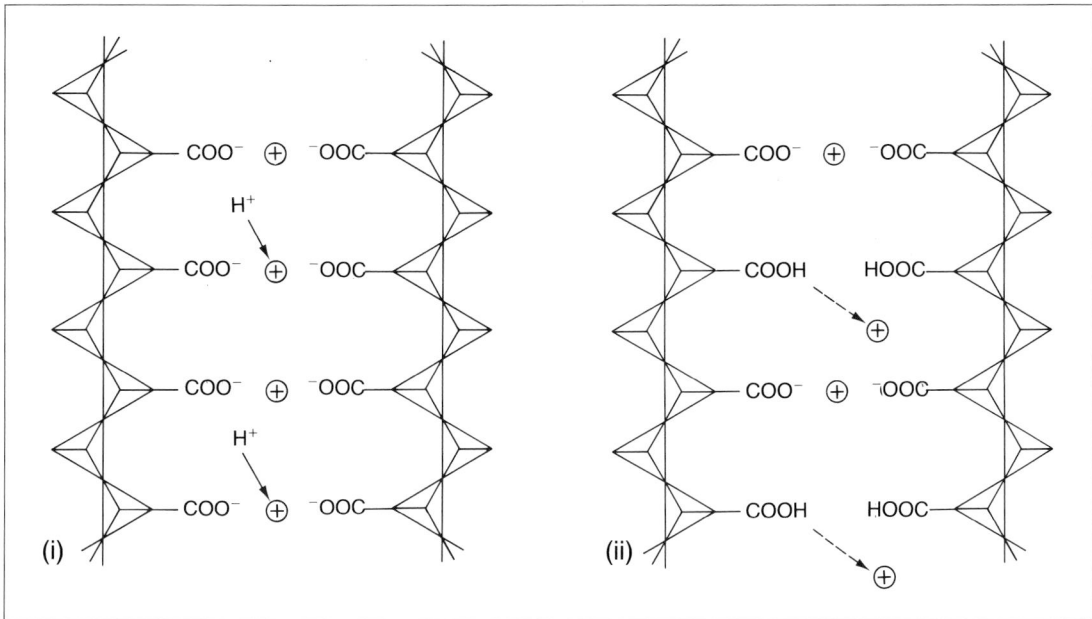

Fig. 7-3b *(i)* Initial stage of acid attack by hydrogen ions (H⁺) on the matrix of a glass-ionomer cement. *(ii)* Removal of some of the cross-linking metal ions does not lead to the disruption of the structure, because sufficient remain to connect the covalent polyacid chains.

Table 7-1 Comparison of the in vivo erosion of dental cements

Investigators	Erosion ranking*
Mitchem & Gronas (1978, 1981)	GI < SP < ZP < PC
Sidler & Strub (1983)	GI < ZP
Mesu & Reedijk (1983)	GI < ZP = PC < ZOE/EBA
Theuniers (1984)	GI < ZP = PC < ZOE/EBA
Pluim (1985)	GI < ZP < PC

*GI = glass-ionomer cement, SP = silico-phosphate cement, ZP = zinc phosphate cement, PC = polycarboxylate cement, ZOE/EBA = zinc oxide–eugenol/o-ethoxybenzoic acid.

Table 7-2 Rate of in vivo erosion of dental cements (μm/week)

Cement	Mitchem & Gronas (1978)	Pluim et al. (1984)
Glass-ionomer	7	0.5–1
Zinc phosphate	23	20–22
Polycarboxylate	36	18–30

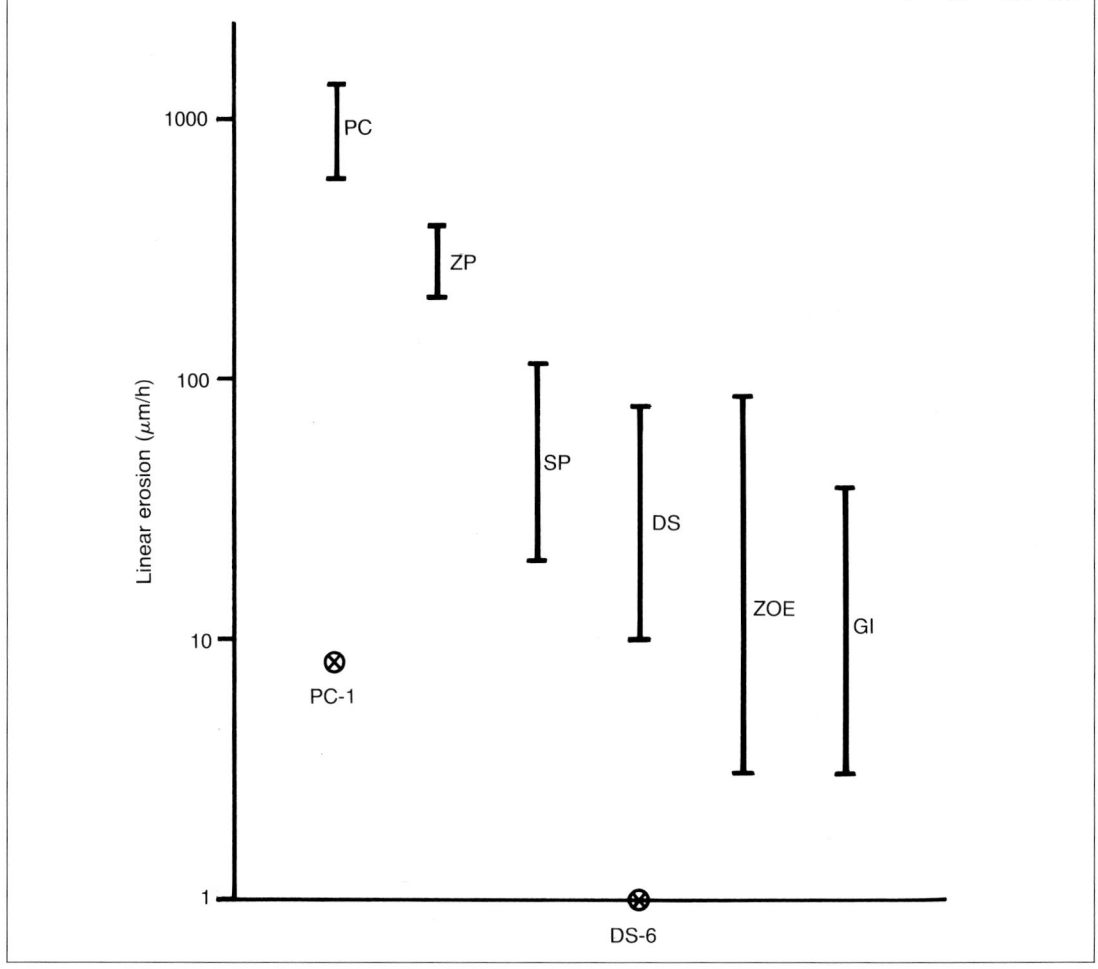

Fig. 7-4 Diagram showing the range of erosion rates of each class of dental cement. Cements were subjected to a jet of lactic acid and this diagram illustrates the durability of glass-ionomer cements. Reprinted with permission from Wilson et al. (1986).

Once the glass-ionomer has fully matured, only nonmatrix elements are leached, namely sodium, fluoride, and silica. These are not matrix-forming species, and the release of fluoride can be considered beneficial. The chief problem with glass-ionomer cements is that they are vulnerable to moisture for a number of minutes after setting. This has long been known (McLean and Wilson, 1977b), and the underlying reasons for the problem are given fully in chapter 3.

Although over the last decade materials have been considerably improved, this fault has yet to be completely eradicated even in recent materials (Öilo, 1984). Thus, the most important factor affecting the durability of glass-ionomer cement is the care devoted to it during the first few minutes of its life.

Early contamination by water involves the imbibition of water followed by swelling and loss of surface material, which leads to surface roughening (Roulet and

Wälti, 1984). Translucency is also impaired (Mount and Makinson, 1982). Paradoxically, the cement is vulnerable to desiccation as well. This is because the best curing condition for the glass-ionomer cement is an environment that is high in humidity (c. 80% relative humidity), but not wet. Desiccation of the cement and contact with moisture alike are to be avoided. Loss of water prevents the cement from curing because it is the reaction medium, and bathing in water removes matrix-forming metal ions. Thus, the most important factor affecting the durability and appearance of the glass-ionomer cement is the care devoted to it during the first few minutes of its life. All of this adds up to a need for temporary protection against adverse conditions until the cement has hardened sufficiently to withstand these conditions.

The correct technique has to thread a careful path through these extremes. Thus, while access of moisture to the restoration during placement has to be prevented, the use of a rubber dam can lead to desiccation. After set, protection by varnish is essential. The period during which protection is required varies. About 30 minutes should suffice to prevent damage by moisture, although for certain recent materials a much shorter period is in order. The cement, however, remains vulnerable to desiccation for a much longer period (Phillips and Bishop, 1985).

Durability and longevity

Although durability and longevity have been touched on in several sections of this book, it is useful to draw all the aspects together at this point. Durability is affected by a number of factors: inadequate preparation of the cement and inadequate protection of the restoration, as well as the variable conditions of the mouth. Not surprisingly, clinical reports on the performance of glass-ionomer cements are conflicting and confused, with failure rates ranging from 0% (over 19 months) to 70% (36 months). From this it would be reasonable to suppose that failure rate is more a measure of a clinician's skill than of the inherent quality of the materials.

The problem of poor instructions has also been cited by Mount (1984) and Smales (1981). Mount (1984) pointed out that problems arising from the slow maturation of the cement, that is, early susceptibility to moisture contamination, were often glossed over. He summarized the results of clinical trials and his summary is reproduced here, brought up to date with reports from more recent studies, in Tables 7-3 and 7-4. It is worth noting that more recent studies report more favourable results, probably as a result of improvements in materials and a better understanding of the techniques required to achieve optimum results.

Mount (1984) also reported a study by two dental practitioners carried out over seven years using several different brands of material mainly in Class V cavities. In view of the importance of this unique study the results are reproduced in full in Table 7-5. Note that there was but a 2% failure rate for Ketac-Fil,* a modern material, compared with 17% for the older De Trey Aspa†—an indication of the progress that has been made in developing glass-ionomer cement.

*ESPE GmbH, Seefeld/Oberbay, West Germany, and Valley Stream, N.Y.
†Amalgamated Dental Co., Weybridge, England.

Table 7-3 Clinical trials of glass-ionomer cements in Class V cavities

Investigator	Cement	Period (months)	Loss %
McLean & Wilson	ASPA IV*	6	8
(1977a)		12	8
		24	9
		36	9
Mount & Makinson (1978)	De Trey Aspa†	12	0
Lawrence (1979)	De Trey Aspa	6	7
		18	9
Smales (1981)	De Trey Aspa	12	43
		24	52
		36	72
Low (1981)	De Trey Aspa	9	5
		15	26
Brandau et al. (1983)	De Trey Aspa	54	10
Brown (1983)	De Trey Aspa	6	0
Mount (1984)	Various	12–24	3
Mount (1984)	De Trey Aspa	24–84	15
	Fuji Ionomer II‡	24–84	3
	Ketac-Fil§	24–84	1
	Total	24–84	7
Knibbs et al. (1986b)	Chem-Fil¶	23–32	3

*Laboratory of the Government Chemist, London.
†Amalgamated Dental Co., Weybridge, England.
‡G-C International Corp., Tokyo, and Scottsdale, Ariz.
§ESPE GmbH, Seefeld/Oberbay, West Germany, and Valley Stream, N.Y.
¶Dentsply International Inc., Weybridge, England, and York, Pa.

Table 7-4 Clinical trials of glass-ionomer cements in Class III cavities

Investigators	Cement	Period	Loss (%)
Mount (1984)	De Trey Aspa*	24–84	8
	Fuji Ionomer II†	24–84	0
	Ketac-Fil‡	24–84	0.1
	Total	24–84	1
Knibbs et al. (1986a)	Chem-Fil§	12	1
		24	3
		36	4
		41	5
Knibbs et al. (1986b)	Chem-Fil	23–32	0

*Amalgamated Dental Co., Weybridge, England.
†G-C International Corp., Tokyo, and Scottsdale, Ariz.
‡ESPE GmbH, Seefeld/Oberbay, West Germany, and Valley Stream, N.Y.
§Dentsply International Inc., Weybridge, England, and York, Pa.

Table 7-5 Seven-year clinical trial of glass-ionomer cements*

	De Trey Aspa†	Fuji Ionomer II‡	Ketac-Fil§	Total
	Restorations placed			
Class V	328	246	802	1376
Class III	28	54	374	466
Others	80	23	155	258
Total	446	323	1331	2100
	Restorations rechecked			
Class V	306	191	421	918
Class III	26	30	183	239
Others	52	18	46	126
Total	384	239	660	1283
	Restorations failed			
Class V	45	8	9	62
Class III	2	0	1	3
Others	19	4	6	29
Total	66 (17%)	12 (5%)	16 (2%)	94 (7%)

*Reprinted with permission from Mount (1984).
†G-C International Corp., Tokyo, and Scottsdale, Ariz.
‡ESPE GmbH, Seefeld/Oberbay, West Germany, and Valley Stream, N.Y.
§Dentsply International Inc., Weybridge, England, and York, Pa.

Clinical performance

The final test of a dental material must be its clinical performance in general practice. However, the gathering of such data and its interpretation is obscured by factors other than the intrinsic merits or demerits of a material, for example, its clinical mishandling. An example from the past is dental silicate cement, which has been shown to be the equal of composite resin in Class III and Class V situations when handled correctly (Robinson, 1971). However, it was widely regarded as unsatisfactory, probably as the result of a disappointing experience that resulted from mishandling and poor materials. By contrast, the composite resin is a robust material, capable of surviving mishandling, provided it is inserted in a dry field.

In between the quantitative but not always relevant laboratory test and the relevant but imprecise impressions of general practice lies the clinical trial, carried out by the trained research clinician. Such studies yield a more focused appreciation of the merits or demerits of a material than do the impressions of general practice. In some cases the clinical trial can be made to yield quantitative answers, but, of course, even these lack the precision of a laboratory test because oral conditions are variable. In the final analysis, a careful qualitative observation can be of as much value as an elaborate clinical trial.

A number of clinical trials have been conducted on the use of glass-ionomer cements in various clinical situations over the years. Gradually a pattern of advantages and limitations is emerging.

Cervical erosion lesions—Class V

A change in pattern of dental health with its reduced incidence of caries early in life has focused attention on the problem of the erosion lesion associated with middle-aged adults. An efficient treatment of such lesions is clearly important. Thus, one of the earliest uses found for glass-ionomer cements was restoring Class V gingival lesions (McLean and Wilson, 1977b). The cement appears well suited for such restoration. Its adhesion to dentine and enamel is compatible with the requirement for minimum cavity preparation, and its aesthetics is acceptable. Moreover, it may be placed in cervical erosion cavities without causing the patient discomfort, despite the sensitivity caused by exposed dentine (Lawrence, 1979). Surprisingly, this reduction of sensitivity is maintained even when the restoration is wholly or partly lost (Low, 1981).

An early three-year study reported a failure rate of only 9% using an early experimental material (see Table 7-3), and concluded that loss occurred either soon after placement by fracture or adhesive failure, or not at all (McLean and Wilson, 1977a). Subsequent clinical trials have yielded varying results (see Table 7-3). Failure rates reported have ranged from 0% (Mount and Makinson, 1978) to 43% (Smales, 1981). However, McLean and Wilson (1977b), Charbeneau and Bozell (1979), and Lawrence (1979) generally agree with each other, finding a 5% to 8% loss in the first six months rising to 9% over longer periods. Other workers are in broad agreement with these findings (Flynn, 1979; Low, 1981; Tyas, 1983; Tyas and Beech, 1985; Knibbs et al., 1986b).

Correct handling of the cement is crucial. Low (1981) noted that increased experience improves clinical results. This point is reinforced by a study of Smales (1981), who, using a variety of operators in a dental hospital, found a 72% failure rate in a three-year study. These poor results were attributed to lack of abuse tolerance, i.e., poor technique on the part of inexperienced operators, and poor manufacturers' instructions. This study underlines the point that glass-ionomer cements must not be put in the hands of inexperienced operators.

Tyas and Beech (1985) compared all the properties of glass-ionomer cement with those of alternative materials and concluded that it remains the material of choice for Class V restorations.

Class III lesions

Glass-ionomer cement can be used in Class III restorations, but some years ago we considered that they would not be aesthetically satisfactory for extensive interproximal carious lesions (McLean and Wilson, 1977a). This restriction has been borne out by later research (Saito, 1979; Mount and Makinson, 1978). However, this view may need to be modified in view of the recent findings of Knibbs and his coworkers (1986a), who recently achieved acceptable aesthetic results in a 42-month trial—a success probably related to the use of one of a new generation of glass-ionomer cements having greater translucency and, hence, better aesthetics (see Table 7-4).

Indications are that the longevity of the glass-ionomer cement as a Class III restorative material is exceptional. Knibbs and his colleagues (1986a) reported a 5% loss in four years, a considerably lower failure rate than those reported by other workers for silicate cements and composite resins (see Table 7-4). Some loss by abrasion and some ditching was encountered by these workers. However, the wear of a glass-ionomer cement

116

proved to be more uniform than that of a composite resin over a two-year period, and its surface remained smoother and more uniform. Although a conservative cavity design was adopted and cavites were not deliberately undercut, only three of 332 restorations placed were lost—suggesting that the adhesion of the glass-ionomer cement alone is sufficient to ensure good retention. No recurrent caries was observed with any of the restorations.

Fissure sealing

Two of the earliest uses envisaged for glass-ionomer cement were fissure sealing and filling (McLean and Wilson, 1974, 1977a). Because the cement could adhere to untreated tooth material, it was thought that it would provide a perfect seal and by virtue of its fluoride-releasing property confer caries resistance on the surrounding tooth enamel. Since that time, these basic assumptions have been confirmed by clinical practice and laboratory experiment. So it is surprising that so little use has been made of glass-ionomer cement as a fissure sealant.

In the earliest days of glass-ionomer cements their use was restricted to fissures that were or had been opened up to more than 100 μm wide (McLean and Wilson, 1974). The treatment proved to be successful, for in a two-year trial 78% of the sealants were fully retained and another 8% partly retained. Most of the losses occurred in the first year. Secondary caries was only observed in those cases where the sealant was completely lost, and then not in all cases. Generally, anatomical form and marginal adaptation of fissure fillings were maintained.

Later, Williams and Winter (1976, 1981) carried out comparative trials on glass-ionomer cement and dimethacry-late resins. No attempt was made to select fissures that were patent, with orifices detectable with a sharp explorer, as recommended by McLean and Wilson (1974). Unfortunately, they also used a phosphoric acid etch throughout, which, while suitable—indeed, essential for successful use of a composite resin—is contraindicated for glass-ionomer cements. Not surprisingly, retention rates for the cement were low (21% after two years). However, they reported no difference in the incidence of caries between cement and composite resin, even though there was a much greater loss of cement restorations. Smales (1981) found 100% retention of glass-ionomer cements after one year but only 14% after two years, findings quite contrary to those of McLean and Wilson (1974). Recently Mount (1984) has reported glass-ionomer cement intact in the base of the fissure after six years.

Minimal cavity techniques

Glass-ionomer cements are well suited to minimal cavity preparation techniques because their adhesion to tooth material frees the clinician from having to shape cavities for mechanical retention. Some mechanical retention will, however, assist in retaining the filling. In high-stress-bearing areas mechanical retention is still advised.

The concept of minimal cavity preparation has undergone steady development over the years and the variety of applications has increased. The earliest of these techniques was to use glass-ionomer cement as a fissure filling, for the prepared fissure can be regarded as a Class I cavity formed by ultra-conservative preparation techniques without undercuts (McLean and Wilson,

1974). No loss of fissure fillings was reported during a two-year study and only 7% lost anatomical form. In no cases were there signs of erosion typical of the silicate and silicophosphate cements. Surface staining was observed in 50% of the restorations but this was of a minor nature. No cases of secondary caries were observed. Later studies have shown that surface roughness of the cement placed in Class I situations increases, with occlusal wear becoming apparent after three years, but without increase in susceptibility to recurrent caries (Saito, 1979; Smales, 1981).

In 1980, McLean described treatment of the early approximal lesion with glass-ionomer cement by use of a buccolingual and lateral marginal ridge approach to cavity preparation (McLean, 1980). Since then Knight (1984) has used a tunnel-like occlusal approach.

While the use of the glass-ionomer cement in conventionally prepared Class II situations is still not recommended (McLean and Wilson, 1977b; Fuks et al., 1984; McLean and Gasser, 1985), minimal cavity preparations have proved successful (Hunt, 1984; Knight, 1984). The carious Class II lesion occurs almost entirely within the body of the tooth, so that the conventional solution involves extensive destruction of sound tooth surface and demands a strong material like amalgam to withstand stresses on a large restoration; Hunt instead removes extensive underlying decay via tunnel-like preparations, and the overlying enamel remains largely intact. This approach is only made possible by the adhesive nature of the glass-ionomer cement, which effectively replaces the role of dentine and bonds the enamel "shell" together, preventing its fracture. The tooth enamel itself provides protection against wear. This technique has yet to be fully proven but it appears to be full of promise.

Deciduous teeth

McLean suggested some years ago that these materials are suitable for restoring deciduous teeth (McLean and Wilson, 1977a). In this application it is essential to avoid thin sections, shallow keyways, and narrow isthmuses (McLean and Wilson, 1977a; Council on Dental Materials and Devices, 1979; Saito, 1979).

Since then, several research workers have reported on the use of glass-ionomer cements in deciduous teeth. Some, such as Satio (1979), encountered difficulties because of the need to protect the cement from moisture, but fairly good results have been reported. In one trial, 75% of restorations were found to be intact after one year, and of these 90% had fair to good marginal adaptation, contour, and surface finish (Plant et al., 1977; Vliestra et al., 1978). Two cavity designs were employed: one without undercuts and with a chamfered margin for low-stress areas, and the other a conventional one. Both designs yielded similar clinical results.

A more recent trial using a new-generation glass-ionomer cement confirmed that the material was satisfactory for the restoration of deciduous teeth even when a matrix was not employed (Knibbs et al., 1986b). The clinical use of Ketac-Silver* has also been described by Croll and Phillips (1986), who recorded the improved wear resistance of the silver-cermet cement.

Luting cements

The first luting cement was developed at the Laboratory of the Government Chemist some years ago by grinding an exist-

*ESPE GmbH, Seefeld/Oberbay, West Germany, and Valley Stream, N.Y.

ing glass used for filling (G-200) down to a fine powder with a maximum particle size of 15 μm (Wilson et al., 1977). Reactivity was slowed down by reducing the powder/liquid ratio; indeed, all luting cements, with the exception of zinc oxide–eugenol cement, employ a low powder/liquid ratio. Little quantitative data is available, but they are at least the equal of other luting agents. They are as strong as silicophosphates and, once hardened, are the most erosion resistant of all cements (Reisbeck, 1981; McComb, 1982; McComb et al., 1984; McCabe, 1982; Mesu, 1982; Finger, 1983; Beech and Bandyopadhyay, 1983; Setchell et al., 1985). Further useful properties will be described under the clinical section dealing with luting cements.

Laminate restorations

We first described the use of a laminate restoration some years ago (McLean and Wilson, 1977a). In this technique the glass-ionomer was used as the "dentine" and a composite resin was laid over it as the "enamel." Although the glass-ionomer was bonded to the dentine, and the composite resin to the enamel (by acid etching), the bond at the glass-ionomer/composite resin interface relied on the retention provided by the surface roughening of the cement. More recently, the technique has been improved by acid etching the glass-ionomer cement and bonding the composite resin to it by micromechanical attachment (McLean et al., 1985; Sneed and Looper, 1985). The result is a laminate restoration with properties superior to both its components. It has the aesthetic appeal and toughness of the composite resin combined with the adhesive, sealing, and fluoride-release properties of the glass-ionomer cement.

The bond strength between the composite resin and the glass-ionomer ce-

ment is considerable and appears to be similar to the tensile strength of the cement. Figures ranging from 6 to 14 MPa have been reported (McLean et al., 1985; Sneed and Looper, 1985). To date no clinical trials have been reported, but the system appears to be very promising and avoids some of the problems of composite resin bonded to dentine with chemical coupling agents. However, an in vitro study by Gordon et al. (1985) indicates that some marginal leakage occurs at the glass-ionomer/dentine surface and is dependent on the particular composite resin/glass-ionomer cement combination used.

Secondary caries

Evidence is accumulating that restorations with glass-ionomer cements may be of considerable importance in preventing secondary caries from developing around restorations and primary caries from forming in surfaces adjacent to a restoration (Table 7-6). Indeed, it would seem that secondary caries is very rarely observed beneath a glass-ionomer restoration. By contrast, secondary caries forming under amalgams and composite resins is the primary reason these restorative materials need replacing (Mjör, 1985; Mjör and Leinfelder, 1985). These favourable clinical characteristics of the glass-ionomer cement are to be attributed to fluoride release and good adhesive and sealing properties. Recent studies have shown that initiation and progression of secondary caries may be reduced significantly when glass-ionomer cements are placed (Kidd, 1978; Hicks et al., 1986). Glass-ionomer cements not only provide protection against caries-like attack at the enamel/restoration interface, but they also significantly reduce lesions in the adjacent surface enamel.

Table 7-6 Secondary caries around glass-ionomer cement restorations

Investigators	Cavity	Cement	Period of study (years)	Fillings Remaining	Fillings Carious
McLean & Wilson (1977b)	Class V	ASPA*	3	90	0
Forsten (1979)	Class V	De Trey Aspa†	2–3	60	
Hunt (1984)	Tunnel	Ketac-Fil‡	2	20	
Brandau et al. (1984)	Class V	De Trey Aspa	4.5	76	0
Osborne & Berry (1986)	Class III	Chelon‡	1	24	
		Ketac-Fil	1	24	
Ngo et al. (1986)	Class III	Ketac-Fil	1	29	
	Class V	Ketac-Fil	1	74	
Mount (1986)	Class III	De Trey Aspa	2–7	26	0
		Fuji Ionomer V§	2–7	30	0
		Ketac-Fil	2–7	183	0
		De Trey Aspa	2–7	306	0
		Fuji Ionomer V	2–7	191	0
		Ketac-Fil	2–7	421	0
Knibbs et al. (1986b)	Class III	Chem-Fil¶	2	63	0
	Class V	Chem-Fil	2	73	1
Knibbs et al. (1986a)	Class III	Chem-Fil	4	232	0

*Laboratory of the Government Chemist, London.
†Amalgamated Dental Co., Weybridge, England.
‡ESPE GmbH, Seefeld/Oberbay, West Germany, and Valley Stream, N.Y.
§G-C International Corp., Tokyo, and Scottsdale, Ariz.
¶Dentsply International Inc., Weybridge, England, and York, Pa.

Colour stability and staining

A comprehensive clinical study on colour stability and staining was carried out by Knibbs et al. (1986b) using Chem-Fil* glass-ionomer cement. They encountered serious colour change in only a few percent of restorations during the 23- to 26-month period of the study (Table 7-7). Most restorations preserved their colour or showed only a slight deterioration. Thus, while glass-ionomer cement is not perfect in this respect, it is good enough and compares favourably with composite resins that frequently develop unsightly marginal staining and colour deterioration in service.

General clinical performance

The general clinical behaviour of the glass-ionomer cement in service is illustrated in Table 7-8. Although few restorations are lost, a significant number lose some surface contour, which is a precursor to failure. Development of surface roughness also has been observed (Charbeneau and Bozell, 1979). This is, perhaps, the most serious deficiency in service. Colour changes and discolouration are minor problems and the development of secondary caries is negligible.

*Dentsply International Inc., Weybridge, England, and York, Pa.

Table 7-7 Optical properties of glass-ionomer restorations after 23 to 26 months*

Optical property	Obvious or gross (%)	Slight (%)
Surface staining	1.0	7.0
Marginal staining	3.1	24.3
Colour mismatch	2.1	40.6
Opacity mismatch	1.0	37.1

*Based on data obtained from Knibbs et al. (1986b).

Table 7-8 General behaviour of glass-ionomer cements in the mouth

Investigators	Cavity	Cement	Period (years)	Loss (%)	Surface contour (%)	Colour change (%)	Marginal discolouration (%)	Caries (%)
McLean & Wilson (1977b)	Class V	ASPA*	3	9	10	6	4	0
Brandau et al. (1984)	Class V	Caulk Aspa†	4.5	10	20	12	9	0
Knibbs et al. (1986b)	Class III & V	Chem-Fil‡	2–2.5	1.4	29	2.1	3.9	1

*Laboratory of the Government Chemist, London.
†L.D. Caulk, Milford, Del.
‡Dentsply International Inc., Weybridge, England, and York, Pa.

References

Beech, D.R., and Bandyopadhyay, S. (1983) A new laboratory method for evaluating the relative solubility and erosion of dental cements. J. Oral. Rehabil. 10:57–63.

Billington, R. (1986) Personal communication.

Brandau, H.E., Ziemieki, T.L., and Charbeneau, G.T. (1984) Restoration of cervical contours on nonprepared teeth using glass-ionomer cement. A four and one half-year report. J. Am. Dent. Assoc. 104:782–783.

Brown, L.B. (1983) Clinical evaluation of glass ionomer retention. J. Dent. Res. 62(Special Issue):664 (abstr. 135).

Charbeneau, G.T., and Bozell, R.R. (1979) Clinical valuation of a glass ionomer cement for restoring of cervical erosion. J. Am. Dent. Assoc. 98:936–939.

Council on Materials and Devices, American Dental Association (1979) Status report on the glass ionomer cements. J. Am. Dent. Assoc. 99:221–226.

Crisp, S., Lewis, B.G., and Wilson, A.D. (1980) Characterisation of glass ionomer cements. 6. A study of erosion and water absorption in both neutral and acidic media. J. Dent. 8:68–74.

Croll, T.P., and Phillips, R.W. (1986) Glass ionomer–silver cermet restorations for primary teeth. Quintessence Int. 17:607–615.

Finger, W. (1983) Evaluation of glass ionomer luting cements. Scand. J. Dent. Res. 91:143–149.

Flynn, M. (1979) Clinical evaluation of Cervident and Aspa in restoring teeth with cervical abrasions. Oper. Dent. 4:118–120.

Forsten, L. (1977) Fluoride release from a glass ionomer cement. Scand. J. Dent. Res. 85:503–504.

Forsten, L. (1979) Personal communication.

Fuks, A.B., Shapira, J., and Bielak, S. (1984) Clinical evaluation of a glass-ionomer cement used as a Class II restorative material in primary molars. J. Pedodon. 8:393–399.

Gordon, M., Plasschaert, A.J.M., Soelberg, K.B., and Bogdan, M.S. (1985) Microleakage of four composite resins over a glass ionomer cement base in Class V restorations. Quintessence Int. 16:817–820.

Henschel, C.J. (1949) Observations concerning in vivo disintegration of silicate cement restorations. J. Dent. Res. 28:528.

Hicks, M.J., Flaitz, C.M., and Silverstone, L.M. (1986) Secondary caries formation in vitro around glass ionomer restorations. Quintessence Int. 17:527–532.

Hunt, P.R. (1984) A modified Class II cavity preparation for glass ionomer restorative materials. Quintessence Int. 15:1011–1018.

Kent, B.E., Lewis, B.G., and Wilson, A.D. (1973) The properties of a glass ionomer cement. Br. Dent. J. 135:322–326.

Kidd, E.A.M. (1978) Cavity sealing ability of composite and glass-ionomer restorations: An assessment in vitro. Br. Dent. J. 144:139–142.

Knibbs, P.J., Plant, C.G., and Pearson, G.J. (1986a) The use of a glass ionomer cement to restore Class III cavities. Rest. Dent. 2:42–48.

Knibbs, P.J., Plant, C.G., and Pearson, G.J. (1986b) A clinical assessment of an anhydrous glass-ionomer cement. Br. Dent. J. 161:99–103.

Knight, G.M. (1984) The use of adhesive materials in the conservative restoration of selected posterior teeth. Aust. Dent. J. 29:324–331.

Lawrence, L.G. (1979) Cervical glass ionomer restorations: A clinical study. J. Can. Dent. Assoc. 45:58, 59, 62.

Low, T. (1981) The treatment of hypersensitive cervical abrasion cavities using ASPA cement. J. Oral Rehabil. 8:81–89.

McCabe, J.F. (1982) Solubility tests for cements. J. Dent. Res. 61(Special Issue):335 (abstr. 1372).

McComb, D. (1982) Retention of castings with glass ionomer cements. J. Prosthet. Dent. 48: 285–288.

McComb, D., Sirisko, R., and Brown, J. (1984) Comparison of the physical properties of commercial glass ionomer luting cement. J. Can. Dent. Assoc. 50: 699–701.

McLean, J.W. (1980) Aesthetics in restorative dentistry: The challenge for the future. Br. Dent. J. 149:368–373.

McLean, J.W., and Gasser, O. (1985) Glass-cermet cements. Quintessence Int. 16:333–343.

McLean, J.W., and Wilson, A.D. (1974) Fissure sealing and filling with an adhesive glass-ionomer cement. Br. Dent. J. 136:269–276.

McLean, J.W., and Wilson, A.D. (1977a) The clinical development of the glass-ionomer cement. II. Some clinical applications. Aust. Dent. J. 22:120–127.

McLean, J.W., and Wilson, A.D. (1977b) The clinical development of the glass-ionomer cement. III. The erosion lesion. Aust. Dent. J. 22:190–195.

McLean, J.W., Powis, D.R., Prosser, H.J., and Wilson, A.D. (1985) The use of glass-ionomer cements in bonding composite resins to dentine. Br. Dent. J. 158: 410–414.

Matsuya, S., Matsuya, Y., Yamamato, Y., and Yamane, M. (1984) Erosion process of a glassionomer cement in organic acids. Dent. Mater. 3:210–219.

Mesu, F.P. (1982) Degradation of luting cements in vitro. J. Dent. Res. 61:665–672.

Mesu, F.P., and Reedijk, T. (1983) Degradation of luting cements measured in vitro and in vivo. J. Dent. Res. 62:1236–1240.

Mitchem, J.C., and Gronas, D.G. (1978) Clinical evaluation of cement solubility. J. Prosthet. Dent. 40: 453–456.

Mitchem, J.C., and Gronas, D.G. (1981) Continued evaluation of the clinical solubility of luting cements. J. Prosthet. Dent. 45:289–291.

Mjör, I.A. (1985) Frequency of secondary caries at various anatomical locations. Oper. Dent. 10:88–92.

Mjör, I.A., and Leinfelder, K.J. (1985) Operative dentistry. pp. 92–123 In I.A. Mjör (ed.) Dental Materials: Biological Properties and Clinical Evaluation. Boca Raton, Fla: CRC Press Inc.

Mount, G.J. (1984) Glass ionomer cements: Clinical considerations. chapt. 20A In J.W. Clark (ed.) Clinical Dentistry. Philadelphia: Harper & Row.

Mount, G.J. (1986) Longevity of glass ionomer cements. J. Prosthet. Dent. 55:682–685.

Mount, G.J., and Makinson, O.F. (1978) Clinical characteristics of a glass-ionomer cement. Br. Dent. J. 145: 67–71.

Mount, G.J., and Makinson, O.F. (1982) Glass-ionomer cements: Clinical implications of the setting reaction. Oper. Dent. 7:134–141.

Ngo, H., Earl, M.S.A., and Mount, G.J. (1986) Glass-ionomer cements: A 12-month evaluation. J. Prosthet. Dent. 55:203–205.

Öilo, G. (1984) Early erosion of dental cements. Scand. J. Dent. Res. 92:534–543.

Osborne, J.W., and Berry, T.G. (1986) Clinical assessment of glass ionomer cements as Class III restorations: A one-year report. Dent. Mater. 2:147–150.

Phillips, S., and Bishop, B.M. (1985) An in vitro study of the effect of moisture on glass ionomer cement. Quintessence Int. 16:175–177.

Plant, C.G., Shovelton, D.S., Vliestra, J.R., and Wartnaby, J.M. (1977) The use of a glass ionomer cement in deciduous teeth. Br. Dent. J. 143:271–274.

Pluim, L.J. (1985) The solubility of dental luting cements. Thesis, University of Groningen, Groningen, The Netherlands.

Pluim, L.J., and Arends, J. (1987) The relation between salivary properties and in vivo solubility of dental cements. Dent. Mater. 3:13–18.

Pluim, L.J., Arends, J., Havinga, P., Jongebloed, W.L., and Stokroos, I. (1984) Quantitative cement solubility experiments in vivo. J. Oral Rehabil. 11:171–179.

Reisbick, M.H. (1981) Working qualities of glass ionomer cements. J. Prosthet. Dent. 46:525–530.

Robinson, A.D. (1971) The life of a filling. Br. Dent. J. 130:206–208.

Roulet, J.-F., and Wälti, C. (1984) Influence of oral fluid on composite resin and glass-ionomer cement. J. Prosthet. Dent. 52:182–189.

Saito, S. (1979) Characteristics of glass ionomer and its clinical aplication. I. Relations between hardening reactions and water. Int. J. Dent. Mater. 8:1–16.

Setchell, D.J., Teo, C.K., and Kuhn, A.T. (1985) The relative solubilities of four modern glass-ionomer cements. Br. Dent. J. 158:220–222.

Sidler, P., and Strub, J.R. (1983) In vivo untersuchung der Löslichkeit und des Abdichtungsvermögens von drei Befestigungzementen. Dtsch. Zahnärztl. Z. 38: 564.

Smales, R.J. (1981) Clinical use of ASPA glass-ionomer cement. Br. Dent. J. 151:58–60.

Sneed, W.D., and Looper, S.W. (1985) Shear bond strength of a composite resin to an etched glass ionomer. Dent. Mater. 1:127–128.

Theuniers, G. (1984) Een onderzoek naar een duurzame afdichting door kroon- enbrugcementen. Thesis, University of Leuven, Leuven, The Netherlands.

Tyas, S. (1983) Clinical performance of adhesive restorative materials for cervical abrasion lesions. J. Dent. Res. 62(Special Issue):646(abstr. S12).

Tyas, M.J., and Beech, D.R. (1985) Clinical performance of three restorative materials for non-undercut cervical abrasion lesions. Aust. Dent. J. 30:260–264.

Vliestra, R.J., Plant, C.G., Shovelton, D.S., and Bradnock, G. (1978) The use of glass ionomer cement in deciduous teeth. Br. Dent. J. 145:164–166.

Walls, A.W.G., McCabe, J.F., and Murray, J.J. (1985) An erosion test for dental cements. J. Dent. Res. 64: 1100–1104.

Williams, B., and Winter G.B. (1976) Fissure sealants: A 2-year clinical trial. Br. Dent. J. 141:15–18.

Williams, B., and Winter, G.B. (1981) Fissure sealants: Further results at 4 years. Br. Dent. J. 150:183–187.

Wilson, A.D. (1976) Specification test for the solubility and disintegration of dental cements: A critical evaluation of its meaning. J. Dent. Res. 55:721–729.

Wilson, A.D., and Batchelor, R.F. (1968) Dental silicate cements: III. Environment and durability. J. Dent. Res. 47:115–120.

Wilson, A.D., Crisp, S., Lewis, B.G., and McLean, J.W. (1977) Experimental luting agents based on the glass-ionomer cements. Br. Dent. J. 142:117–122.

Wilson, A.D., Groffman, D.M., Powis, D.R., and Scott, R.P. (1986) An evaluation of the significance of the impinging jet method for measuring the acid erosion of dental cements. Biomaterials 7:55–60.

Chapter 8

Biocompatibility

The biocompatibility of glass-ionomer cements with living tissue is a subject of some importance, more so than for the traditional nonadhesive cements. Glass-ionomer cements have to be in direct contact with dentine because they were designed to adhere to tooth materials by molecular bonding. It follows that any intervening protective layer, such as a zinc oxide–eugenol or calcium hydroxide cement, will interfere with this adhesion. Fortunately, clinical experience has shown that the adverse effects of glass-ionomer cement on living tissues are minor, so that protective liners are rarely required. Perhaps the most serious problem that arises is the occasional sensitivity encountered with certain luting agents.

The glass-ionomer cements are therapeutic materials. Their adhesion to tooth material ensures that they provide an excellent and enduring marginal seal, thus eliminating secondary caries, while the sustained release of fluoride confers resistance to caries on adjacent tooth material. Hicks and coworkers (1986) indicated that such beneficial effects are to be expected. The positive effect the material has when used as a bone cement on promoting bone growth has prompted Jonck (1986) to remark that these materials are not only biocompatible but bioactive.

Effects on pulp and cells

We do not propose to review all the literature on the biocompatibility of glass-ionomer cements. The literature on this subject is large and often contradictory. The effect of the cement on cells is one example. Whereas both Dahl and Tronstad (1976) and Meryon and coworkers (1983) found that freshly mixed glass-ionomer cements were cytotoxic, Kawahara and his coworkers (1979) reported that, although the freshly mixed cement inhibited cellular proliferation, it was not cytotoxic. All of these authors found that the set cement had no effect upon cell cultures.

While the effects of the cement on cells and small animals is of scientific interest, studies that have recently appeared on the pulpal response in human subjects are the most relevant for the clinician (Tobias et al., 1978; Cooper, 1980; Plant et al., 1984). Research workers found that glass-ionomer cement causes greater inflammatory response than zinc oxide–eugenol cement, but less (according to Plant et al., 1984) than zinc phosphate cement and the related dental silicate cement (Tobias, 1978; Kawahara et al., 1979; Pameijer et al., 1981). The inflammatory response of pulpal tissues toward glass-ionomer cement resolves within 30 days and there is no enhancement of reparative or secondary dentine formation.

The response of gingival tissues towards the cement in Class V cavities is minimal (Garcia et al., 1981).

The possible reasons for the blandness of poly(acrylic acid) were given by McLean and Wilson as long ago as 1974. They may be expanded upon:

1. Poly(acrylic acid) is a weak acid.
2. Even dissociated H^+ ions are constrained to remain in the neighbourhood of the polyanion chain because of electrostatic attraction arising from a multiplicity of negative charges.
3. When partly neutralized, the tendency of poly(acrylic acid) to dissociate into hydrogen and polyacrylate ions is reduced because of the increase in the negative charge on the chain. In effect, it becomes a weaker acid.
4. Diffusion of the polyacid, with its train of associated H^+ ions down the dentinal tubules, is unlikely because of its high molecular weight and chain entanglement.
5. Poly(acrylic acid) will be readily precipitated by calcium ions in the tubules. Thus, the thinnest layer of dentine should be sufficient to bind poly(acrylic acid) as insoluble salts.

McLean and Wilson (1977b) also cautioned against the use of citric acid in sensitive dentine areas where tubules have been opened, a view that has apparently been unheeded for it is still echoed today. Tobias and his coworkers (1978) and Cotton and Siegel (1978), indeed, found greater inflammatory response when citric acid was used as a cleansing agent on cut dentinal tubules. The use of less reactive agents, which do not remove the smear layer and open dentinal tubules, is therefore advisable (see chapter 6). These agents are referred to as *surface conditioners*.

Reports of sensitivity under glass-ionomer luting cements can no longer be regarded as anecdotal; possible causes will be discussed in a section dealing with luting cements. Most probably, this phenomenon is related to faulty technique rather than to the chemistry of the cement.

Although the glass-ionomer cements cannot be regarded as totally bland materials, current pulp studies confirm the view of McLean and Wilson (1977a, 1977b) some ten years ago: linings of zinc oxide–eugenol or calcium hydroxide cement are only required where less than 1 mm of sound dentine remains over the pulp. These linings should be used sparingly to avoid the reduction of bonding sites, which would occur if large areas of peripheral dentine were overlaid.

Fluoride release

Glass-ionomer cement has a cariostatic effect. The spread of caries is arrested at the restoration/cavity wall margin. Protection is conferred on the enamel of the crown for some distance from the restoration. The influence of fluoride is found in a zone of resistance to demineralization which is at least 3 mm thick around a glass-ionomer restoration (Kidd, 1978; Hicks et al., 1986; Hötz, 1979; Wesenberg and Hals, 1980). This favourable result has been attributed to the release of fluoride from the cement and its movement into adjacent enamel.

Fluorine is the first member of the halogens and differs considerably from other members of the group. The fluoride ion forms strong complexes with a number of metal ions, and hydrogen bonds to it are the strongest known. Not surprisingly, the fluoride ion exerts a powerful

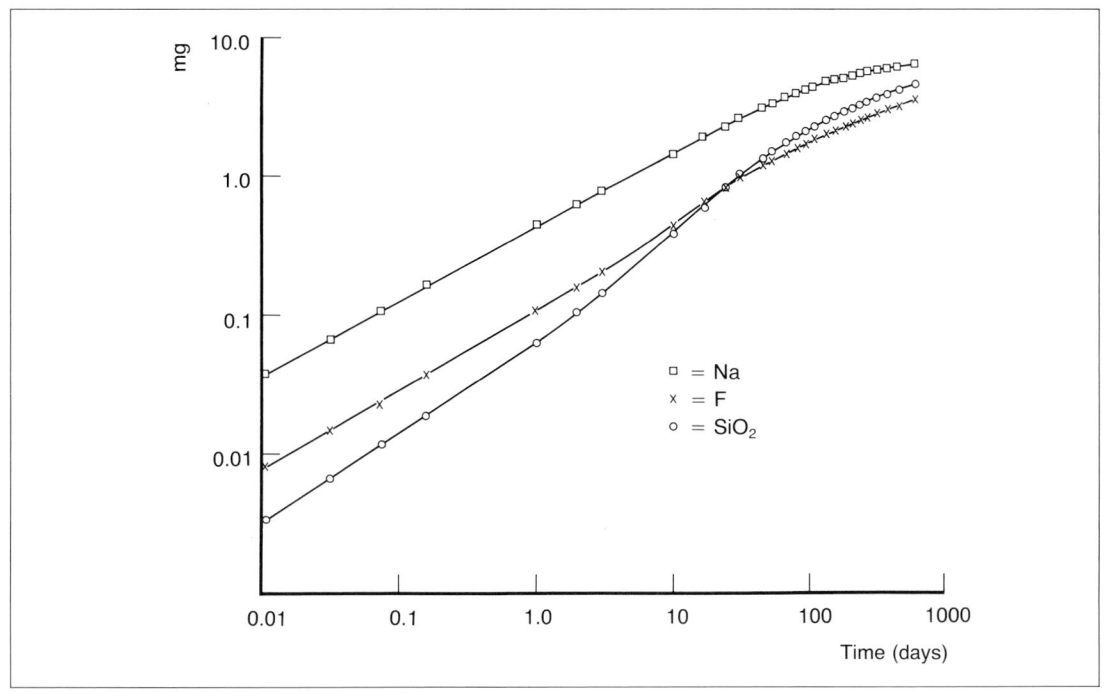

Fig. 8-1 The release of fluoride and sodium from a glass-ionomer cement. Reprinted with permission from Wilson et al. (1985).

effect on chemical and biological processes. The ionic radius of the fluoride ion (1.36 Å) is similar to that of the hydroxyl ion (1.40 Å), and this has important consequences because the fluoride ion can replace the hydroxyl ion in the apatite lattice.

Fluoride released from a restorative material has a clinical importance, for fluoride has long been known to have a caries-preventive effect (Dean et al., 1942; Bibby, 1942; Horowitz, 1973).

The action of fluoride in preventing caries is complex and imperfectly understood. Several explanations have been advanced (e.g., Smith and Peltoniemi, 1982). The anti-caries effect has been attributed to the uptake of fluoride by enamel apatite at hydroxyl sites, and high fluoride levels at the enamel surfaces do appear to increase resistance to plaque acids (Brundevold et al., 1967; McLundie and Murray, 1972; Muhler, 1956; Moreno et al., 1977). Also, the surface energy of apatite is reduced, making it more difficult for dental plaque to adhere to tooth enamel surfaces (Glantz, 1969). And, almost certainly, fluoride aids the remineralization of damaged enamel (Silverstone, 1978).

There is another kind of explanation. Fluoride effects changes in the composition of the bacterial plaque and plaque biochemistry and may exert its effect by altering the carbohydrate metabolism of dental plaque (Horowitz et al., 1977; Silverstone, 1978; Mellberg, 1977; Ingram and Nash, 1980; Capozzi et al., 1967; Cimasoni, 1972; Norman et al., 1972). These mechanisms are not mutually exclusive—more than one is almost certainly implicated.

Fluoride is released from glass-ionomer cements for a sustained period of time—at least 18 months, according to Wilson and coworkers (1985). The pattern of release is depicted in Fig. 8-1. There is a considerable body of work to support this conclusion of Wilson and his coworkers (Crisp et al., 1976; Forsten, 1977; Maldonado et al., 1978; Causton, 1981; Swartz et al., 1984; Shimokobe et al., 1987). The fluoride originates from that used in preparing the aluminosilicate glasses, which can contain up to 23% fluoride (Kent et al., 1979). Thickly mixed cements used for restorations release more fluoride than thinly mixed ones used for luting because they contain proportionately more glasses, and, hence, more fluoride (Meryon and Smith, 1984).

Not all the fluoride is available for release (Causton, 1981). In the case of a glass-ionomer cement examined by Wilson and coworkers (1985), the fluoride was found to be released as sodium fluoride. More recent work has shown that some calcium, too, is released with fluoride (Powis and Wilson, 1987). So it would seem that fluoride release is restricted by the sodium and, to some extent, the calcium content of the glass, and not by the total fluoride content of the glass. This conclusion may explain the observation of Meryon and Smith (1984), who found that the fluoride released bears no relationship to the fluoride content of the glass. Not unexpectedly, sodium fluoride tends to be preferentially released from the matrix rather than the filler (Matsuya et al., 1984).

The mechanism of fluoride release is complex, but it is dominated by a diffusion mechanism where the rate of release is proportional to the inverse of the square root of time (Wilson et al., 1985; Kuhn and Wilson, 1985). Substantial amounts of fluoride are taken up by enamel, dentine, and cementum in cavity walls adjacent to the cement and become resistant to acid attack (Maldonado et al., 1978; Wesenberg and Hals, 1980; Retief et al., 1984; Shimokobe et al., 1987).

Fluoride, as we have seen, is leached mainly as the sodium salt, which is not a matrix-forming species. Thus, the cement is not weakened by the loss of fluoride; indeed, the cement increases in strength as it ages.

Thornton and his coworkers (1986) found that the pattern of fluoride release for a cermet-ionomer cement differs from that of its conventional parent. Thus, there is an initial washout of fluoride from Ketac-Fil* that is not found in Ketac-Silver.* After a few days the rates of release from both cements were similar. The clinical implications of these findings is uncertain. Possibly, this is a surface effect and the burnished silver particles in the cermet cement form a barrier that curtails initial fluoride release.

Fluoride is not the only ion to be released from aluminosilicate cements. Aluminium ions are released for a short period and can be absorbed by tooth enamel, conferring acid-resistance upon it (Halse and Hals, 1976; Putt and Kleber, 1985). However, it must be emphasized that this is only a temporary phenomenon—release of aluminium ceases once the cement has fully hardened.

*ESPE GmbH, Seefeld/Oberbay, West Germany, and Valley Stream, N.Y.

References

Bibby, B.G. (1942) Preliminary report on the use of sodium fluoride applications in caries prophylaxis. J. Dent. Res. 21:314.

Brundevold, F., McCann, H.G., Nilsson, R., Richardson, B., and Coklica, V. (1967) The chemistry of caries inhibiting problems and challenges in topical treatments. J. Dent. Res. 46:37–45.

Capozzi, L., Brunetti, P., Negri, P.L., and Migliorini, E. (1967) Enzymatic mechanism of action of some fluoride compounds. Caries Res. 1:69–77.

Causton, B.E. (1981) The physico-mechanical consequences of exposing glass ionomer cements to water during setting. Biomaterials 2:112–115.

Cimasoni, G. (1972) The inhibition of enolase by fluoride in vitro. Caries Res. 6:93–102.

Cooper, I.R. (1980) The response of the human dental pulp to glass ionomer cements. Int. Endod. J. 13:76–88.

Cotton, W.R., and Siegal, R.L. (1978) Human pulpal response to citric acid cavity cleanser. J. Am. Dent. Assoc. 96:639–644.

Crisp, S., Lewis, B.G., and Wilson, A.D. (1976) Glass-ionomer cements: Chemistry of erosion. J. Dent. Res. 55:1032–1041.

Dahl, B.L., and Tronstad, L. (1976) Biological tests of an experimental glass ionomer (silicopolyacrylate) cement. J. Oral Rehabil. 3:19–24.

Dean, H.T., Arnold, F.A., and Elvove, E. (1942) Domestic water and dental caries. Public Health Rep. 57: 1155–1181.

Forsten, L. (1977) Fluoride release from a glass ionomer cement. Scand. J. Dent. Res. 85:503–504.

Garcia, R., Caffesse, R.G., and Charbeneau, G.T. (1981) Gingival tissue response to restoration of deficient cervical contours using a glass-ionomer material: A 12-month report. J. Prosthet. Dent. 46:393–398.

Glantz, P.-O. (1969) On wettability and adhesiveness. Odontol. Revy. 20(suppl. 17).

Halse, A., and Hals, E. (1976) Electron probe microanalysis of secondary caries lesions adjacent to silicate fillings. Calcif. Tissue Res. 21:183–193.

Hicks, M.J., Flaitz, C.M., and Silverstone, L.M. (1986). Secondary caries formations in vitro around glass ionomer restorations. Quintessence Int. 17:527–532.

Horowitz, H.S. (1973) A review of systemic and topical fluorides for the prevention of dental caries. Community Dent. Oral Epidemiol. 1:104–114.

Horowitz, H.S., Heifetz, S.B., Myers, R.J., Driscoll, W.S., and Korts, D.C. (1977) Evaluation of a combination of self-administered fluoride procedures for control of dental caries in a non-fluoride area: Findings after two years. Caries Res. 11:178–185.

Hötz, P.R. (1979) Experimental secondary caries around amalgam, composite and glass ionomer cement filling in human teeth. Helv. Odont. Acta 23:9–39.

Ingram, G.S., and Nash, P.F. (1980) A mechanism for the anti-caries action of fluoride. Caries Res. 14:298–303.

Jonck, L.M. (1986) Personal communication.

Kawahara, H., Imanishi Y., and Tomioka, K. (1977) Dental applications of a glass ionomer cement. Dent. Outlook 50:623–633.

Kawahara, H., Imanshi, Y., and Oshima, H. (1979) Biological evaluation of glass-ionomer cements. J. Dent. Res. 58:1080–1086.

Kent, B.E., Lewis, B.G., and Wilson, A.D. (1979) Glass ionomer formulations: I. The preparation of novel fluoroaluminosilicate glasses high in fluorine. J. Dent. Res. 58:1607–1619.

Kidd, E.A.M. (1978) Cavity sealing ability of composite and glass ionomer restorations: An assessment in vitro. Br. Dent. J. 144:139–142.

Kuhn, A.T., and Wilson, A.D. (1985) The dissolution mechanisms of silicate and glass-ionomer dental cements. Biomaterials 6:378–382.

McLean, J.W., and Wilson, A.D. (1974) Fissure sealing and filling with an adhesive glass ionomer cement. Br. Dent. J. 136:269–276.

McLean, J.W., and Wilson, A.D. (1977a) The clinical development of the glass-ionomer cement. II. Some clinical applications. Aust. Dent. J. 22:120–127.

McLean, J.W., and Wilson, A.D. (1977b) The clinical development of the glass-ionomer cement. III. The erosion lesion. Aust. Dent. J. 22:190–195.

McLundie, A.C., and Murray, F.D. (1972) Silicate cements and composite resins—A scanning electron microscopic study. J. Prosthet. Dent. 27:544–551.

Maldonado, A., Swartz, M.L., and Phillips, R.W. (1978) An in vitro study of certain properties of a glass ionomer cement. J. Am. Dent. Assoc. 96:785–792.

Matsuya, S., Matsuya, Y., Yamamato, Y., and Yamane, M. (1984) Erosion process of a glass ionomer cement in organic acids. Dent. Mater. 3:210–219.

Mellberg, J.R. (1977) Enamel fluoride and its anti-caries effects. J. Prev. Dent. 4:8–20.

Meryon, S.D., and Smith, A.J. (1984) A comparison of fluoride release from three glass ionomer cements and a polycarboxylate cement. Int. Endod. J. 17:16–24.

Meryon, S.D., Stephens, P.G., and Browne, R.M. (1983) A comparison of the in vitro cytotoxicity of two glass-ionomer cements. J. Dent. Res. 62:769–773.

Moreno, E.C., Kresak, M., and Zahradnick, R.T. (1977) Physicochemical aspects of fluoride apatite systems relevant to the study of dental caries. Caries Res. 11: (suppl. 1) 142–171.

Muhler, J.C. (1956) Effects of fluorides and other solutions on solubility of powdered enamel in acid. Proc. Soc. Exp. Biol. Med. 92:849–851.

Norman, R.D., Mehra, R.V., Swartz, M.L., and Phillips, R.W. (1972) Effects of restorative materials on plaque composition. J. Dent. Res. 51:1596–1601.

Pameijer, C.H., Segal, E., and Richardson, J. (1981) Pulpal response to a glass ionomer cement in primates. J. Prosthet. Dent. 46:36–40.

Plant, C.G., Browne, R.M., Knibbs, P.J., Britton, A.S., and Sorhan, T. (1984) Pulpal effects of glass ionomer cements. Int. Endod. J. 17:51–59

Powis, D.R., and Wilson, A.D. (1987) Unpublished data.

Putt, M.S., and Kleber, C.J. (1985) Dissolution studies of human enamel treated with aluminium solutions. J. Dent. Res. 64:437–440.

Retief, D.H., Bradley, E.L., Denton, J.C., and Switzer, P. (1984) Enamel and cementum fluoride uptake from a glass ionomer cement. Caries Res. 18:250–257.

Shimokobe, H., Komatsu, H., and Matsui, I. (1982) Fluoride content in human enamel after removal of the applied glass ionomer cement. J. Dent. Res. 66(Special Issue):131 (abstr. 196).

Silverstone, L.M. (1978) Preventive Dentistry. Fort Lee, N.J.: Update Books.

Smith, D.C., and Peltomiemi, A. (1982) chapt. 8 In D.C. Smith and D.F. Williams (ed.) Biocompatibility of Dental Materials. Vol I. Characteristics of Dental Tissues and Their Response to Dental Materials. Boca Raton, Fla: CRC Press Inc.

Swartz, M.L., Phillips, R.W., and Clark, H.E. (1984) Long-term F release from glass ionomer cements. J. Dent. Res. 63:158–160.

Thornton, J.B., Retief, D.H., and Bradley, E.L. (1986) Fluoride release from and tensile bond strength of Ketac-Fil and Ketac-Silver to enamel and dentin. Dent. Mater. 2:241–245.

Tobias, R.S., Browne, R.M., Plant, C.G., and Ingram, D.V. (1978) Pulpal responses to a glass ionomer cement. Br. Dent. J. 144:345–350.

Wesenberg, G., and Hals, E. (1980) The in vitro effect of a glass ionomer cement on dentine and enamel walls. J. Oral Rehabil. 7:35–42.

Wilson, A.D., Groffman, D.R., and Kuhn, A.T. (1985) The release of fluoride and other chemical species from a glass-ionomer cement. Biomaterials 6:431–433.

Chapter 9

Clinical Uses

The clinical development and use of glass-ionomer cements was first described by McLean and Wilson (1977a, 1977b, 1977c) in the 1970s. Certain properties, such as their hydrophilic nature, adhesion to tooth structure, and ability to release fluoride ions, made them very attractive materials as "preventive restorations" or for lining and luting purposes. With the passage of time their use has been expanded and the glass-ionomer cements are now recognized as playing a major role in restorative dentistry.

Indications for use

Restorative materials

1. Restoration of erosion/abrasion lesions without cavity preparation
2. Sealing and filling of occlusal pits and fissures
3. Restoration of deciduous teeth
4. Restoration of Class V carious lesions
5. Restoration of Class III carious lesions, preferably using a lingual approach
6. Repair of defective margins in restorations
7. Minimal cavity preparations; approximal lesions buccal and occlusal approach (tunnel preparations)
8. Core buildup
9. Provisional restorations where future veneer crowns are contemplated
10. Sealing of root surfaces for overdentures

Fast-setting lining cement and bases

1. Lining of all types of cavities where a biological seal and cariostatic action are required
2. Replacement of carious dentine for the attachment of composite resins using the acid-etch technique
3. Sealing and filling of occlusal fissures showing early signs of caries

Luting cements

Fine-grain versions of the glass-ionomer cement are now available for luting purposes. Because of their fluoride leach, these cements are particularly useful in patients with high caries incidence. In addition, the translucency of the glass-ionomer cement is of great value where porcelain margins are used for cosmetic reasons.

Contraindications for use

In their present stage of development, glass-ionomer cements are brittle materials with a low tensile strength and therefore must be used in bulk and in low-stress-bearing cavity preparations. They also have insufficient translucency and lack polishability, thus making them less suitable than composite resins for restoring large areas of labial enamel. They are not recommended for the following restorative applications:

1. Class IV carious lesions or fractured incisors
2. Lesions involving large areas of labial enamel where aesthetics is of major importance
3. Class II carious lesions where conventional cavities are prepared; replacement of existing amalgam restorations
4. Lost cusp areas

Clinical procedures for placement

Clinical procedures for placing glass-ionomer cements have been given by a number of authors and have been well summarized by Mount (Mount and Makinson, 1978; 1982; Mount, 1984):

1. Select the appropriate shade of cement.
2. Isolate the tooth with a rubber dam where there is any risk of gingival seepage or bleeding.
3. Prepare the cavity:
   (a) Erosion-abrasion lesion: clean only.
   (b) Carious lesion: conventional instrumentation to remove caries and provide some mechnical retention.
4. Where there is less than 0.5 mm of remaining dentine, line the cavity with a setting calcium hydroxide.
5. Apply a surface conditioner to the cavity to remove the smear layer and improve adhesion.
6. Dispense the cement on a refrigerated glass slab and mix quickly: 30 seconds for hand mixing, ten seconds for machine mixing.
7. Wash and lightly dry the cavity. Do not dehydrate the dentine because this will tend to reduce wettability. Insert the cement, preferably using a syringe.
8. Place a matrix wherever possible.
9. Allow to set for the recommended manufacturer's setting time, which is generally at least four minutes from start of mix.
10. Remove the matrix and immediately apply a waterproof varnish or light-cured bonding agent. *Do not delay application of varnish* since this is the most critical point in the procedure.
11. Using magnification, trim any excess material *external* to the cavity with sharp scalpel blades or excavators. If the matrix has been correctly applied it is possible to achieve a very accurate marginal adaptation. Do not use rotary instruments at this stage of setting.
12. Reapply varnish or light-cured bonding agent.
13. If the marginal adaptation is good the final polishing of the restoration should be delayed until the patient's next visit. Alternatively, the modern fast-setting glass-ionomers may be finished within ten to 15 minutes.
14. Reapply varnish or bonding agent after polishing.

In the remaining chapters of this book the clinical use of glass-ionomer cement will be described. It is appropriate that its most valuable use as an adhesive restorative in the Class V restoration be given first (see chapter 10).

The various brands of materials will be described under the following classification:

Type I: Luting cements
Type II: Restorative materials
    (a) aesthetic
    (b) reinforced
Type III: Fast-setting lining materials and fissure sealants

The types and brands of materials with their physical and mechanical properties are given in Tables 4-1 and 4-2.

Questions often arise with regard to the clinical use of glass-ionomer cements. The most common are the following:

• What are the best methods for dispensing and mixing the cement?
• What is the effect of early water contamination and what is the best method of protecting the surface during early setting?
• How can the clinician optimize translucency?
• Does the cement shrink on setting and does it leak?
• What are the best methods of selecting shades?
• When fluoride is leached from the cement, does it weaken the structure?
• How do we maximize adhesion?
• What are the best finishing techniques?

Although many of the answers to the above questions have already been covered in this text, it will, at this stage, help to clarify the reader's thoughts if each question is answered briefly. A fuller understanding of the chemical and clinical problems in handling glass-ionomer cements may then be achieved prior to describing detailed clinical procedures.

Dispensing and mixing techniques

In all dental cements manipulation time is at a premium and, if there are no disadvantages, any dental cement should be mixed as rapidly as possible in order to gain working time. However, traditional dental cements generate too much heat to be mixed rapidly, and in order to dissipate heat on the mixing block the powder is introduced into the liquid progressively.

Little heat is generated when a glass-ionomer cement is mixed, and the low exotherm means that all the powder can be incorporated into the liquid at the same time. Mixing must not be hurried excessively, however, because it is important that the paste be thoroughly mixed.

Other points of mixing need to be noted. For restorations the rule still holds: mix the paste as thickly as possible. Judgement here is difficult when mixing a cement with the highest possible powder content—it appears at one stage as if the mix is too dry and a paste is not going to form. However, a rheological change occurs at this stage and the mix suddenly forms a smooth paste. A careful check on the manufacturer's recommended powder/liquid ratio should be made to avoid adding too little powder.

Devices to ensure correct proportions are not easy to devise. The liquid can be precisely measured using a microsyringe (Fig. 9-1), but the powder is not as easy

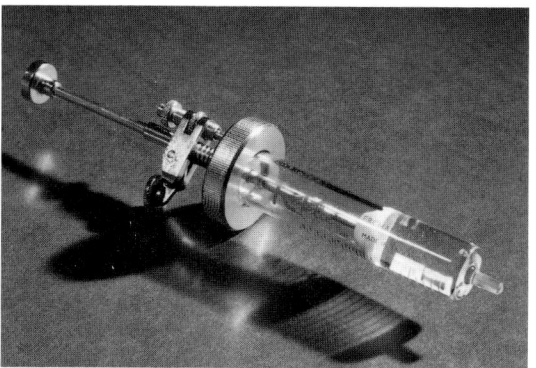

Fig. 9-1 Microsyringe for dispensing liquid.

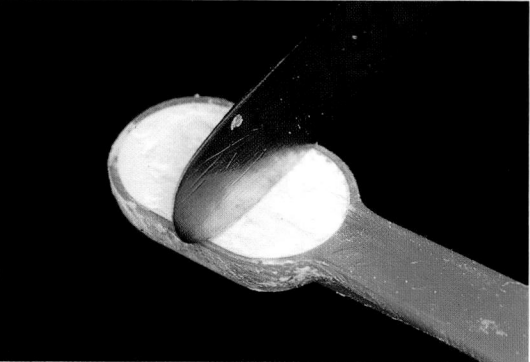

Fig. 9-2 Powder leveled with spatula in the measuring spoon.

Table 9-1 Variations in the mass of powder when using measuring sticks*

Material	Recommended ratio	Measured ratio
Chem-Fil†	6.8:1.0	6.64:1.0
Fuji Ionomer II‡	2.2:1.0	2.38:1.0
Shofu Hy-Bond Restorative§	2.5:1.0	2.60:1.0

*Based on Mount (1984).
†Dentsply International Inc., Weybridge, England, and York, Pa.
‡G-C International Corp., Tokyo, and Scottsdale, Ariz.
§Shofu Dental Corp., Kyoto, Japan, and Menlo Park, Calif.

Table 9-2 Setting times (mins) at different temperatures*

Material	Temperature of slab	
	21.5°C	37.0°C
Chem-Fil†	6.30	3.40
Fuji Ionomer II‡	6.31	3.45
Ketac-Fil§	6.00	3.00
Shofu Hy-Bond Restorative¶	4.45	2.35

*Based on Mount (1984).
†Dentsply International Inc., Weybridge, England, and York, Pa.
‡G-C International Corp., Tokyo, and Scottsdale, Ariz.
§ESPE GmbH, Seefeld/Oberbay, West Germany, and Valley Stream, N.Y.
¶Shofu Dental Corp., Kyoto, Japan, and Menlo Park, Calif.

to measure because of variations in packing densities (Mount, 1984; Table 9-1). As yet, no simple method has been devised except for weighing the powder and dispensing it in sachets or capsules.

When hand mixing a glass-ionomer cement, the dispensation of both powder and liquid is critical. Where a measuring spoon or stick is applied the scoop should be firmly filled but not deliberately compacted. Level the powder with a spatula and make sure that the spoon or stick is completely filled (Fig. 9-2).

Where polyacid liquids are supplied, the bottle should be held horizontally until all air has escaped from the nozzle; it may then be inverted and the correct dosage delivered. High-viscosity liquids may easily gel at the nozzle entrance, so cleanliness is vital—carefully wipe the nozzle after each use. When distilled water or tartaric acid solution are supplied for use with freeze-dried polyacid powder, dispensation is easier providing the bottle is held vertically. To avoid risk of overdosage a calibrated laboratory microsyringe is the delivery system of choice (see Fig. 9-1).

Mixing on a chilled slab can significantly prolong working and setting time (Mount, 1984; Table 9-2). The use of old-fashioned thick glass slabs is recommended because they do not heat up quickly and moisture condensation can be observed. Hand-mixing should be carried out rapidly, as explained above; the main object is to wet out all the powder particles as quickly as possible. Stainless steel, plastic, or agate spatulas should be used. For fast mixing, stainless steel is best. By dividing the powder into two or three parts, according to the size of the mix, it is possible to complete mixing within 20 to 30 seconds. However, make certain that a smooth plastic paste is produced by spreading the mix across the slab and then regathering it. This method also reduces entrapped porosity.

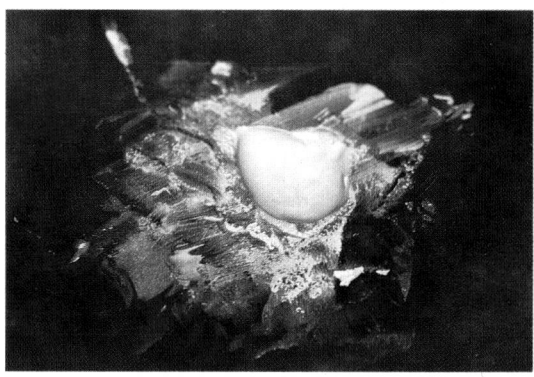

Fig. 9-3 Ideal mix of cement should be a stiff paste that has retained its gloss.

A word of warning about using a chilled slab is appropriate. The danger of condensation of water vapour is real on a hot and humid summer's day and will give rise to a weak cement. When a glass slab, rather than a plastic pad, is used for mixing this condensation can be seen and is a signal that a film of moisture will condense on the powder. Chilled glass slabs should not be used under such atmospheric conditions. These problems do not arise when air-conditioning is available.

A further note of warning should be made on the dangers of using too dry a mix. Good adhesion of glass-ionomer cements is very dependent on sufficient wetting of the tooth structure, which can only be achieved if the cement is glossy and provides free surface polyacid for ion-displacement at the enamel/dentine interface. Dehydration of the dentine may also be detrimental.

The ideal hand-mixed cement should be a stiff paste that has retained its gloss and packing consistency (Fig. 9-3). When hand mixing cements for use in syringes, or when using fast-setting lining cements, a slightly lower powder/liquid ratio may be needed to achieve sufficient

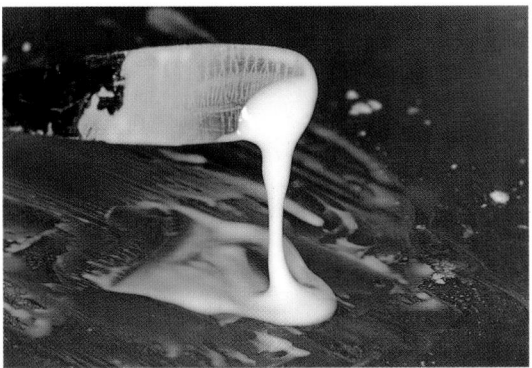

Fig. 9-4 Fast-setting lining cements may be applied as a more fluid mix. Thinner mixes are also needed when syringes are used.

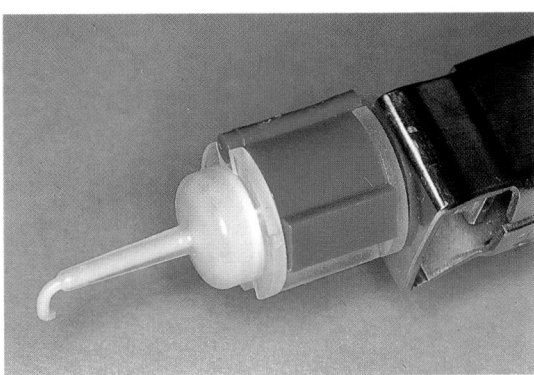

Fig. 9-5 Capsulated cement ejected through applicator.

fluidity (Fig. 9-4). However, such a mix will always be weaker; it is for this reason that capsulated cements are preferable when syringe techniques are being used.

Capsulated mixing

Capsulated mixing is highly recommended. It is well worth using such materials despite their expense. All of the mixing problems outlined above are eliminated, since the manufacturer has accurately dispensed both powder and liquid, which allows the clinician to avoid the difficulty of judging the proper consistency of the mix (Fig. 9-5). There are no problems of moisture condensation, and mixing is thorough and extremely rapid, ensuring maximum manipulation time. The clinician is assured of a uniform and correctly mixed paste with a high powder/liquid ratio giving optimum mechanical strength and water resistance.

Early water contamination and protection

Although the glass-ionomer cement when fully hardened is impervious to oral fluids, it is vulnerable to moisture while setting and hardening. This vulnerability occurs while cement-forming ions (Ca^{2+}, Al^{3+}) from the glass are being transferred to the polyacid, where ultimately they are locked up in a resistant gel.

If water comes into contact with this surface before it has hardened, the cement-forming ions calcium and aluminium will be washed out and lost. The damage is permanent. Water will be absorbed, the cement will lose its translucency, and the weakened surface will erode. To prevent this from occurring, the clinician must take steps to protect the freshly placed restoration against oral fluids. Where a dry field cannot be obtained, for example with cotton rolls and gingival packing cord, then a rubber dam should be used. However, a rubber dam can create conditions that dehydrate the cement, resulting in loss of water needed for cement formation (see "Chemistry of the setting reaction" in chapter 3).

For the above reasons it is vital not to lose water needed for hydration, but at the same time not to allow ingress of excess water which could wash out the vital cement-forming ions. In simple terms, there is a critical water balance at the interface between water needed for cement formation and excess water absorbed from saliva. One way of preventing dehydration of the cement under the rubber dam is to apply a varnish or bonding resin immediately after removal of the matrix. To apply a protective coating under moist conditions is of dubious value—analogous to painting a house when it is raining—so that surface water contamination from gingival seepage prior to final set is a disaster for glass-ionomer cements.

Earl and coworkers (1985) have done a considerable amount of work on the effect of varnishes on water movement across glass-ionomer cement surfaces and concluded that:

1. Varnishes recommended by the manufacturers to protect glass-ionomer cement are reasonably effective, but some proprietary varnishes that were not developed especially for this purpose are ineffective.
2. Light-curing bonding resins of very low viscosity, and giving low contact angles on the cement, are the most effective in reducing water outflow from glass-ionomer cement for the first hour of setting reaction.
3. Chemically activated bonding resins do not control water outflow to a significant degree.

It may be said that there is no protective coating material that is entirely satisfactory. Ideally, a water-based emulsion would seem to be the most appropriate material, but no suitable ones are available. Wax or petroleum jelly only afford brief protection because they are easily washed off.

At present the most effective materials for protecting glass-ionomer cements are low-viscosity, light-curing bonding agents and proprietary varnishes specially prepared for sealing glass-ionomer cements.

Translucency

Translucency is largely controlled by the manufacturer, and if the glass is formulated correctly the modern glass-ionomer cement has good aesthetics. Type II restorative cements are the most translucent, as will be described later. The clinician should try to preserve the inherent translucency in these cements by not infringing basic rules of technique. Dry mixes will appear more opaque because of increased porosity. Removing the matrix too early will cause rapid loss of translucency if the freshly set surface is damaged by moisture. Translucency will be preserved if the surface is protected during set by varnishes or light-cured bonding resins. Accurate proportioning of the powder and liquid will also ensure a mix which produces both optimum strength and optimum translucency. For this reason, capsulated materials will always leave less room for error unless the clinician is conversant with all of the clinical requirements for hand mixing.

One of the reasons for the limited use of glass-ionomer cements for anterior restorations in the past has been its rather poor colour match to enamel, arising from poor translucency. The darker shades, too, are more opaque than the lighter ones because they reflect less light (Crisp et al., 1979; Asmussen, 1983). However, their colour stability has always been good, so that modern glass-ionomer cements have arrived with such considerably improved transluency and colour match that they are often the material of choice for Class III and Class V restorations.

Shade selection

The translucency of a glass-ionomer cement does not reach its maximum for about a day after insertion. This increase in translucency means that reliance on matching to a plastic shade guide supplied by the manufacturer at the time of insertion can be misleading. For this reason, experience is vital. It is possible to make a glass-ionomer cement shade guide in which the cement is coated with a light-curing bonding agent to prevent dehydration and crazing. These shade guides should be stored in water.

Shade guides can only be used as an aid, however. In general, cervical restorations will be in the dark brown, yellowish brown, or grey-brown areas. Familiarization with the manufacturer's shades will soon enable the clinician to make a reasonably accurate choice. In more extensive restorations when the middle third of the tooth is involved, such as in a Class III restoration, shade-matching becomes more critical. The yellow, grey, and pinkish yellow colours are preferred. If the optimum in aesthetics is required, then veneering of the glass-ionomer base with a microfilled composite resin could be the procedure of choice. Guidelines for selection of either glass-ionomer restorations or glass-ionomer/composite resin laminates will be given in subsequent chapters for each type of anterior restoration.

Shrinkage

All cements tend to shrink on setting, unless other factors come into play; for example, plaster of Paris expands because of the formation of crystals. Glass-ionomer cements shrink slightly on setting, except under conditions of high humidity, when they pick up water and expand. Slight expansion is to be preferred; this will normally occur, except in mouth-breathers. The coefficient of thermal expansion for glass-ionomer cements is close to that for tooth structure and its thermal diffusivity is low. For this reason microleakage at the tooth/cement interface is minimal compared with other types of direct restoratives.

Fluoride release

Glass-ionomer cements contain 12% to 18% of fluoride as F, depending on the exact nature of the cement. Some of this fluoride is available for leaching; studies have shown that fluoride is released continuously for at least 18 months, though in ever-diminishing amounts (Maldonado et al., 1978; Wilson et al., 1985). The transfer of fluoride to adjacent tooth enamel has been demonstrated—fluoride replaces hydroxyl ions in apatite. The action of fluoride is complex; it enhances the resistance of apatite to acids and disrupts the mechanisms of plaque carbohydrates (Smith and Peltoniema, 1982).

Fluoride is released as a sodium salt. In this form, matrix-forming cations, calcium and aluminium, are not lost, so that the strength of the cement is unaffected.

The anticariogenic properties of glass-ionomer cements are now being exploited for treatment of the early carious lesion, and new types of cavity design are revolutionizing our approach to the preservation of the enamel cap, as will be described in chapter 12.

Adhesion

Glass-ionomer cements are capable, under moist conditions, of permanently adhering to reactive or polar substrates (including enamel, dentine, and base metals). This is an important attribute for a filling material and, to a lesser extent, for a luting agent.

The principal barrier to effective adhesion to dental tissue is water. Water will compete with a potential adhesive for the surface of a substrate and can also hydrolyse adhesive bonds. Dentine is permeated by aqueous fluids transported from the pulp, and the enamel surface contains both firmly and loosely bound water. Nonpolar polymers are unable to compete successfully with water, for the polar enamel surface and polymers tend to form hydrolyzable bonds. However, glass-ionomer cement is a highly ionic polymer that can compete successfully with water because of the multiplicity of carboxyl groups that can form strong hydrogen bonds to apatite. Glass-ionomer cements will adhere to untreated enamel or dentine. In the case of enamel, the cement may adhere to the acquired pellicle or penetrate this layer, bonding directly to the enamel.

Adhesion to both enamel and dentine can be improved if substrate surfaces are first treated and cleaned with agents such as aqueous solutions of tannic acid, poly(acrylic acid), or dodicin. Their effect on enamel and dentine surfaces is mild. McLean and Wilson (1977a, 1977b) first used the term "surface conditioning" to differentiate this treatment from acid etching, which is used in the preparation of enamel for attachment of composite resins. Dentine tubules are revealed but not opened, and enamel surfaces are only sightly etched. Adhesive bonding almost equals the tensile strength of the cement. Solutions of 25% poly(acrylic) or tannic acid may be used as surface conditioners—at the present time these are regarded as the most effective agents. Poly(acrylic acid) may be used to condition cavities, while tannic acid is preferred for conditioning large areas of exposed dentine which can occur, for example, in crown preparations. In such cases the use of poly(acrylic acid) could open up tubules and produce postoperative sensitivity.

Finishing technique

The best surface obtainable is that produced when the cement is allowed to set against the matrix. Unfortunately, during finishing, this smooth gel surface, which rarely has porosity (Fig. 9-6), is destroyed. Where access can be gained, carving the cement external to the cavity margins with sharp knives or scalers after initial set is the best technique for finishing, thus preserving the gel surface (Fig. 9-7). If this cannot be done, then finishing becomes an exercise in damage limitation. The general requirement is that the finest abrasive should be used to minimize tearing of the surface. Gross finishing of bulk surfaces with rotary instruments after initial set is strongly deprecated. Whenever possible, margins should be smoothed with hand instru-

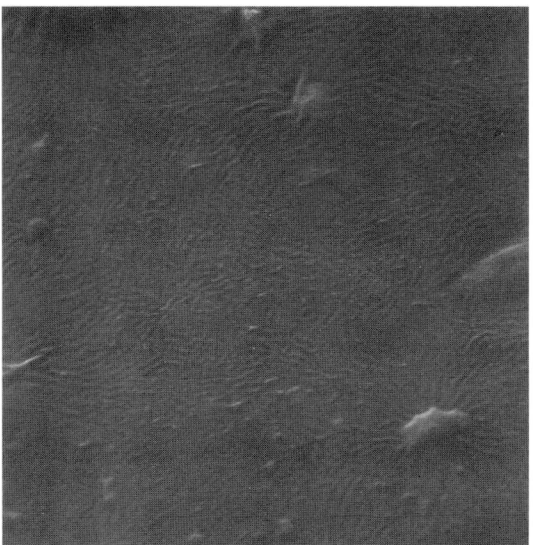

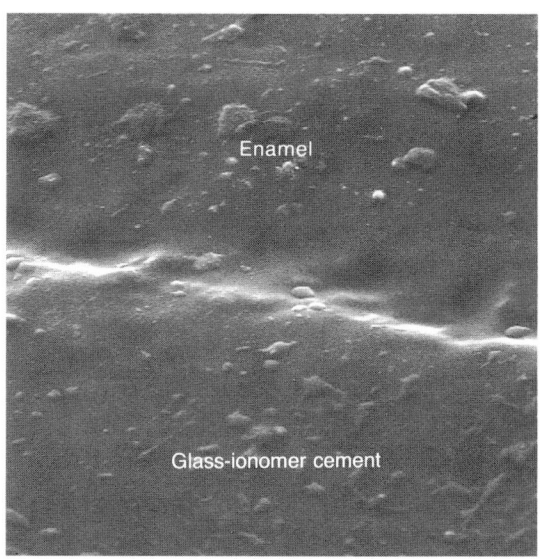

Fig. 9-6 Intact smooth gel surface. SEM × 1,000.

Fig. 9-7 Margin of glass-ionomer cement after carving with sharp knife. SEM × 200.

ments and the bulk of the cement left with its protective coating intact. Finishing with rotary instruments and final polishing can be undertaken at a subsequent visit. Glass-ionomer cements should never be finished under dry con-ditions; a petroleum lubricant may be used to prevent desiccation.

Details for finishing glass-ionomer cements in various types of cavity preparations are given in later chapters of this book.

References

Asmussen, E. (1983) Opacity of glass ionomer cements. Acta Odontol. Scand. 41:155–157.

Crisp, S., Abel, G., and Wilson, A.D. (1979) The quantitative measurement of the opacity of aesthetic dental filling materials. J. Dent. Res. 58:1585–1596.

Earl, M.S.A., Hume, W.R., and Mount, G.I. (1985) Effect of varnishes and other surface treatments on water movement across the glass-ionomer cement surface. Aust. Dent. J. 30:298–301.

McLean, J.W., and Wilson, A.D. (1977a) The clinical development of the glass-ionomer cement. I. Formulations and properties. Aust. Dent. J. 22:31–36.

McLean, J.W., and Wilson, A.D. (1977b) The clinical development of the glass-ionomer cement. II. Some clinical applications. Aust. Dent. J. 22:120–127.

McLean, J.W., and Wilson, A.D. (1977c) The clinical development of the glass-ionomer cement. III. The erosion lesion. Aust. Dent. J. 22:190–195.

Maldonado, A., Swartz, M.L., and Phillips, R.W. (1978) An in vitro study of certain properties of a glass ionomer cement. J. Am. Dent. Assoc. 96:785–792.

Mount, G.J. (1984) Glass ionomer cements: Clinical considerations. chapt. 20A In J.W. Clark (ed.) Clinical Dentistry. Philadelphia: Harper & Row.

Mount, G.J., and Makinson, O.F. (1978) Clinical characteristics of a glass-ionomer cement. Br. Dent. J. 145:67–71.

Mount, G.J., and Makinson, O.F. (1982) Glass-ionomer cements: Clinical implications of the setting reaction. Oper. Dent. 7:134–141.

Smith, D.C., and Peltoniemi, A. (1982) Release and enamel retention of fluoride from tooth coatings and other dental materials. chapt. 8 In D.C. Smith and D.F. Williams (ed.) Biocompatibility of Dental Materials. Vol. I. Characteristics of Dental Tissues and Their Response to Dental Materials. Boca Raton, Fla.: CRC Press Inc.

Wilson, A.D., Groffman, D.M., and Kuhn, A.T. (1985) The release of fluoride and other chemical species from a glass-ionomer cement. Biomaterials 6:431–434.

Chapter 10

Class V and Class III Restorations

The erosion/abrasion lesion

Erosion lesions in teeth have become very common with the change in the pattern of dental health. Their incidence increases with age and they are associated with patients in middle life. A study of over 10,000 extracted teeth by Sognnaes and coworkers (1972) using random sampling found typical erosion patterns in 18% of these. In another study, based on five months of in vitro observation, Xhonga and coworkers (1972) estimated that the erosion advancement rate was approximately 7 μm per week for untreated and fluoride-treated teeth. When the lesions were restored, the rate of erosion was decreased to about half. Clearly, if erosion lesions can be restored without cavity preparation, then the preservation of both tooth structure and pulp vitality can be achieved.

Classification of erosion/abrasion is generally based on physical form and location (Gilmore, 1967), because often one cannot readily identify any obvious mechanical or chemical agent involved, or any unusual habits or health conditions. The dentist is presented with a complexity of shapes to restore, ranging from the typical V-shaped notch to the "hour-glass" pattern of erosion.

Erosion lesions generally present two types of finishing lines. The V-shaped notch with knife-edges, or the more saucer-shaped lesion with no clearly defined edges (Fig. 10-1). Of the two types, the V-shaped notch is easier to restore because of the definite finishing line, which is more satisfactory for a brittle cement. By contrast, the acid-etch composite resin is easily bonded to an enamel edge, but often fails at the dentine surface because of its hydrophobic nature and loss of adhesion with time (Fig. 10-2). This failure rate can be reduced by the use of glass-ionomer linings, which can be acid etched for the attachment of the composite resins. The restoration of Class V erosion/abrasion lesions falls into two categories: *(1)* total restoration with glass-ionomer cement, and *(2)* the laminated glass-ionomer/composite restoration.

Figs. 10-1a and b   Finishing lines on erosion lesions.

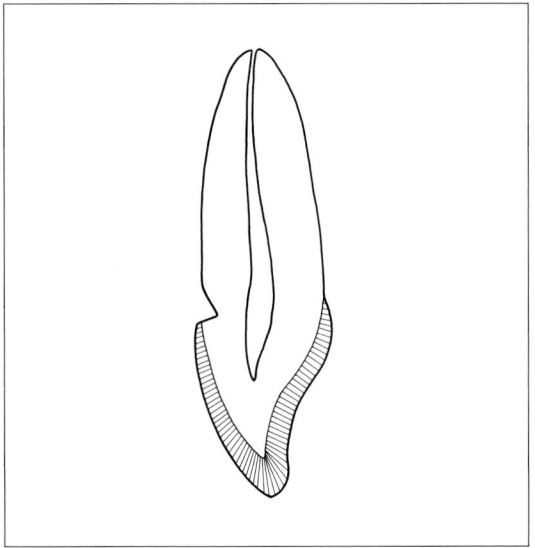
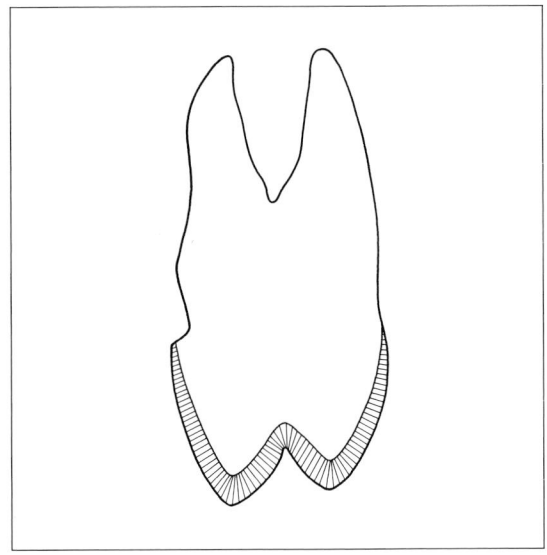

Fig. 10-1a   V-shaped notch.

Fig. 10-1b   Saucer-shaped lesion.

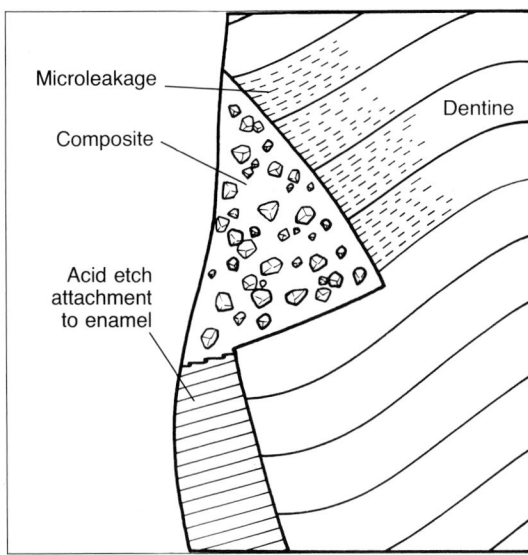
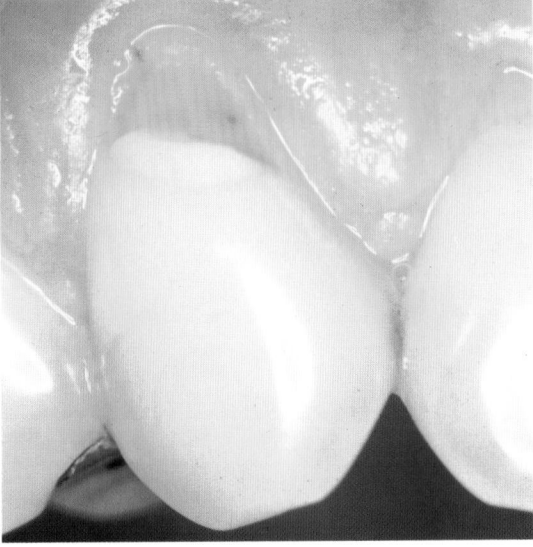

Fig. 10-2a   Diagram of failure of composite resin at dentine interface.

Fig. 10-2b   Composite resin failed at dentine interface due to microleakage. Restoration was only lost when enamel bond failed.

The Class V glass-ionomer cement restoration

The success of the Class V glass-ionomer restoration depends on five main factors:

1. Geometry of the erosion lesion
2. Thickness and structure of the tooth
3. Cleanliness of the dentine surface
4. Wettability of the glass-ionomer cement
5. Aesthetics

Geometry and structure of the tooth

The lesion should preferably have a depth of at least 1 mm to provide sufficient bulk of cement to resist fracture or erosion. Well-defined cavosurface margins are more easily restored, since a finishing line is provided for the cement (see Fig. 10-1a).

The structure of the tooth also plays a major role in the success rate. Thin teeth such as mandibular incisors can flex more than maxillary incisors and, despite good chemical bonding, the cement restoration can be dislodged under sudden occlusal loading (Fig. 10-3). In teeth where cervical erosion is extensive the dentist should appreciate that the remaining dentine is often less than is revealed in a quick clinical examination. The modulus of elasticity of dentine is quite low, and flexure of teeth can play a major part in debonding and loss of glass-ionomer restorations in the cervical region.

Dentine surface

The importance of securing clean and uncontaminated surfaces to dentine has already been emphasized in chapter 6.

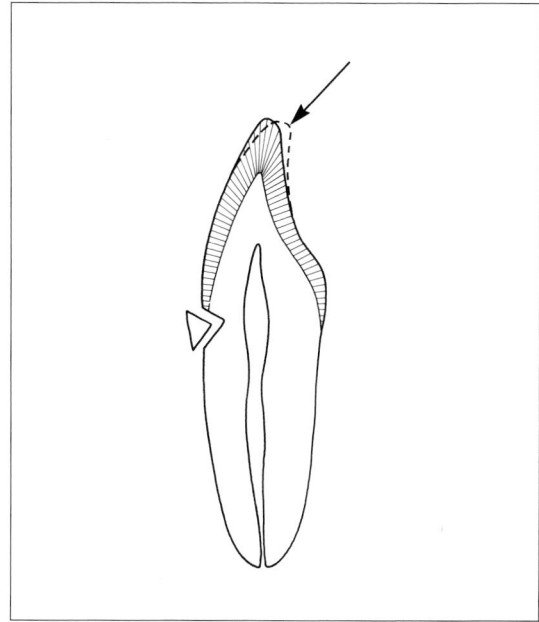

Fig. 10-3 Diagram of loss of cervical glass-ionomer restoration in a mandibular incisor due to flexing of dentine.

In the case of the erosion lesion where no mechanical preparation is involved, a clean surface is vital to long-term success. The dentinal tubules in these lesions are almost obliterated, so there will be minimal dentine fluid flow (Fig. 10-4). In addition, plaque and pellicle will be present and must be removed. Decalcified dentine may also be present in some areas. This must also be removed mechanically if a good bonding surface is to be achieved. Lack of calcium in the surfaces means there will be insufficient bonding ions for attachment.

Wettability of the cement

If there is not enough free polyacid on the surface of the mixed cement the chances of securing good chemical bonding are remote. The mechanism for this bonding has already been described

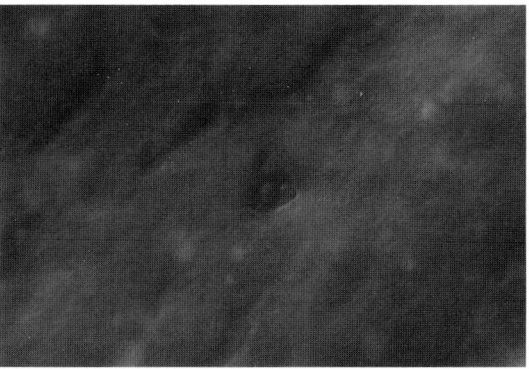

Fig. 10-4 SEM of the dentine surface of an erosion lesion showing tubules obliterated.

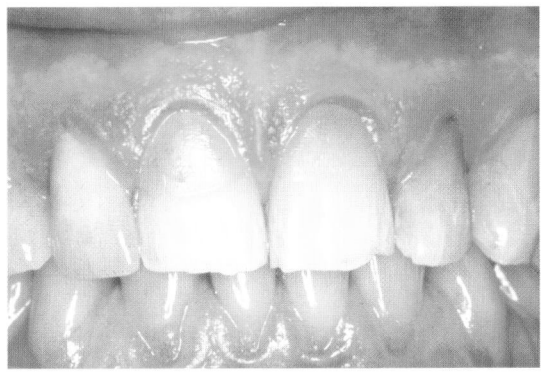

Fig. 10-5 Extensive lesions in anterior incisors restored with glass-ionomer cement showing loss of smooth surface after four years and lack of aesthetic appeal. These surfaces could be veneered with a composite resin using the acid-etch technique. The glass-ionomer cement should be removed to a depth of only 1 mm.

in chapter 6. Dry mixes of cement will not wet out the dentine, and the bonding sites will be considerably reduced.

Aesthetics

The translucency of the modern glass-ionomer Type II restorative materials has been considerably improved. However, their polishability leaves something to be desired, so that attempts to restore large areas of labial or buccal enamel with glass-ionomer cement can be disappointing (Fig. 10-5). A useful rule to observe is that if the erosion/abrasion area extends from the cervical margin by more than one third, then a composite resin material may be the restoration of choice. On the average maxillary central incisor, this recommendation indicates a cervicoincisal length of filling of not more than 3 to 4 mm. Even then, anterior teeth may present a greater problem because light reflection is at a maximum.

Clinical placement

Saliva control

Because of the hydrophilic nature of glass-ionomer cement, routine use of a rubber dam is not necessary when restoring a Class V erosion/abrasion lesion. However, when there is gingival haemorrhage arising from poor periodontal condition or when saliva control is difficult, a rubber dam should be used. *Excessive dehydration of teeth is undesirable* when using glass-ionomer cements, since wettability can be reduced and dehydration of the cement can produce crazing and weakening of the set cement matrix. Isolation with cotton rolls and gingival cord can help avoid dehydration.

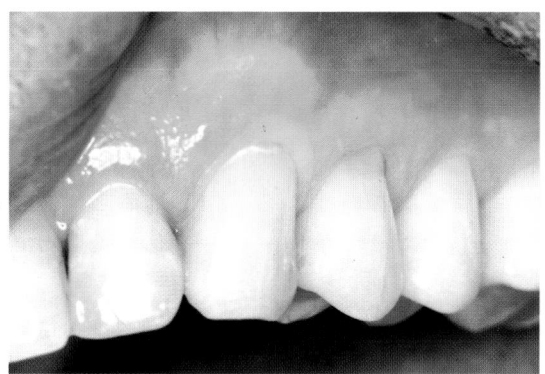

Fig. 10-6 Class V erosion lesion in tooth 24 after cleaning with pumice and water.

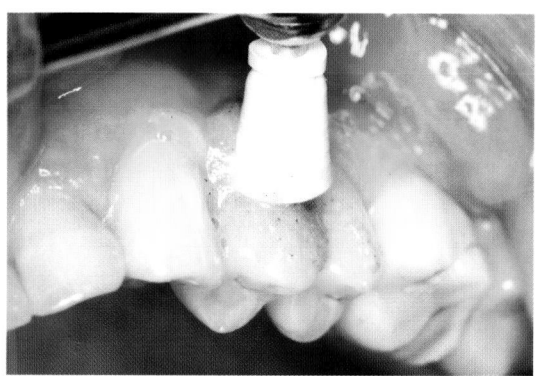

Fig. 10-7 Erosion lesion may be conditioned with a 25% solution of poly(acrylic acid) and fine pumice flour for ten seconds.

Tooth preparation

Any plaque, pellicle, or stain in the lesion should be removed by scrubbing lightly for about ten seconds with a slurry of fine pumice flour in water on a soft rubber cup. Do not use proprietary polishing pastes, because they may contain contaminants. Cleaning can usually be done without the use of local anaesthesia (Fig. 10-6). Alternatively, both cleaning and surface conditioning may be done simultaneously using a 25% solution of poly(acrylic acid) mixed with fine pumice flour and polishing the tooth for ten seconds (Fig. 10-7).

Lining

Where the lesion is deep, a small quantity of calcium hydroxide should be placed at the tip of the notch. It must not be extended further, since it will prevent adhesion of the glass-ionomer cement (Fig. 10-8).

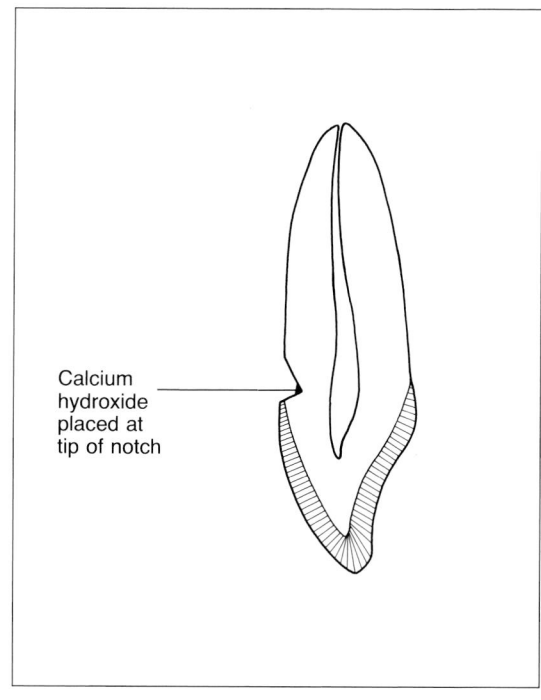

Calcium hydroxide placed at tip of notch

Fig. 10-8 Diagram showing ideal placement of a calcium hydroxide lining in a typical erosion lesion. Only the deepest portion of the notch should be covered.

Shade selection

Details for selecting shades of glass-ionomer cements are given in chapters 5 and 9. The most useful shades for the Class V restoration lie in the dark brown, yellow-brown, and grey-brown ranges.

Surface conditioning

If the cleaning and conditioning have not been done in one operation, it is essential to use a separate conditioner. Apply a solution of 25% poly(acrylic acid) for ten seconds on a pledget of cotton wool. Wash off and lightly dry the tooth. Do not dehydrate.

The matrix

Prior to placement of the cement it is essential to apply a matrix. Not only will it protect the cement during setting, but, more importantly, it allows pressure to be applied to the cement to bring it into intimate atomic contact with the dentine and to reduce porosity. The cement surface produced under a matrix is the smoothest possible. Useful matrices for Class V erosion lesions are of the soft-metal type, such as the Hawe Matrices* (Fig. 10-9). These are made in several shapes and sizes and can be adapted accurately to the margins of the cavity. Initially the matrix is tucked under the gingival margin then burnished to position. A useful procedure that has become popular with many clinicians is to hold the matrix in a pair of tweezers and lift the incisal edge prior to injecting the cement (Fig. 10-10). The matrix is then closely burnished over the cavity margins (Fig. 10-11).

*Hawe Matrices, Hawe-Neos Dental Co., Gentilino, Switzerland.

Insertion of the cement

Trapped air in the mixed cement, which can result in surface porosity, is a major problem with all powder/liquid formulae. Injecting the cements into the cavity with a syringe can minimize this problem.

The tip of the syringe should be placed into the base of the cavity and withdrawn slowly while still syringing. Watch for any air inclusions or folding of material. Magnification is recommended for this procedure.

Initial set

The initial set of the glass-ionomers will vary according to the material selected, mixing technique, temperature, and the powder/liquid ratio. If a little of the cement is left around the matrix it may be tested with an explorer. The cement should feel rock-hard before removing the matrix; usually a period of five minutes from start of mix is adequate for capsulated materials.

Removing matrix and protecting cement

After the initial set, the removal of the matrix is a critical procedure. At this stage the cement is extremely vulnerable to moisture contamination and dehydration. The matrix should be lifted gently from one edge while securing the main bulk with finger pressure, and then peeled off. In this way there is no risk of removing the entire filling before it has a chance to develop physicochemical adhesion. A waterproof varnish must be applied immediately because seconds count—any delay can cause crazing of the cement. Ideally, as the matrix is removed, a light-curing bonding resin should be applied in one operation and then light cured

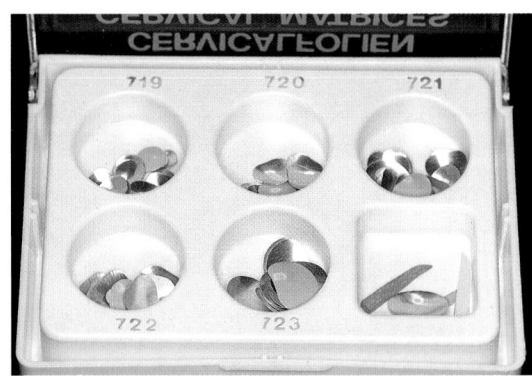

Fig. 10-9 Soft-metal-type cervical matrices.

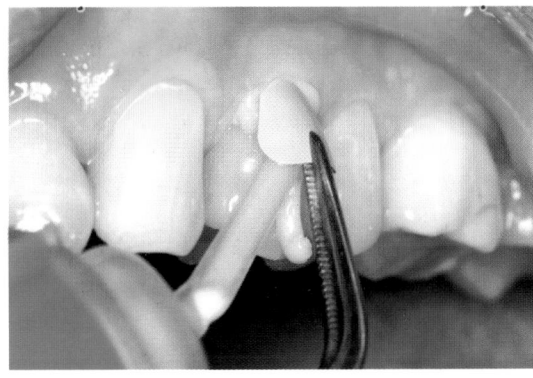

Fig. 10-10 Soft-metal matrix tucked under the gingiva and glass-ionomer cement injected under the matrix.

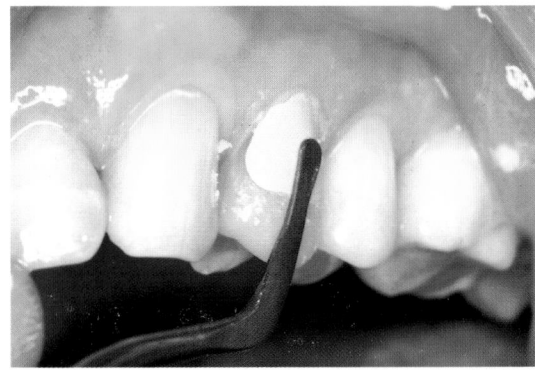

Fig. 10-11 Matrix burnished closely to the cavity margins to avoid excess cement.

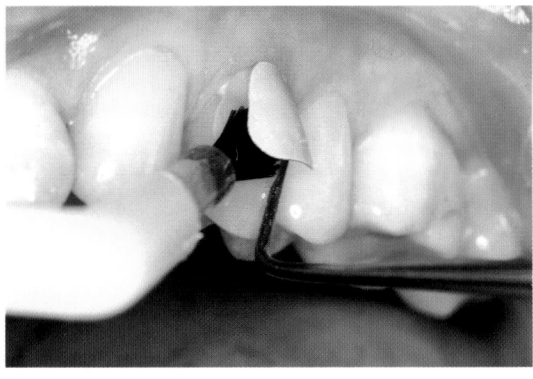

Fig. 10-12 Light-curing bonding resin applied immediately after lifting the matrix. The bonding agent will act as a lubricant during trimming of excess cement from the margins and can be cured *after* finishing the edges.

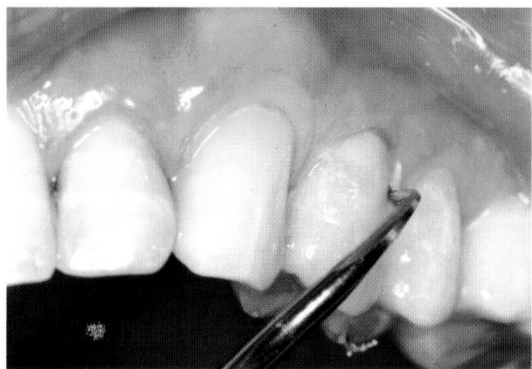

Fig. 10-13 Avoid the use of rotary instruments. Wherever possible, use sharp knives, scalers, or excavators to trim externally to the margin. *Do not destroy* the main bulk of the filling, but confine the finishing operation to the margins. Always use magnification.

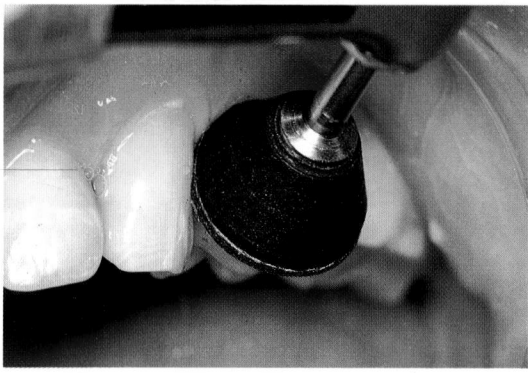

Fig. 10-14 Abrasive rubber cup used with a slurry of fine polishing-grade alumina to polish restoration.

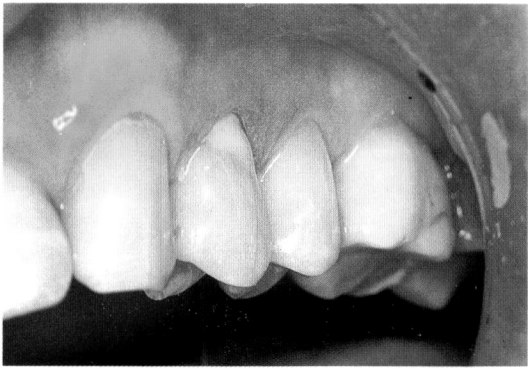

Fig. 10-15 Completed restoration of an erosion lesion in tooth 24.

(Fig. 10-12). If a varnish is used, a second coat should then be applied to ensure sealing of the cement surface and to prevent drying. The role of varnishes and light-curing bonding resins has been discussed in chapter 3.

Finishing

Premature finishing of a glass-ionomer cement restoration with rotary finishing instruments is one of the main causes for ruining the surface. Dehydration during finishing can also be disastrous. By contrast, the composite resin filling materials can stand more abuse. However, provided that the practitioner appreciates the setting mechanism of the glass-ionomer cements, excellent results can be obtained with these materials. As explained in chapter 3 the glass-ionomers develop their resistance to solution in water once the calcium and aluminium ions released from the glass are fully fixed as insoluble polyacrylates. Before the cement hardens soluble calcium and aluminium ions in the matrix (aluminium is precipitated rather slowly) render the cement vulnerable. Varnishing or, preferably, an application of a light-curing bonding agent to the surface will prevent any deleterious effects either due to moisture or to dehydration—but the trimming of margins or cement surfaces is the critical procedure. By using magnification of up to 3× the practitioner should be able to clearly identify the cavosurface margins. With a sharp knife or scaler, and using a very light touch, excess cement outside the cavity margin can be removed (Fig. 10-13). Accurate contouring of the cervical matrix should make gross trimming of the filling surface unnecessary, thus avoiding the use of rotary finishing instruments. The argument over which types of rotary burs or stones to use can be irrelevant when considering the Class V restoration. Accurate matrix technique combined with sharp carving instruments used under good lighting and magnification can produce a glass-ionomer restoration that is undamaged on the surface. At a later visit these surfaces can be polished with soft abrasive rubber cups and a slurry of fine-grained alumina (Fig. 10-14). Completed restorations should never be allowed to dry out. If other operative work is contemplated, existing restorations should be protected with varnish.

Gross excess on the surface of the filling can be removed with fine diamond-plated stones or fluted carbide burs. Finishing discs lubricated with petroleum jelly also provide a useful adjunct. But since in the Class V restoration any inadvertent cutting of the cementum can result in hypersensitivity, trimming of these margins is better left to hand instrumentation. The complete restoration is shown in Fig. 10-15.

Class V carious lesions

Carious lesions at the cervical region of teeth generally indicate an active caries rate, prevalent in geriatric patients or adolescents with high sugar consumption. Figure 10-16 shows a patient who sucked on large quantities of hard mints supplemented with evening drinks of Coca-Cola. Within five weeks a lesion developed in tooth 34. Glass-ionomer cements are ideal for the treatment of lesions when dietary habits cannot be changed, because the cement offers some caries protection through fluoride release (Fig. 10-17). As discussed previously, cervical restorations may fail due to flexure of the tooth, and amalgam,

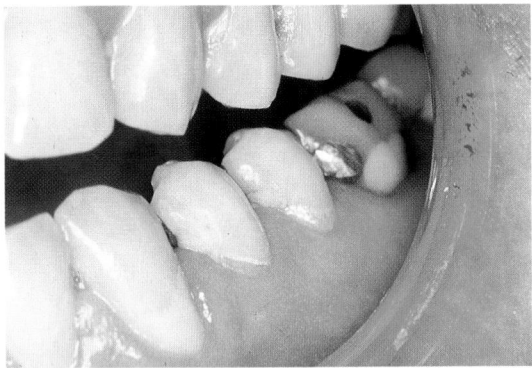

Fig. 10-16 Class V carious lesion in tooth 34 due to poor dietary habit and high sugar intake.

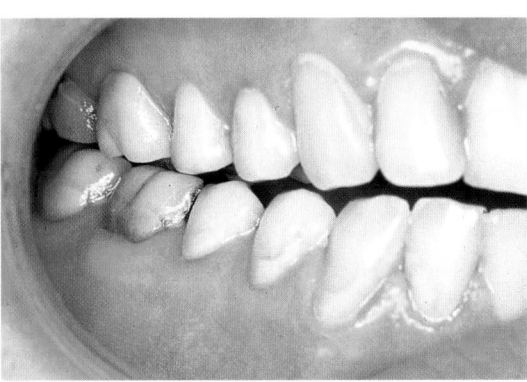

Fig. 10-17 Class V lesions in teeth 43, 44, 45, 46, and 47 three years after restoration with glass-ionomer cement, showing excellent protection against secondary caries due to leaching of fluoride.

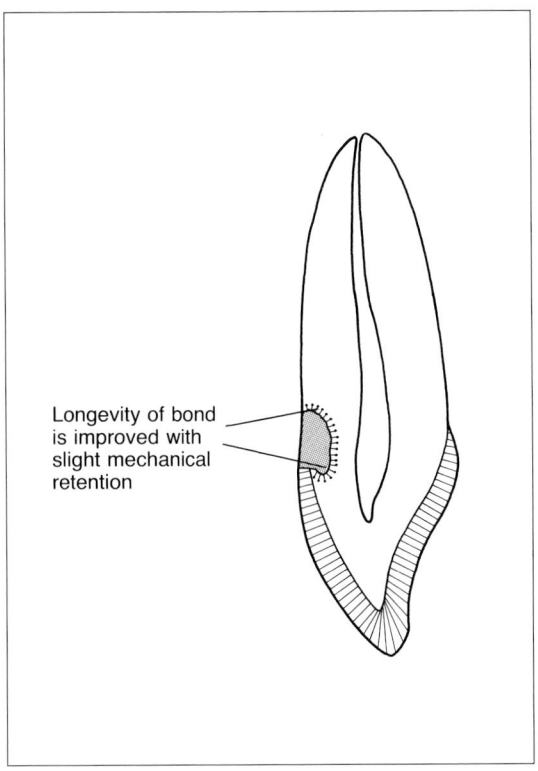

Longevity of bond is improved with slight mechanical retention

Fig. 10-18 Diagram of an ideal cavity preparation for a Class V carious lesion in a maxillary incisor.

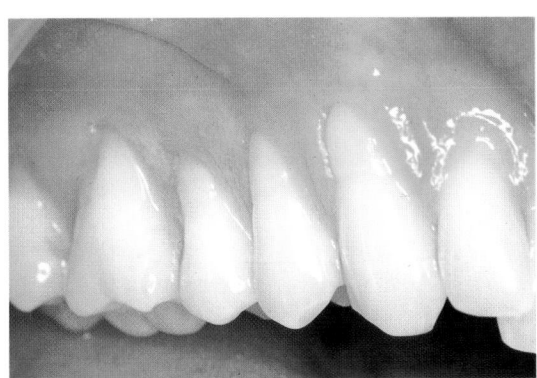

Fig. 10-19 Glass-ionomer cement restorations in teeth 13, 14, 15, and 16 after four years.

gold, or porcelain restorations may leak. An adhesive cement can offer better long-term resistance to percolation of fluids.

Clinical techniques for the Class V carious lesion should follow the principles set out for the erosion/abrasion lesion, including the use of calcium hydroxide linings in the deepest part of the cavity. Although the adhesion of the glass-ionomer cements will allow the preparation of nonundercut cavities, retention can be improved by providing small undercuts in the dentine, as illustrated in Fig. 10-18.

The translucency of glass-ionomer cements has been greatly improved; often the aesthetic results in a Class V cavity can be better than composite resin restorations, which may exhibit staining at margins or a colour shift over time. Class V restorations using Chem-Fil* are illustrated in Fig. 10-19. Excellent appearance has been maintained over four years.

The Class III glass-ionomer restoration

Glass-ionomer cements are still not as translucent as composite resin restorations, and where more than 1 mm of the approximal enamel is involved, the appearance of labial restorations can meet with criticism from the patient. A lingual approach to the restoration of these lesions is preferred.

Cavity preparation

A small round diamond stone is used to gain access to the lesion and the lingual surface is opened enough to see quite clearly the extent of the dentine caries. Magnification and good lighting should be used, since the main objective of the procedure should be micro-, not macro-, cutting of the tooth (Fig. 10-20).

A 244 discoid Excavator* may be used to remove the caries or, alternatively, an F. G. (Friction grip) no. 1 or 2 round bur

*Dentsply International Inc., Weybridge, England, and York, Pa.

*Cottrell, Ltd., London, and Parker, Colo.

153

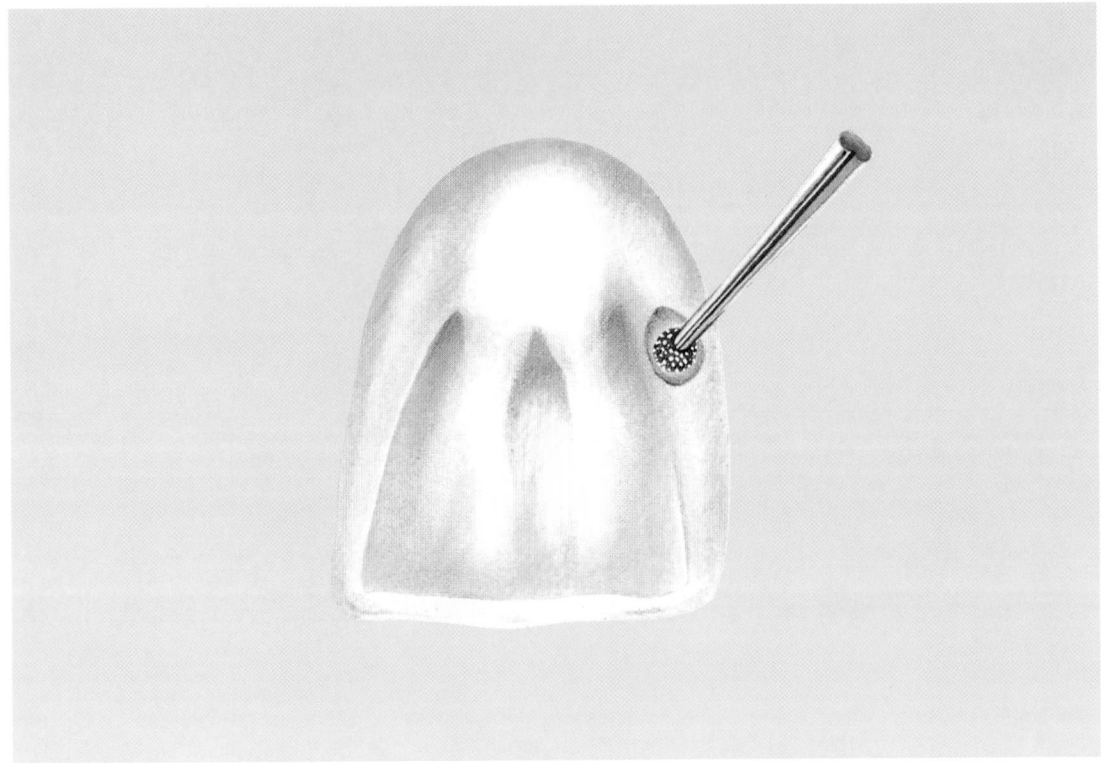

Fig. 10-20 Diagram of Class III carious lesion. Lingual access gained with small round diamond. This access point is suitable for either a tunnel or standard Class III cavity preparation.

at slow speed will remove the softened dentine. Removal of labial enamel should seldom be necessary and the early carious lesion is easily dealt with in this way.

Many approximal cavities will extend into cervical dentine. In these cases the glass-ionomer cements are particularly useful. The Class III glass-ionomer restoration is strongly recommended, either as a base or complete restorative, when there is active caries present, because resin-based materials are very prone to leakage at approximal dentine cavosurface margins. In deep cavities a lining of setting calcium hydroxide should be placed.

Knight (1984) has also suggested a "tunnel" approach to the Class III lesion, in which access is gained via an internal lingual approach (Fig. 10-20). Only the carious dentine is removed and all the approximal enamel is left intact, except for any area that is cavitated. After removal of the carious dentine and surface conditioning with polyacrylic acid, the glass-ionomer cement is injected into the cavity and adjusted to position with a mylar strip.

This type of cavity approach is only suitable for early Class III lesions. It is essential to leave the approximal ridge of enamel intact. Magnification and fibreoptic lighting are essential for such a fine operation.

The clinical procedures for placement of Class III glass-ionomer restorations, including internal or tunnel preparations, are shown in Figs. 10-21 to 10-26.

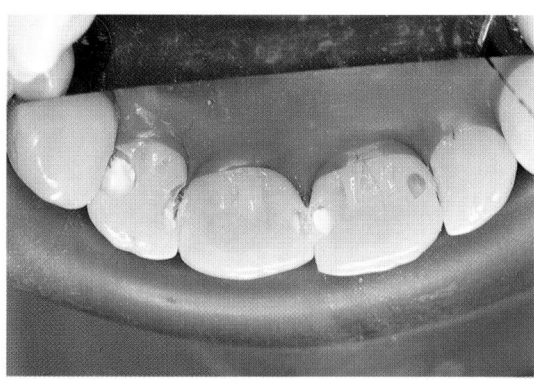

Fig. 10-21 Class III cavities prepared in teeth 12, 11, and 21 for restoration either with glass-ionomer cement or a glass-ionomer cement/composite resin laminate. Details of cavity preparation are as follows: distal tunnel or internal preparation in tooth 21; mesial Class III preparation in tooth 21 lined with calcium hydroxide; mesial and distal Class III preparations in tooth 11; mesial and distal Class III preparations in tooth 12, which is lined with glass-ionomer cement for attachment of an acid-etched composite resin, because the facial surface is involved.

Figs. 10-22a and b After surface conditioning with 25% poly(acrylic acid) solution for ten seconds, cavity preparations are washed and lightly dried and mylar strips inserted. A syringe is inserted at the base of the cavity to avoid entrapping air. In tunnel preparations the mylar strip can be inserted after injection of the glass-ionomer cement.

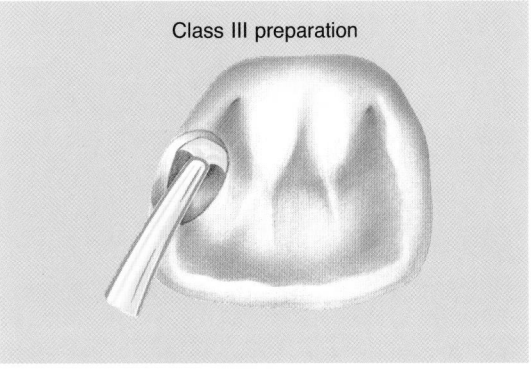

Class III preparation

Fig. 10-22a Glass-ionomer cement is injected into the mesial cavity in tooth 21.

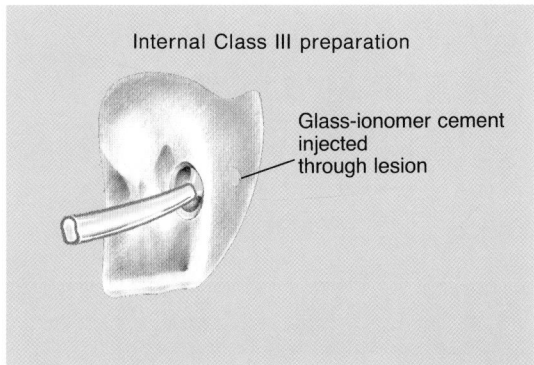

Internal Class III preparation

Glass-ionomer cement injected through lesion

Fig. 10-22b Glass-ionomer cement is injected into the distal internal preparation in tooth 21.

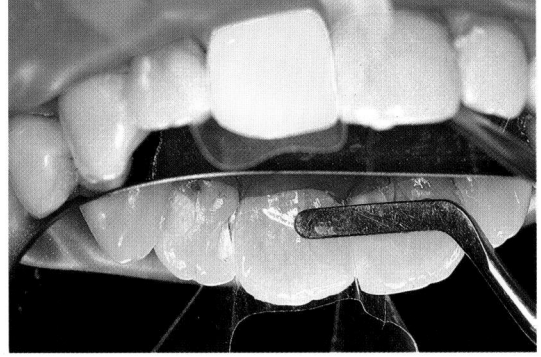

Fig. 10-23 After filling the cavities in tooth 21, the Class III cavities in tooth 11 are filled with glass-ionomer cement and a matrix strip is tightly adapted and burnished into position in order to eliminate as much excess cement as possible.

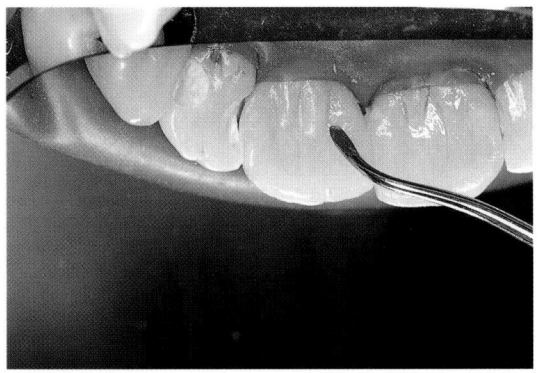

Fig. 10-24 Matrix strips removed and light-cured bonding agent applied immediately. Excess cement external to the cavity trimmed with sharp excavators. Trimming of the external margin of the cement may be done *before curing the bonding agent,* which acts as a protective lubricant.

Figs. 10-25a and b Mesial and distal cavities in tooth 12 etched with 37% phosphoric acid for 20 seconds, washed, and dried. Light-cured bonding agent applied, followed by an anterior composite resin applied by the standard procedure (see chapter 11).

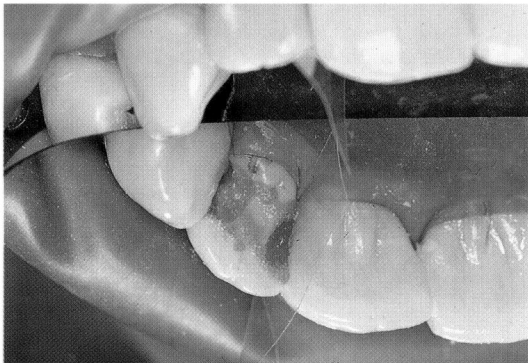

Fig. 10-25a

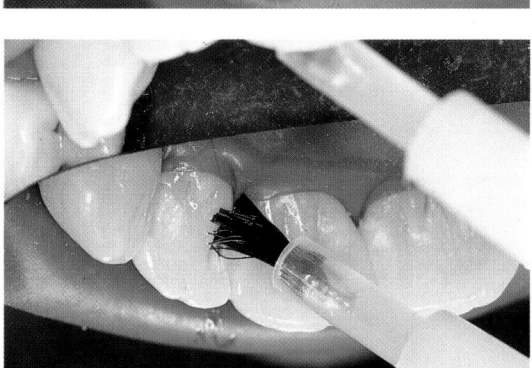

Fig. 10-25b

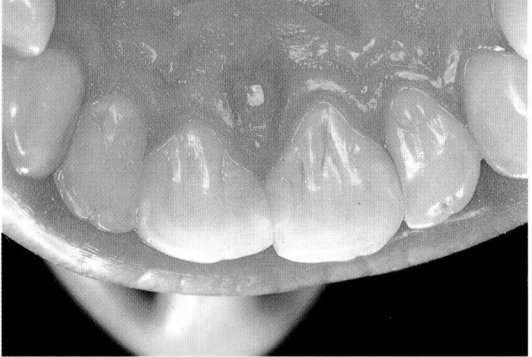

Fig. 10-26 Complete restorations in teeth 12, 11, and 21. The distal tunnel preparation in tooth 21 filled with glass-ionomer cement is hardly visible, illustrating the importance of treating dentinal caries at an early stage before the destruction of the enamel becomes too severe.

References

Gilmore, M.W. (1967) Textbook of Operative Dentistry. St. Louis: C.V. Mosby Co.

Knight, G.M. (1984) The use of adhesive materials in the conservative restoration of selected posterior teeth. Aust. Dent. J. 29:324–331.

Sognnaes, R.F., Wolcott, R.B., and Xhonga, F.A. (1972) Dental erosion. I. Erosion-like patterns occurring in association with other dental conditions. J. Am. Dent. Assoc. 84:571–576.

Xhonga, F.A., Wolcott, R.B., and Sognnaes, R.F. (1972) Dental erosion. II. Clinical measurements of dental erosion progress. J. Am. Dent. Assoc. 84:577–582.

Chapter 11

Laminate Restorations

The principles of attaching composite resins to glass-ionomer cements have been described in chapter 6. The clinician should regard the cement as a *replacement dentine,* the surface of which may be treated similarly to enamel. *Clinical success with this technique is enhanced with increasing thickness of cement. The use of thin linings of glass-ionomer cement is strongly deprecated, since the cement may be destroyed by acid etching, or polymerization shrinkage of the composite resin may break the adhesive bond.* A minimum thickness of 0.5 mm of glass-ionomer cement will also prevent penetration of phosphoric acid into the dentine during etching (Walker et al., 1986). If a lining of glass-ionomer cement cannot be placed with a minimum thickness of 0.5 mm then etching with phosphoric acid could displace the cement or cause severe crazing. An alternative restoration should be considered.

Clinical technique

The glass-ionomer/composite resin laminate is particularly useful where aesthetics is of prime importance and when extensive areas of labial enamel have been destroyed. The modern composite resin filling material is recognized as the most aesthetic restorative material. The acid-etch technique enables it to be attached to enamel with a well-defined prism structure. However, the effectiveness of the marginal seal can be affected by the anatomical position and structural surface conditions of the tooth enamel (Van Noort, 1983). Cervical enamel is thinner and more irregular in prism structure and the surface can be devoid of characteristic prism markings (Gwinnett, 1967). Marginal seal may be established by etching enamel walls in butt and bevel preparations in the incisal and body areas of the tooth, but the Class V carious lesion and caries extending into dentine or areas of structureless cervical enamel present greater problems: microleakage may occur in the dentine area (Fig. 11-1). Using dentine bonding agents does not always mitigate the problem. The use of glass-ionomer cement to seal these dentine areas offers a solution. A rubber dam should be placed when the cavity extends subgingivally; the attachment of composite resins to glass-ionomer-coated dentine surfaces must be made under dry conditions.

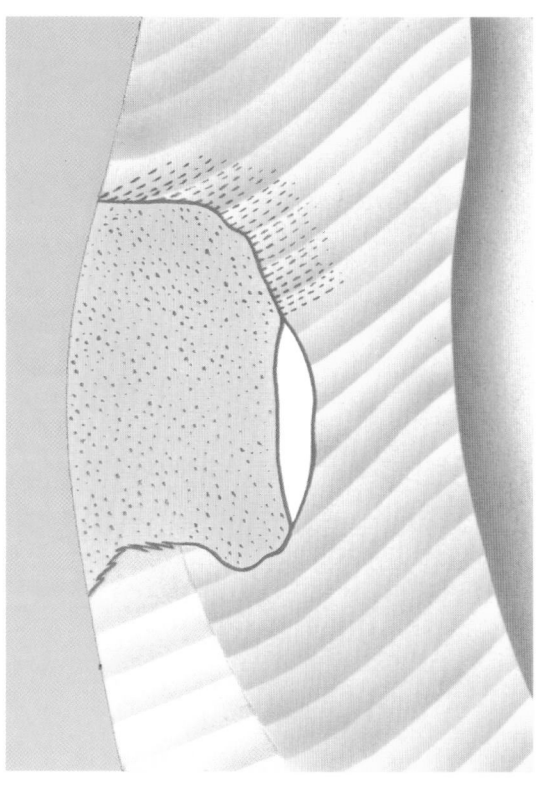

Fig. 11-1 Microleakage in the cervical dentine produced by failure of dentine bond.

Fig. 11-2 *(right, above)* A Class V restoration using the glass-ionomer cement/composite resin laminate showing correct placement of calcium hydroxide lining.

Fig. 11-3 *(right, below)* Incorrect placement of calcium hydroxide lining. Only the immediate pulpal floor should be covered.

The Class V restoration

Cavity preparation

A standard Class V cavity is prepared and any cavosurface margin involving dentine is finished to a butt joint. Enamel margins should be bevelled where structureless enamel is present, to increase the surface area for bonding of the composite resin (Fig. 11-2). Only where a near-exposure is observed with less than 0.5 mm of remaining dentine should a calcium hydroxide liner be used. Even then, it must not cover an area large enough to interfere with glass-ionomer bonding (Fig. 11-3). Margins should be finished with fine diamond stones or sintered diamond stones. A Class V cavity preparation in a maxillary lateral incisor is illustrated in Fig. 11-4.

Surface treatment

The cavity is washed and a 25% solution of poly(acrylic acid) is applied for ten seconds.

Insertion of cement

Fast-setting Type III glass-ionomers are now available.* The colour of the cement should be selected to match the dentine colour. Fast-setting glass-ionomer cements should be mixed on a refrigerated

*Chem-Fil Express (Dentsply International Inc., Weybridge, England, and York, Pa.); Ketac-Bond (ESPE GmbH, Seefeld/Oberbay, West Germany, and Valley Stream, N.Y.); Fuji Lining Cement (G-C International, Tokyo, and Scottsdale, Ariz.); Glass Ionomer Liner (3M Dental Products, St. Paul, Minn.); Shofu Lining Cement (Shofu Dental Corp., Kyoto, Japan, and Menlo Park, Calif.).

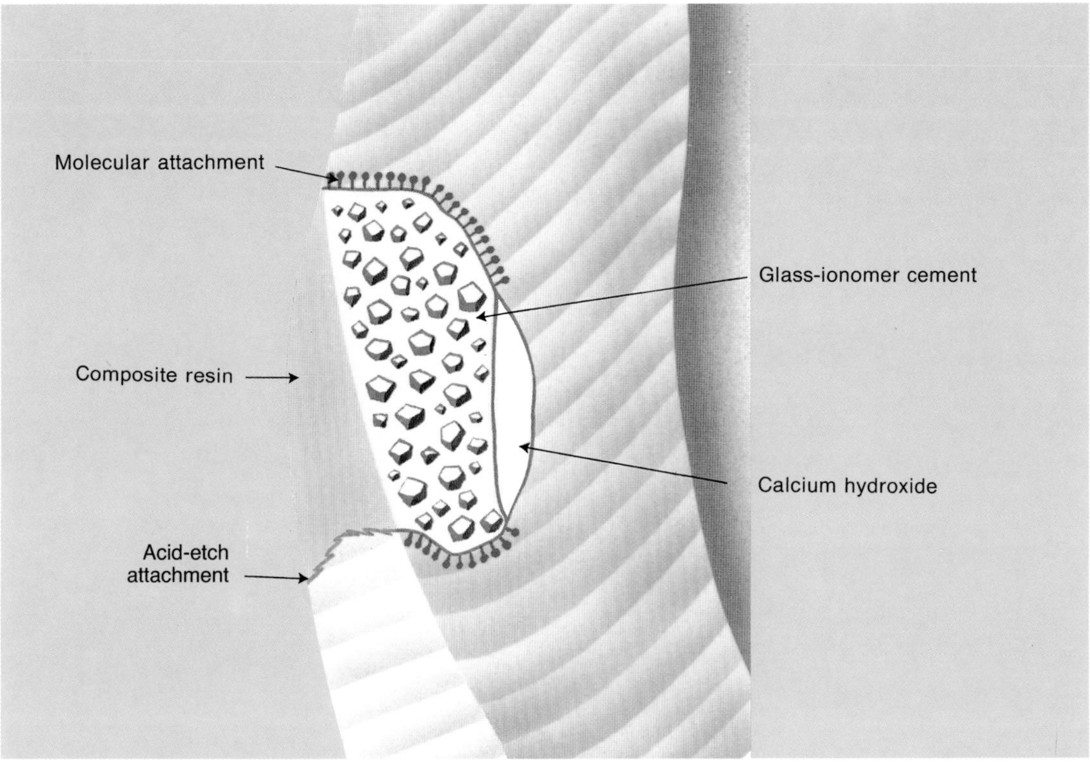

Molecular attachment

Composite resin

Acid-etch attachment

Glass-ionomer cement

Calcium hydroxide

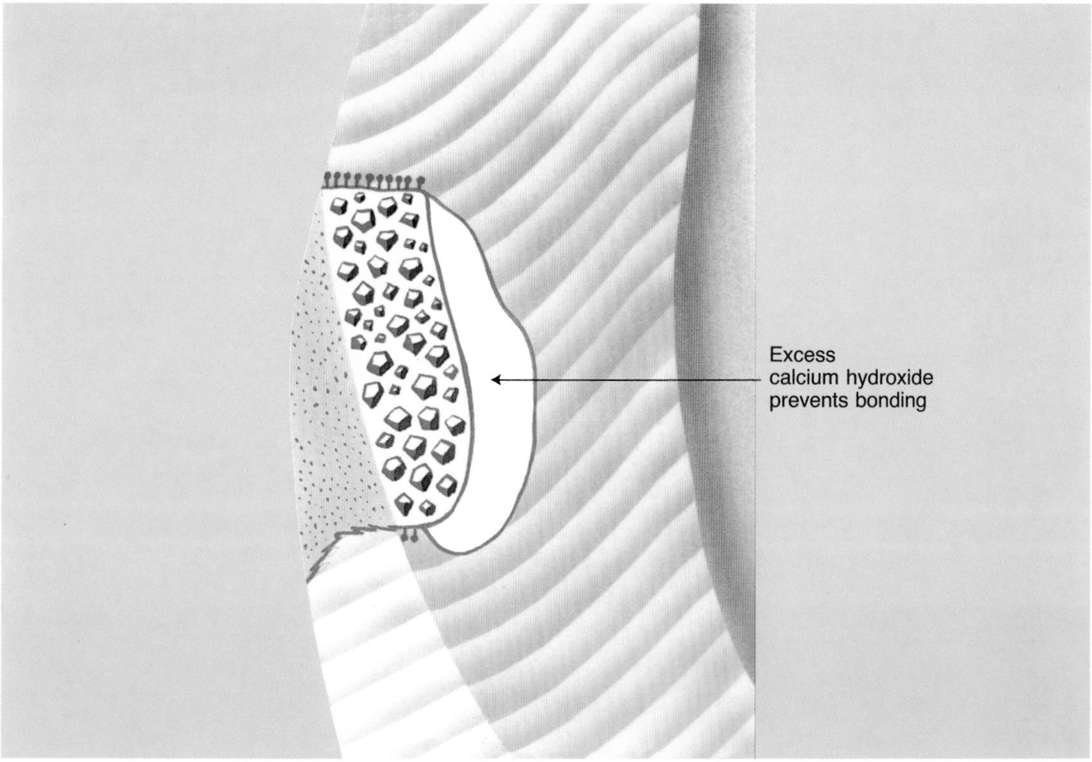

Excess calcium hydroxide prevents bonding

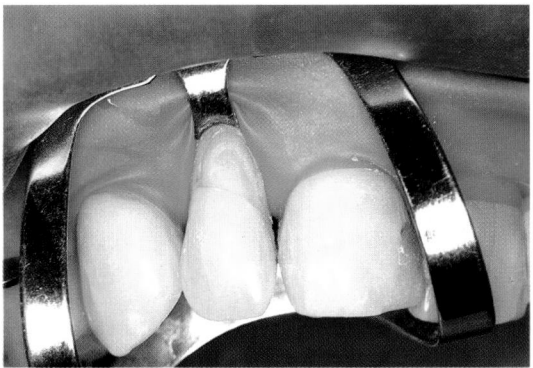

Fig. 11-4 Class V cavity prepared in tooth 12. A butt joint is cut in the dentine and the enamel is beveled.

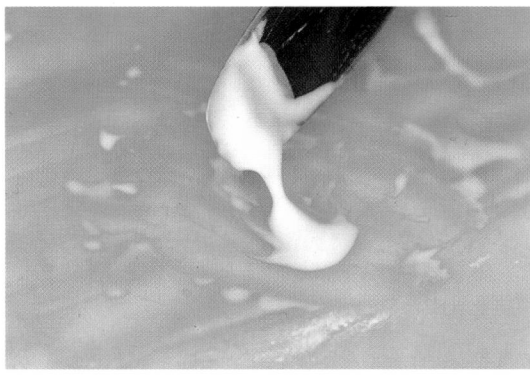

Fig. 11-5 Fast-setting glass-ionomer cement mixed to a creamy consistency.

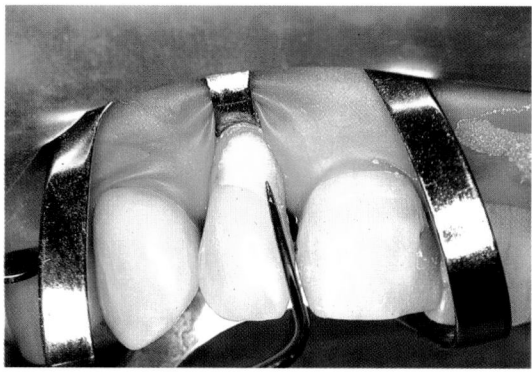

Fig. 11-6 Cement applied to a depth of at least 0.5 mm. Where space is limited, the more translucent Type II cements should be used. A fine explorer is a useful instrument to remove any cervical excess from the dentine margins.

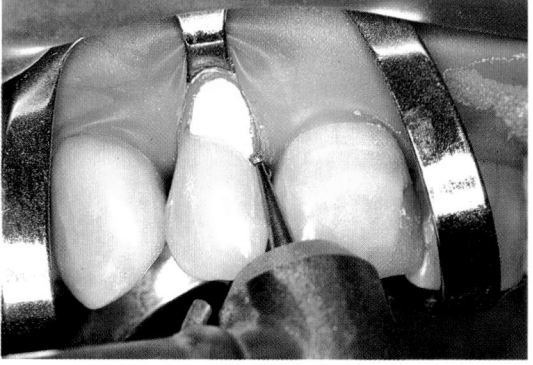

Fig. 11-7 Any excess cement is removed from the enamel wall with a small round diamond stone.

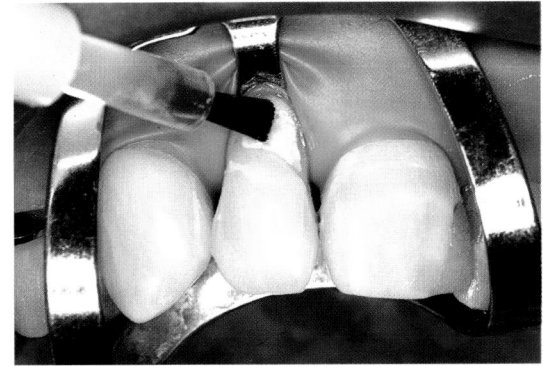

Fig. 11-8 Enamel and cement etched for 30 seconds with 37% phosphoric acid. After washing and drying, a thin coat of light-cured bonding agent is applied to the surface.

glass slab as rapidly as possible (Fig. 11-5). A fluid consistency can be achieved in 15 seconds, but a maximum time of 30 seconds is permissible. The cavity is washed and dried and the cement applied to the dentine surface with a fine, ball-ended instrument. Provided that magnification is used, it is possible to apply the cement exactly to the dentine margins without smearing it over the enamel. A fine explorer may be used for final and delicate smoothing of the margins (Fig. 11-6). After three to four minutes of setting, any excess cement should be removed from the enamel margins (Fig. 11-7). It is essential that the cement should be fully hard to the touch prior to acid etching. Too early application of phosphoric acid is a common cause of failure.

Acid etching

A solution of 37% phosphoric acid or a coloured acid gel is applied to the cement and enamel margins for 30 seconds, then washed for ten seconds and thoroughly dried. The new fast-setting glass-ionomer cements when applied in 0.5-mm thickness do not appear to be weakened by acid etching, as explained in chapter 6. However, these cements are more opaque—at least 1-mm thickness of composite resin is required to mask them. Where this is not possible, a standard Type II glass-ionomer filling material should be used and allowed to set for a longer period. Generally, a minimum period of ten minutes is required. The greater translucency of the filling materials will improve aesthetics where such dimensions are critical.

Application of bonding resin

After washing and drying, a light-cured liquid resin bonding agent must be applied immediately. Rapid application eliminates the possibility of contamination. Provided the resin is immediately light cured for 20 seconds, both the enamel and glass-ionomer surfaces will be totally protected. The bonding resin coat should be as thin as possible to prevent pooling (Fig. 11-8).

Application of bulk composite resin

A microfilled composite resin is usually the preferred material to apply to the cavity surface, because it will produce the best aesthetics and polishability. The

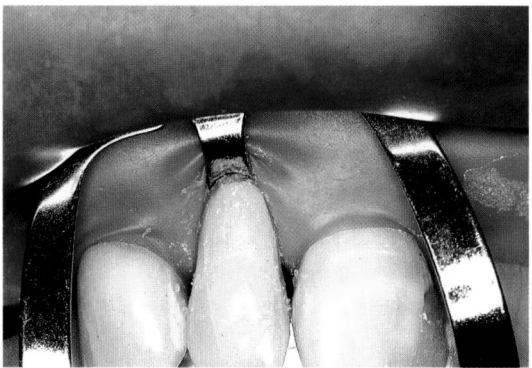

Fig. 11-9 Bulk composite resin applied and contoured to position.

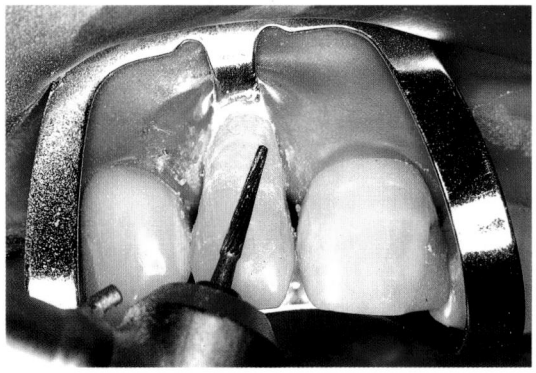

Fig. 11-10 Margins of restoration finished with fluted carbide burs. Trimming should be directed along the line of the cavosurface margins, not across enamel and composite resin. This will prevent damage to the enamel margin, which otherwise could produce a white line.

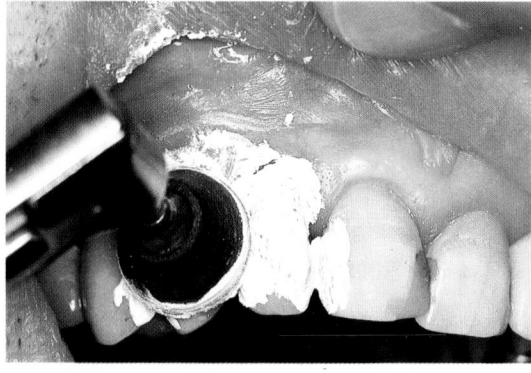

Fig. 11-11 Composite surface polished with abrasive rubber polishing cups and a slurry of fine aluminium oxide.

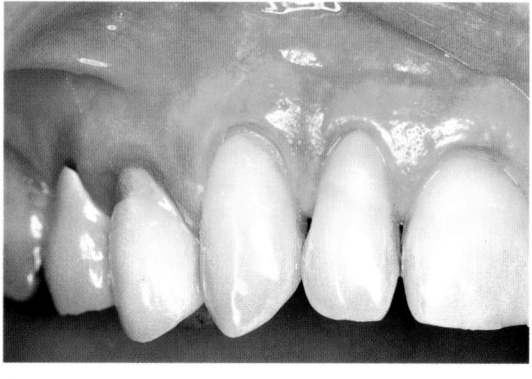

Fig. 11-12 Completed glass-ionomer cement/composite resin laminate restorations in teeth 13 and 12.

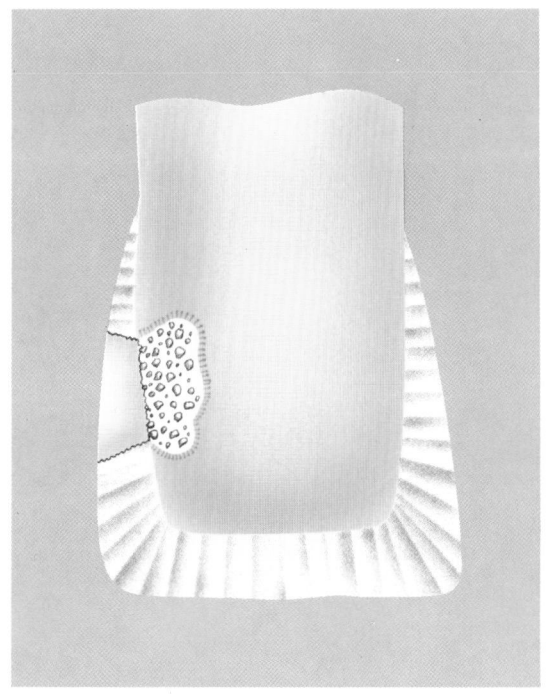

Fig. 11-13 A Class III glass-ionomer cement/composite resin laminate restoration.

paste is applied using either plastic- or Teflon-coated instruments. A stiff brush will also assist in smoothing the composite resin to position. Accurate adaptation may avoid the use of clear plastic matrices (Fig. 11-9).

Finishing

After light-curing for 20 seconds, the restoration should be finished with fluted 12- or 16-bladed carbide burs (Fig. 11-10). Polishing of the restoration can then be completed using abrasive rubber polishing cups and a slurry of fine aluminium oxide (Fig. 11-11).

After polishing, a further light cure of 20 seconds is recommended to ensure that maximum monomer conversion is achieved. The complete restorations are shown in Fig. 11-12.

The Class III restoration

The glass-ionomer acid-etch technique is particularly suitable for the very large Class III restoration because it can provide a biological seal for the tooth. The cement should be applied in bulk and should totally seal the dentine area (Fig. 11-13). The chemical bond and leaching of fluoride will give long-term protection to the surrounding enamel against microleakage and secondary decay. In this way the optimum properties of both composite resin and glass-ionomer cement are used to their maximum advantage: the composite resin for its excellent aesthetics and strong bond to enamel, and the glass-ionomer cement for its long-term adhesion and cariostatic action.

The clinical use of the glass-ionomer cement/composite resin laminate restoration in a Class III carious lesion is illustrated in Figs. 11-14 to 11-21.

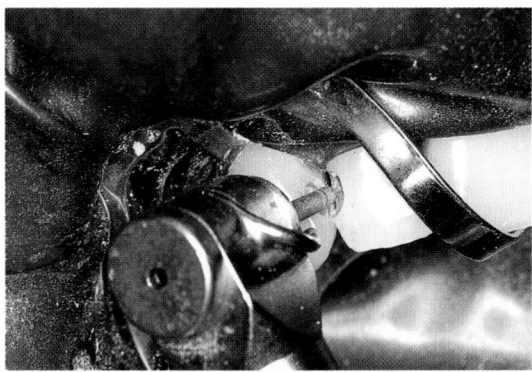

Figs. 11-14 to 11-21 Laminate restorations in Class III carious lesions.

Fig. 11-14 Class III cavity prepared in distal surface of tooth 12. Margins finished to butt joint with fine sintered diamonds.

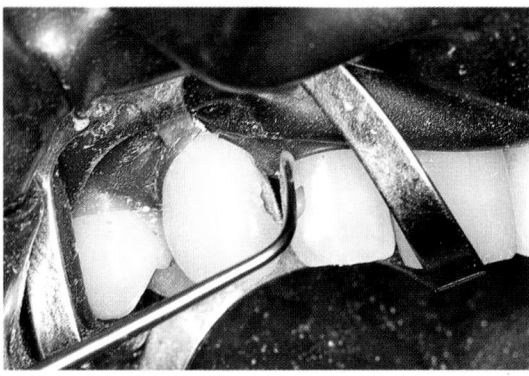

Fig. 11-15 Type III fast-setting lining used to restore the missing dentine.

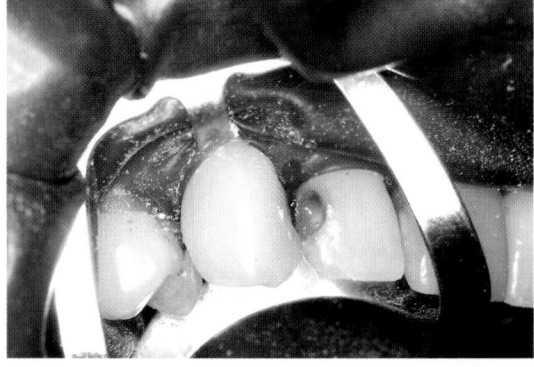

Fig. 11-16a Enamel and base etched for 30 seconds with 37% phosphoric acid.

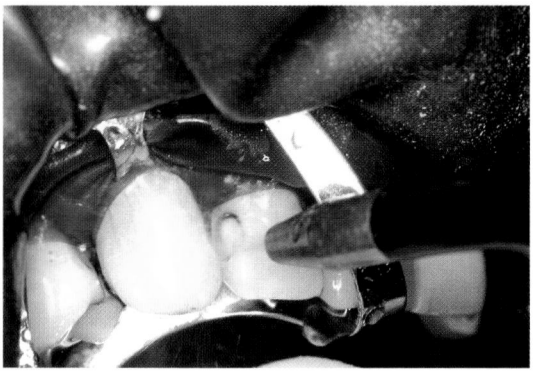

Fig. 11-16b Thoroughly washed.

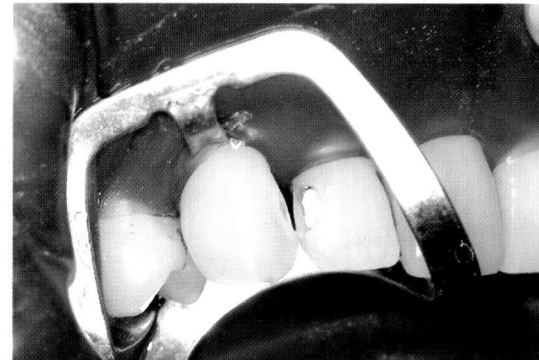

Fig. 11-16c Dried so that the enamel appears frosted.

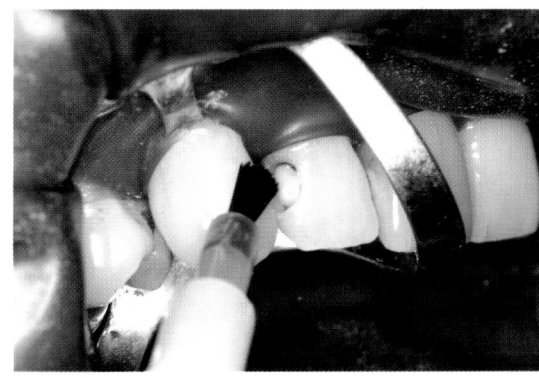

Fig. 11-17 Light-cured bonding resin applied.

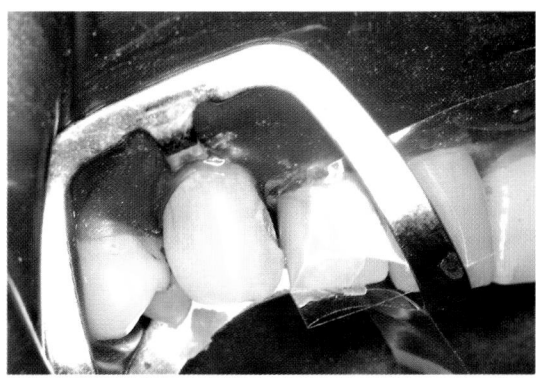

Fig. 11-18 Composite resin applied and matrix tightly adapted prior to light curing.

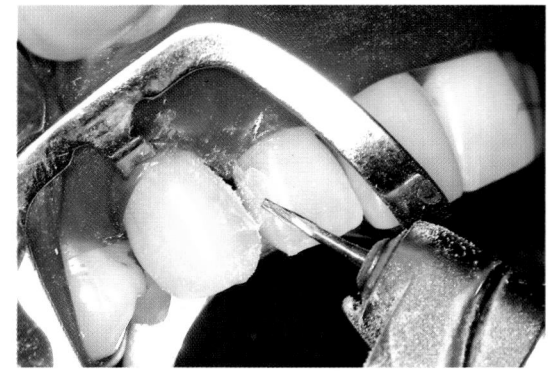

Fig. 11-19 Composite resin finished with fluted carbide burs run along the cavosurface margins (not across the restoration/enamel edges) in order to prevent damage to enamel prisms, which could produce a white line.

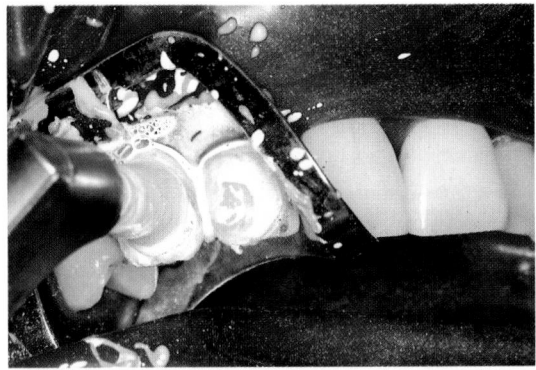

Fig. 11-20 Composite resin polished with a slurry of 30 μm aluminium oxide and rubber cup.

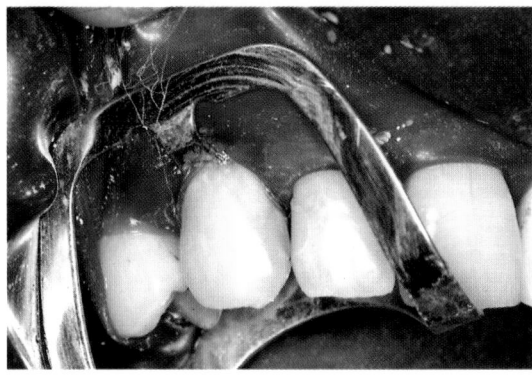

Fig. 11-21 Completed restorations in teeth 13 and 12.

The Class IV restoration

Glass-ionomer cements are brittle materials lacking high flexural strength. They are unsuitable for use in high-tensile–stress-bearing areas. However, like many brittle materials, their compressive strength is adequate where the main occlusal forces place the cement in compression. For this reason, small occlusal restorations perform very well.

The main use for the glass-ionomer cements in the Class IV restoration is as a lining for the dentine. Even in these cases, reliance on the adhesive properties of the cement as the sole means of retention should not be expected. Comparison of the flexural strengths of the various restorative materials in Table 11-1 shows clearly that the composite resin materials are far better suited for the restoration of the Class IV carious lesion. Even in these cases, certain rules should be followed:

Table 11-1 Comparison of flexural strengths

Material	Breaking stress (MPa)
Glass-ionomer Type II	9–30
Glass-ionomer Type II cermet	32–40
Composite resin microfil	60–80
Composite resin hybrid and small particle size	110–135

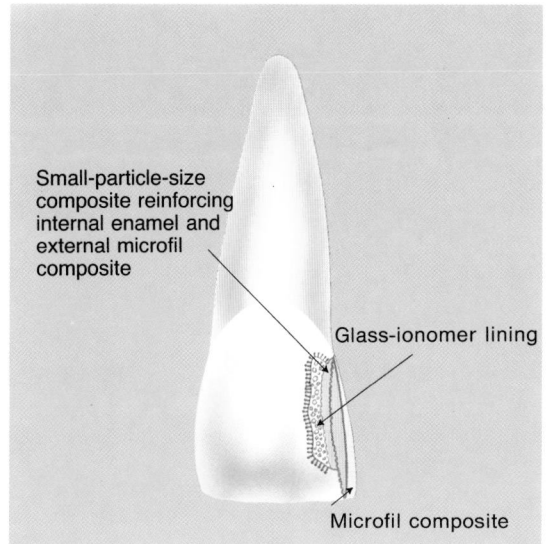

Small-particle-size composite reinforcing internal enamel and external microfil composite

Glass-ionomer lining

Microfil composite

Fig. 11-22 Diagram of minimum thickness (0.5 mm) of glass-ionomer cement lining for a Class IV restoration.

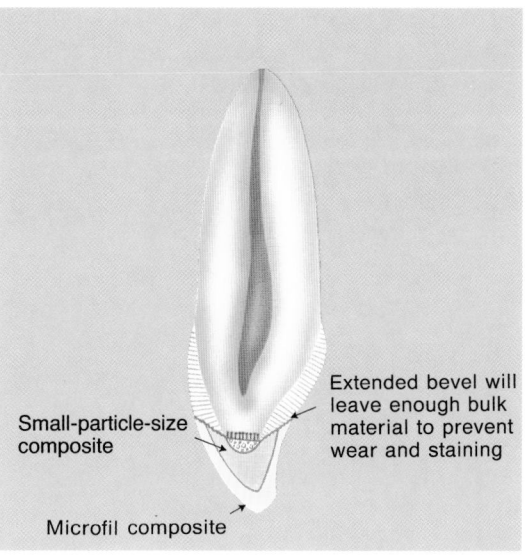

Small-particle-size composite

Extended bevel will leave enough bulk material to prevent wear and staining

Microfil composite

Fig. 11-23 Composite resin should be attached to enamel using extended bevels. Use the higher-strength small-particle-size or hybrid composite to reinforce the veneer material.

1. Glass-ionomer cement linings should be placed only on dentine and should be at least 0.5 mm thick (Fig. 11-22). Where insufficient space is available and the lining is thin, the use of acid etching may weaken the cement and is therefore not advised.
2. Composite resin materials should be attached to enamel using extended bevels to increase surface areas for attachment (Fig. 11-23).
3. Stress on the glass-ionomer cement/ composite resin laminate restoration will be reduced where there is still some supporting incisal enamel left to maintain incisal edge-to-edge contact and incisal guidance (Fig. 11-24).
4. The main bulk of the composite resin restoration should be composed of higher-strength hybrid or small-particle-size materials. Microfilled compos-

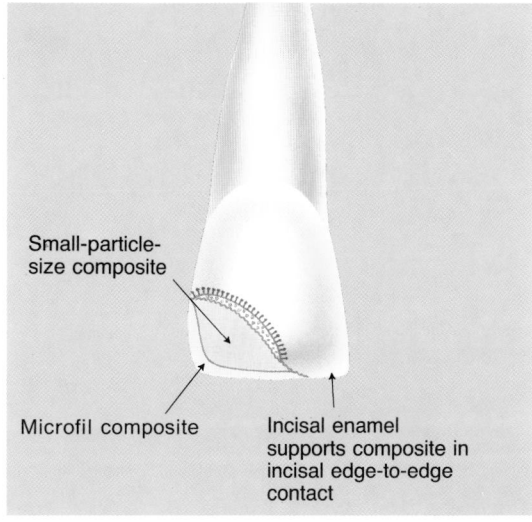

Small-particle-size composite

Microfil composite

Incisal enamel supports composite in incisal edge-to-edge contact

Fig. 11-24 Diagram showing how incisal enamel may support the composite resin in incisal edge-to-edge contact. Hybrid or small-particle-size composite resins should be used to reinforce the main body.

Figs. 11-25a and b The least favourable types of Class IV restorations.

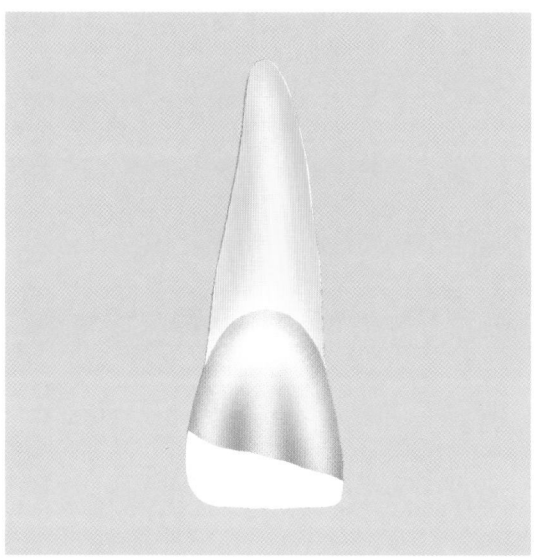

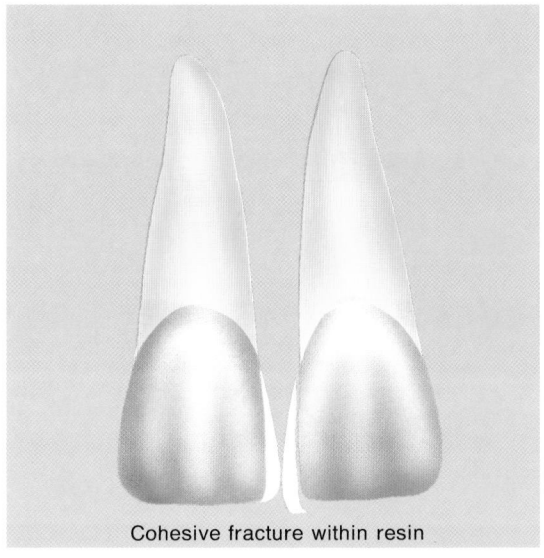

Cohesive fracture within resin

Fig. 11-25a Stress on the restoration will be greater without natural enamel support.

Fig. 11-25b Where teeth are to be widened for cosmetic reasons, support for the approximal composite diminishes with increasing thickness, and the risk of cohesive fracture within the resin is high.

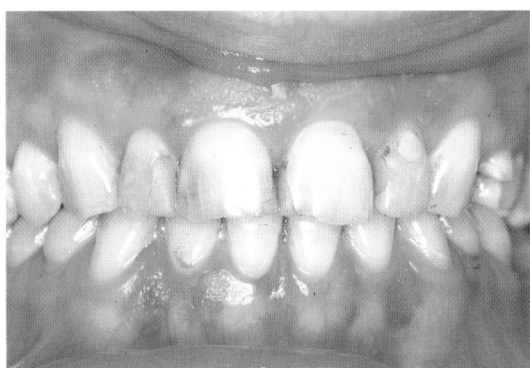

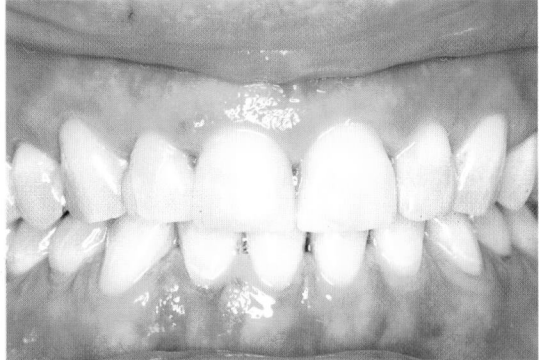

Fig. 11-26a Anterior restorations prior to replacement with glass-ionomer cement/composite resin laminates.

Fig. 11-26b Anterior glass-ionomer cement/composite resin restoration in teeth 12, 11, 21, and 22.

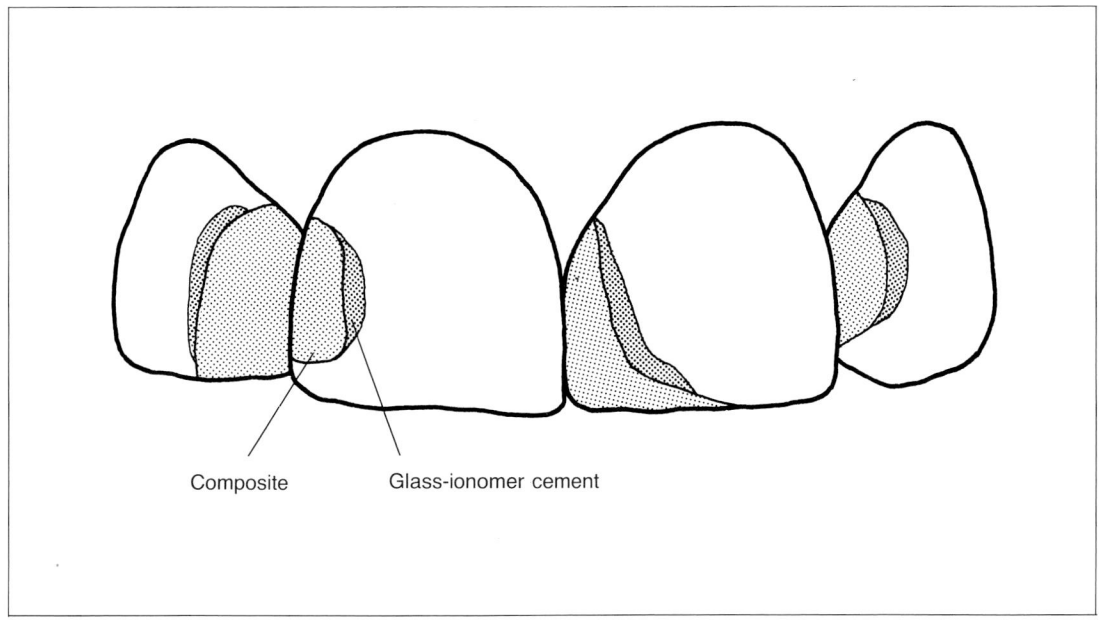

Composite   Glass-ionomer cement

Fig. 11-27 Outline tracing of teeth in Fig. 11-26 showing that incisal area will still provide some natural support. The glass-ionomer cement used as a dentine replacement is also shown in cross section.

ite resins, because of their susceptibility to fatigue fractures, should only
be used as thin veneers to improve
surface finish (Fig. 11-24).

The most favourable type of Class IV
carious lesions for restoration with glass-
ionomer cement/composite resin laminates is shown in Figs. 11-22 and 11-24,
and the least favourable in Figs. 11-25a and
b. Clinical use of the materials is illustrated in Fig. 11-26. Although on a long-
term basis the patient would probably be
better served by the insertion of porcelain veneer crowns, the remaining incisal
enamel in this case is favourable for the
support of composite resin restorations
(Fig. 11-26b). Examination of the outline
tracing of these teeth in Fig. 11-27 shows
that the entire incisal area will still provide some natural enamel support. Only

in the case of tooth 12 is there a likeli-
hood of failure through shear stresses.
Class III composite resin restorations can
benefit aesthetically with glass-ionomer
cement acting as a dentine replacement,
thereby preventing the halo effect that
can occur with the more translucent
composite resin alone (see Fig. 11-26, in
particular, tooth 11).
  It is not within the scope of this book to
give detailed procedures for placement
of Class IV composite resin restorations;
the reader is referred to other texts on
the subject (Simonsen, 1978; Albers,
1985; Jordan, 1987).

Laminate veneers

Increasing interest in the use of labial veneers made in either porcelain or composite resin has led to demands for better dentine-bonding agents. At present neither the resin bonding agents or glass-ionomer cements can be regarded as a complete answer to securing long-term adhesion, particularly where tensile or shear stresses prevail. Permanent adhesion to dentine by glass-ionomer cements attached either to laboratory processed composite resin veneers or porcelain laminates depends not only on the quality of the mechanical bond produced by acid etching of the cement, but also on the cohesive strength of the cements. In simple terms, the bond is only as strong as the cement.

The cohesive strength of glass-ionomer cement is between 4 and 30 MPa (Prosser et al., 1984), and bond strengths to dentine have been assessed at 2 to 7 MPa (Powis et al., 1982). By contrast, bond strengths of composite materials to enamel can be as high as 20 MPa (Rider et al., 1977). Clearly, attachment of laminate veneers to enamel surfaces is preferable but is limited by the space available for the laminate. A study of Fig. 11-28 shows the average thickness of enamel covering a maxillary central incisor. Provided that the tooth to be veneered is close to these figures, then a bulk of 0.6 mm of laminate can be applied, except at the cervical aspect (Fig. 11-28). Even then it should be recognised that when using porcelain, reduction of the wall thickness plays a significant part in the longevity of the restoration. All dental ceramics tend to fail at the same critical strain, of the order of 0.1% (Jones, 1983). For this reason, any increase in strength and toughness can only be achieved by an increase in stiffness (elastic modulus).

Crystalline materials such as aluminous porcelains or glass-ceramics are therefore better materials for use in laminate construction. Aluminous porcelain is too opaque to be used as the main veneer and is only suitable as a thin opaquer. Even with this improvement in toughness, the clinician should be aware that the strength of a laminate is related to thickness and conforms to the law of beams. A laminate of 1.0 mm would therefore be eight times stronger than a laminate of 0.5 mm. If the laminate is attached only to enamel, then the enamel's higher elastic modulus will provide better support. By contrast, if the major part of the labial face involves dentine, then a glass-ionomer base, although being firmly bonded to the laminate, may be subject to increased stress and result in bond failure or fracture of the porcelain laminate (Fig. 11-29).

Certain recommendations can therefore be made in relation to the use of porcelain or reinforced plastic laminates bonded to glass-ionomer cement bases.

Porcelain laminates

1. Where possible, the laminate should be bonded only to enamel (Fig. 11-30).
2. Where dentine is exposed, the laminate should be bonded to at least 1 mm of peripheral enamel (Fig. 11-31). Do not rely on glass-ionomer bases as the sole means of retention.
3. If the dentine area exposed exceeds 50% of the facial surface and incisal enamel is missing, then full-veneer porcelain crowns should be used (Fig. 11-31).
4. Where cervical enamel is removed or missing and only peripheral dentine remains for attachment, a cervical fill-

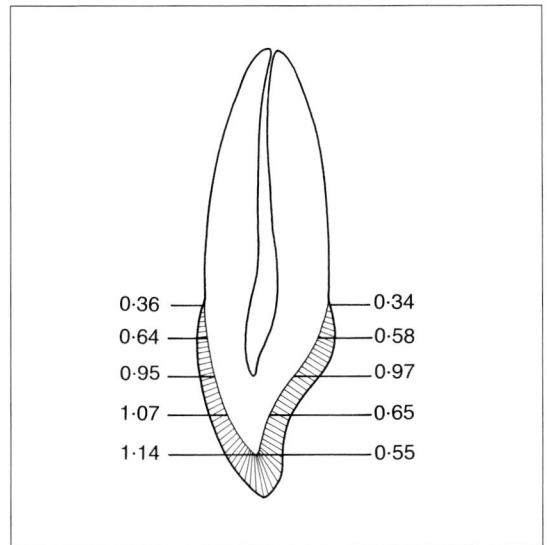

Fig. 11-28 Average thickness (mm) of enamel on a maxillary central incisor.

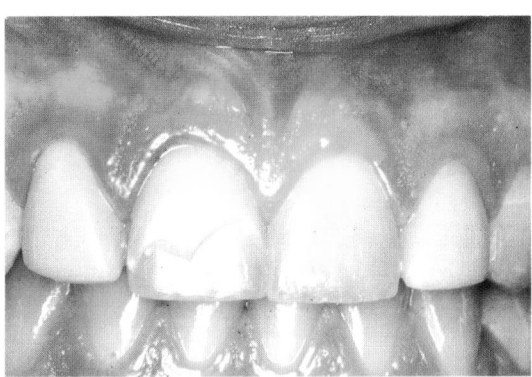

Fig. 11-29 Horizontal fracture of porcelain veneer facing on tooth 11, and debonding of facing on tooth 21.

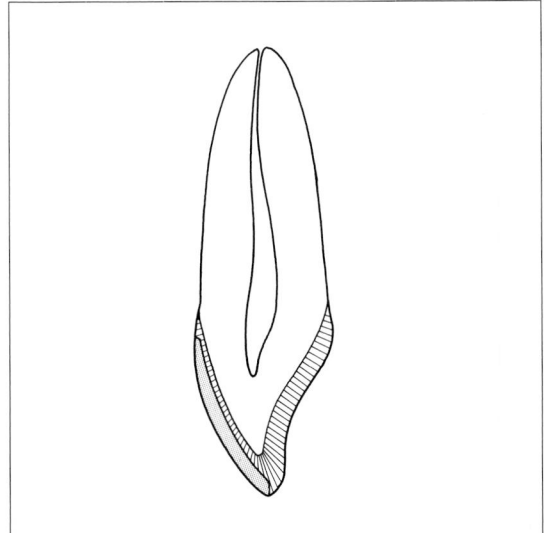

Fig. 11-30 The ideal preparation for a porcelain laminate, where all the porcelain is bonded to enamel and the preparation ensures complete support for the porcelain. However, many teeth are too thin to allow a finish line to be placed internally, and an incisal butt joint is necessary. See Fig. 11-35, *d*.

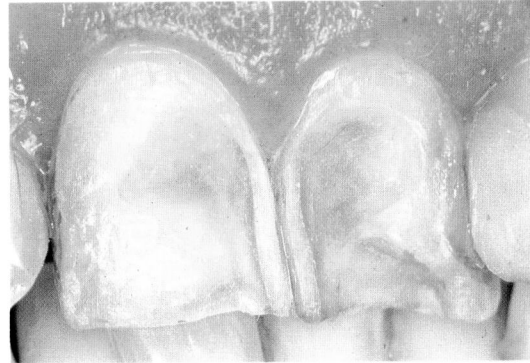

Fig. 11-31 Remaining structure on tooth 11 is just sufficient to support a porcelain veneer but the dentine should be carefully lined with glass-ionomer cement. Remaining structure on tooth 21 unfavourable for placement of porcelain veneer due to loss of incisal support and excessive exposure of dentine.

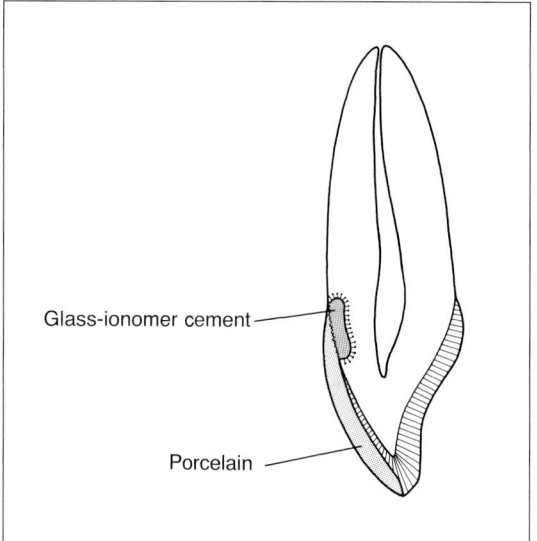

Fig. 11-32 Diagram showing replacement of cervical dentine with glass-ionomer cement prior to bonding with a porcelain veneer. Ideally the glass-ionomer cement should be at least 0.5 mm thick.

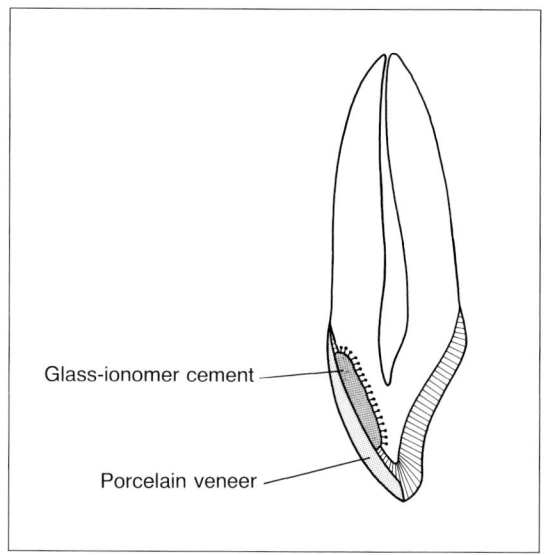

Fig. 11-33 The use of Type II glass-ionomer cements as replacements for heavily discoloured dentine.

ing of glass-ionomer cement must be made and the laminate finished to the glass-ionomer cement/dentine junction (Fig. 11-32). This procedure is the least favourable for maintaining permanent adhesion.

5. Where dentine is involved and glass-ionomer bases are contemplated, a minimum thickness of 0.5 mm of glass-ionomer cement should be applied (Fig. 11-32).

6. Where optimum aesthetics is required and the dentine is heavily stained, it should be removed to a depth of 0.5 mm and restored with a glass-ionomer cement that acts as a *dentine replacement,* restoring both contour and colour background. Type II restorative glass-ionomer cements are more translucent than the base cements, but will need a minimum setting period of ten minutes prior to acid etching (Fig. 11-33). They are better

applied prior to impression taking and only acid etched at the final visit for cementation of the porcelain laminate.

The design of tooth preparations for porcelain veneers and their limitations has been well covered (Albers, 1985; Horn, 1983; Calamia, 1985). At present the aesthetics on anterior teeth leave much to be desired when compared with full-veneer porcelain crowns. New methods of building full-veneer crowns involving lateral segmental building of porcelain powder and the use of dentin-oenamels and high-chroma cervical porcelains has transformed the standards of cosmetic dentistry (Fig. 11-34). It is difficult to create colour in depth in a thin porcelain veneer; greater reliance has to be placed on the use of coloured resin cements.

Constructing porcelain veneers without tooth preparation is not advised since the

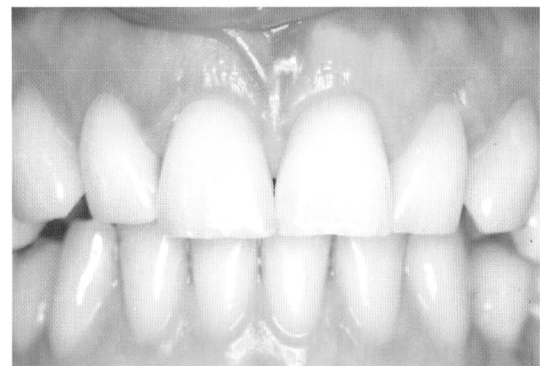

Fig. 11-34a Anterior aluminous porcelain crown on tooth 11.

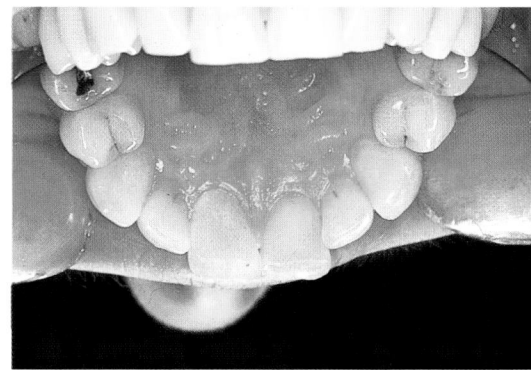

Fig. 11-34b Lingual view of anterior aluminous porcelain crown on tooth 11.

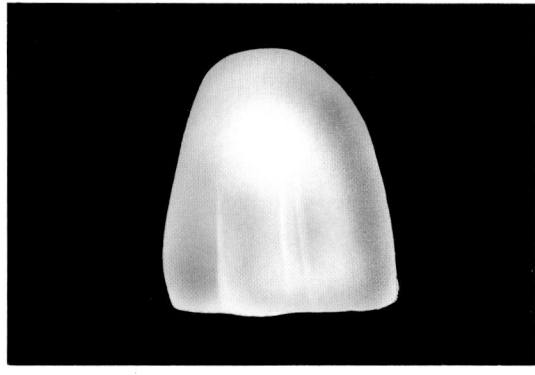

Fig. 11-34c Diagram of method of building colour using internal segmental enamel techniques on tooth 11.

resultant overcontour of the laminate may cause serious periodontal problems. Even when the tooth is prepared many veneers do not fit accurately and are doomed to failure. The design of incisal edges also plays a major role in the incidence of fracture (Fig. 11-35). Thin labial faces placed in tension are very likely to exceed the 0.1% strain level, causing failure. Success with porcelain laminates is therefore very dependent upon first-rate technical support and a thorough knowledge of the design of tooth preparations. These can be excellent restora-

175

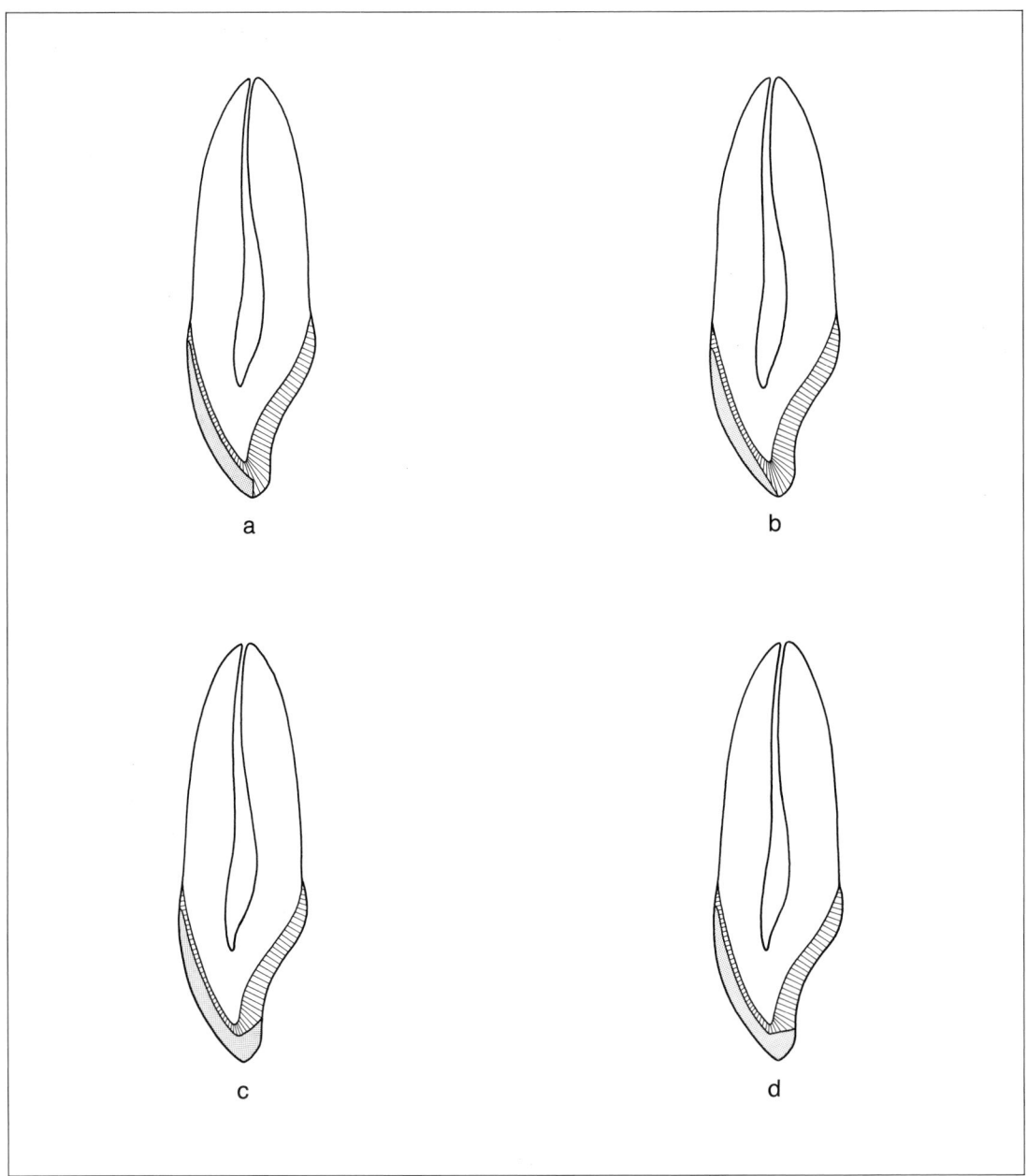

Fig. 11-35 Types of preparations used for porcelain veneer facings, showing the most likely order of magnitude of stresses to produce fracture, in descending order: *(a)* intraenamel preparation; *(b)* feather-edge preparation; *(c)* acute incisal bevel preparation; *(d)* butt joint incisal preparation.

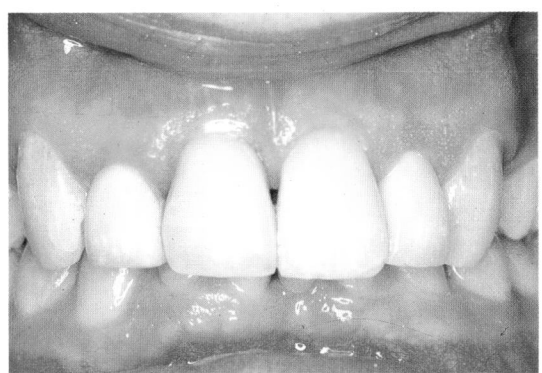

Fig. 11-36a Porcelain veneer facing on tooth 12 with aluminous porcelain crowns on teeth 11 and 22. Facing used to realign tooth 12, which is lingually retruded.

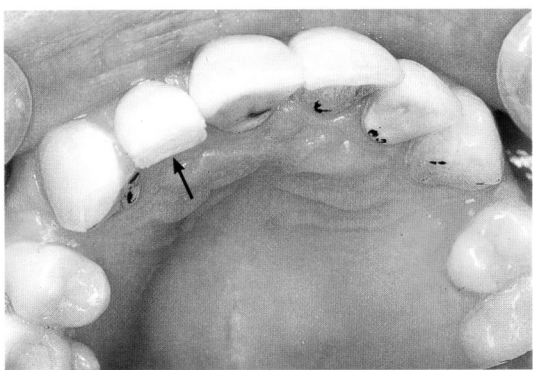

Fig. 11-36b Lingual mirror view showing occlusal contacts giving full support for porcelain veneer facing (arrow) on tooth 12. Note the thickness of the facing for better development of internal colour. Thinner facings would need to rely on coloured cements to achieve a good aesthetic effect.

tions for replacing discoloured enamel or malaligned teeth (Fig. 11-36), but if used indiscriminately, the risk of long-term staining at the margins and possible fracture should be explained to the patient.

Many adult teeth are either worn or deficient in critical stress-bearing areas, so that their restoration needs careful thought and a knowledge of occlusion. In most cases the full-veneer porcelain crown with lingual metal backing provides a better long-term result.

Composite resin laminate veneers

Indirect veneers made in resin are not new. They were first used in the 1930s by Pincus (Albers, 1985) to improve the appearance of actors. These veneers were cemented temporarily into position using denture adhesives and were only used during performances.

Two types of veneer are now available: prefabricated acrylic resin veneers such as Mastique,* which are available in several preformed shapes and shades, and laboratory-processed veneers made to an impression of the labial face of a patient's tooth. Their use has been described in a number of texts (Albers, 1985; Jordan, 1987; Garber et al., 1988).

The laboratory-cured materials that are now becoming more popular are generally made from microfilled composite-type resins and may be cured under vacuum (Visio-Gem†) or pressure (Isosit‡). Custom-made composite resin veneers are generally easier to fit than porcelain laminates and can be finished and polished to a high degree of accuracy. Their main defects are that, as highly cross-linked materials, they are brittle and do not form strong bonds to the resin luting cements, and they lack the abrasion resistance of porcelain laminates. They are

*L.D. Caulk Co., Milford, Del.
†ESPE GmbH, Seefeld/Oberbay, West Germany, and Valley Stream, N.Y.
‡Vivadent Inc., Tonawanda, N.Y.

cheaper to produce than porcelain laminates, but still do not compare with the lower costs of directly bonded composite resins. The recommendations for use of porcelain laminates with glass-ionomer cement bases are also applicable to the composite resin laminate veneers. However, one difference in property should be emphasized. Composite resin veneers are more flexible materials (low modulus), and under occlusal load will deform more easily than ceramics. Their use in high-stress-bearing areas may therefore cause loss of seal of the glass-ionomer cement/dentine bond. If this occurs, then the enamel bond remains the sole means of retention. For this reason, composite resin laminate veneers perform better where the peripheral enamel is intact.

References

Albers, H.F. (1985) Tooth-Coloured Restoratives. 7th ed. Cotati, Calif.: Alto Books.

Calamia, J.R. (1985) Etched porcelain veneers: The current state of the art. Quintessence Int. 16:5–12.

Garber, D.A., Goldstein, R.E., and Feinman, R.A. (1988) Porcelain Laminate Veneers. Chicago: Quintessence Publ. Co.

Gwinnett, A.J. (1967) The ultrastructure of prismless enamel of permanent human teeth. Arch. Oral Biol. 12:381–389.

Horn, H. (1983) Porcelain laminate veneers bonded to etched enamel. Dent. Clin. North Am. 27:671–684.

Jones, D.W. (1983) The strength and strengthening mechanisms of dental ceramics. pp. 83–141 In J.W. McLean (ed.) Dental Ceramics: Proceedings of the First International Symposium on Ceramics. Chicago: Quintessence Publ. Co.

Jordan, R.E. (1987) Esthetic Composite Bonding: Techniques and Materials. St. Louis: C. V. Mosby Co.

McLean, J.W., Powis, D.R., Prosser, H.J., and Wilson, A.D. (1985) The use of glass-ionomer cements in bonding composite resins to dentine. Br. Dent. J. 158:410–414.

Powis, D.R., Folleras, T., Merson, S.A., and Wilson, A.D. (1982) Improved adhesion of a glass-ionomer cement to dentine and enamel. J. Dent. Res. 61:1416–1422.

Prosser, H.J., Powis, D.R., Brant, P., and Wilson, A.D. (1984) The characterization of glass-ionomer cements. 7. The physical properties of cement materials J. Dent. 12:231–240.

Rider, M., Tanner, A.N., and Kenny, B. (1977). Investigation of the adhesive properties of dental composite materials using an improved tensile test procedure and scanning electron microscopy. J. Dent. Res. 56: 368–372.

Simonsen, R. (1978) Clinical Application of the Acid Etch Technique, Chicago: Quintessence Publ. Co.

Van Noort, R. (1983) Controversial aspects of composite resin restorative materials. Br. Dent. J. 155:383–385.

Walker, T.M., Jensen, M.E., and Chan, D.C.N. (1986) Acid penetration through glass-ionomer bases. J. Dent. Res. 64:(Special Issue):345 (abstr. 1580).

Chapter 12

Treatment of Early Carious Lesions

The diagnosis and treatment of early dental caries remains an area of controversy and arouses great emotion among clinicians and academicians. Phrases such as "overprescription" and "supervised neglect" are good examples of the divergence of opinion.

Kidd (1983) has given a masterly survey of the problems involved in the diagnosis and management of the early carious lesion in permanent teeth and explained the importance of making an accurate diagnosis.

Dental caries is a dynamic process of alternating demineralization and remineralization (Figs. 12-1 and 12-2). As Kidd (1983) has stated:

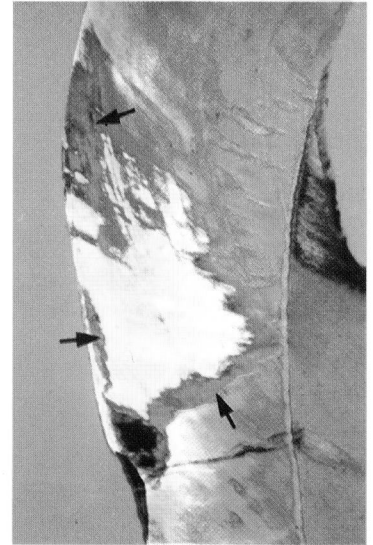

Fig. 12-1 Ground section of a carious lesion viewed in polarized light after imbibition with quinoline (original magnification ×60). Dark zones *(arrows)* indicating partial healing are obvious at the advancing front of the lesion, within the lesion, and at the surface of the lesion. Reprinted with permission from Kidd (1984).

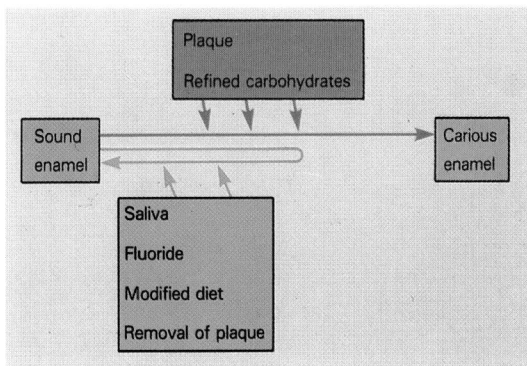

Fig. 12-2 The balance between sound and carious enamel. Reprinted with permission from Kidd (1984).

Sound enamel may become carious in time if plaque bacteria are given the sugary substrate they need to produce acid. However, saliva is an excellent remineralising fluid particularly if it contains the fluoride ion. . . . If the disease can be diagnosed in its earliest stages the balance can be tipped in favour of repair by use of fluoride, modifying diet and attempting to remove plaque.

In this chapter we are more concerned with the treatment of the carious lesion that has reached a stage where demineralization is considered to be irreversible. However, a discussion of the role of glass-ionomer cements as fissure sealants in the prevention of fissure caries is also pertinent.

The role of fissure sealants in arresting caries

In a recent joint report on fissure sealants (1986) the British Dental Association/Department of Health and Social Security Working Party defined a sealant restoration as:

The restoration of the fissured surface of a tooth, in which removal of caries has been limited and with no extension into noncarious tissue, the cavity being filled with a suitable adhesive material in conjunction with a fissure sealant which extends over the remainder of the fissured surface of the tooth.

Some of the conclusions and recommendations made in the report were:

1. Fissure sealants, if properly applied and maintained, are effective in preventing dental caries in pits and fissures.

2. Fissure sealant materials should be nontransparent or coloured to facilitate subsequent inspection and maintenance.

3. The use of fissure sealants is recommended as an alternative to amalgam fillings to treat questionable or early carious lesions in pits and fissures. It will sometimes be appropriate for the dentist to explore the extent of the lesion and to remove caries before applying the fissure sealant, in which case a filled composite resin or polyalkenoate (glass-ionomer) cement in a combined sealant restorative technique may be required.

The report also considered the fate of potentially pathogenic bacteria sealed in dental cavities and in a review of the literature confirmed that the number of viable bacteria left beneath restorations decreases with time. The microbiological implications of sealing carious lesions have been reviewed by Handelman and coworkers (1986), who conclude that bacteria have great difficulty in surviving beneath an intact seal. A limited number of organisms may persist in some lesions but do not appear capable of continued destruction of tooth structure under these circumstances. Indeed, the carious lesion may ultimately become sterile. There is therefore convincing evidence that fissure sealants are capable of arresting the carious process.

Fissure sealing with glass-ionomer cements

A cariostatic action on the tooth is an essential property of a caries-preventive material. One way in which this favourable result may be achieved is by topical release of fluoride, although the mechanism is not fully understood. It has variously been suggested that fluoride converts hydroxyapatite to the less soluble fluorapatite by ion-exchange; that it promotes formation of well-ordered crystals of apatite; and that it inhibits glycolysis and the corresponding conversion of sugars to acids (Levine, 1976). The glass-ionomer cement continually releases fluoride ions from the matrix and the filler as the sodium salt, as explained in chapter 8. Because the cement becomes attached to the enamel via ionic and polar bonds, the intimate molecular contact facilitates fluoride ion exchange with the hydroxyl ions in the apatite of the surrounding enamel in the fissure. By contrast, a filling material that does not adhere by molecular interactions would leave gaps between the filling and tooth, so that if it released fluoride, ion exchange would be hindered. Clearly, dynamic materials such as the glass-ionomer cements offer a better chance of preventing recurrent caries than composite resin fissure sealants, which are inert.

However, when resins are attached to enamel by acid-etching techniques they provide stronger mechanical bonds than the molecular bonds of glass-ionomer cements. For this reason, glass-ionomer cements, when used as fissure sealants, are not successful when placed in fissures that have no orifice. Although the cement may be applied to such a fissure, it will soon be lost through erosion/abrasion (Fig. 12-3). By contrast, when glass-ionomer cement is used in patent fissures as sealants they are very successful (McLean and Wilson, 1974). In an individual clinical study spanning some two years McLean and Wilson reported a failure rate of only 10% in the first year and 4% in the second year. More recently, Mount (1984), in a limited clinical

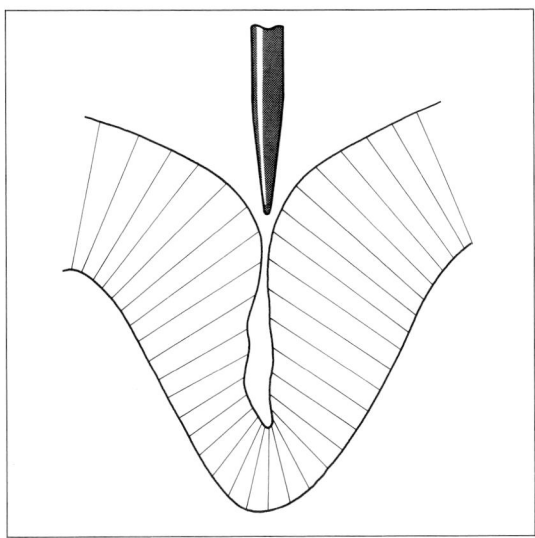

Fig. 12-3 Fissure that is not wide enough to retain glass-ionomer cement.

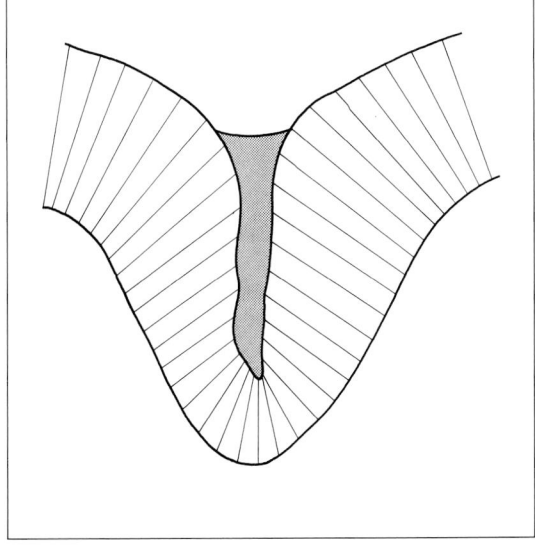

Fig. 12-4 Fissure that is suitable for sealing with glass-ionomer cement. A sharp explorer tip should enter the fissure.

study, found retention in the depth of the fissures beyond six years. The cement penetrated into narrow fissures and tended to wear away evenly rather than peel away in bulk, as composite resin is prone to do.

From these studies certain recommendations can be made:

1. Glass-ionomer cements are only suitable as fissure sealants where the pit or fissure orifice is patent. This size of fissure should allow a sharp explorer tip to enter the crevice, and is thus clinically detectable. The fissure orifice is generally in excess of 100 μm wide (Fig. 12-4).
2. Fissures or pits that are not patent and provide no crevice for entry by the cement are better treated with light-curing resin sealants.

Glass-ionomer cement fissure sealant technique

A number of rapid-setting glass-ionomer cements are now available as fissure sealing materials (see chapter 2). These cements should be applied as low-viscosity mixes. The following clinical technique is recommended:

1. Isolate the tooth or teeth in one quadrant with cotton rolls and dry the surface. Swab a solution of 25% poly-(acrylic acid) into the fissures and work the solution into the depth of the crevices with a sharp explorer. Debris may be raked out with the explorer. The cleaning treatment should not exceed 30 seconds (Fig. 12-5). Do not use prophylactic pastes or pumice because these materials can block the fissure entrance or contaminate the surface.

2. Clean off the debris and poly(acrylic acid) solution with air/water spray and dry the tooth with warm air.
3. While the fissure is being cleaned, dispense the glass-ionomer cement onto a mixing pad and mix according to the manufacturer's instructions. Using a refrigerated glass slab will prolong working time, but this may be undesirable if quick setting is required in the more difficult cases where saliva control is a problem.
4. Pick up a small bead of the cement on the end of the explorer (Fig. 12-6) and work it up and down the fissures. The low viscosity of the glass-ionomer water-based cements allow excellent wetting and easy penetration of the fissures (Fig. 12-7). Add more cement as required.
5. Immediately after application of the cement apply a thin sheet of wax (such as Kerr's green occlusal indicator wax*) to the occlusal surface of the tooth and press it firmly into position (Fig. 12-8). This technique will provide a very effective seal, allowing the child to relax and thereby avoid the discomfort of muscle fatigue.
6. After setting, remove the wax and immediately apply a coat of varnish or a light-cured bonding agent to the sealant. Check occlusion and remove any excess cement with sharp excavators or a slow-running small round bur. Apply another coat of varnish or, preferably, a light-cured bonding agent (Fig. 12-9).

Use of capsulated cements and syringes for applying sealants

Where multiple applications of sealant are required it is often preferable to use a modern capsulated glass-ionomer cement as a fissure sealant that can be in-

*Kwik-Wax, Kerr Mfg. Co., Div. of Sybron Corp., Romulus, Mich.

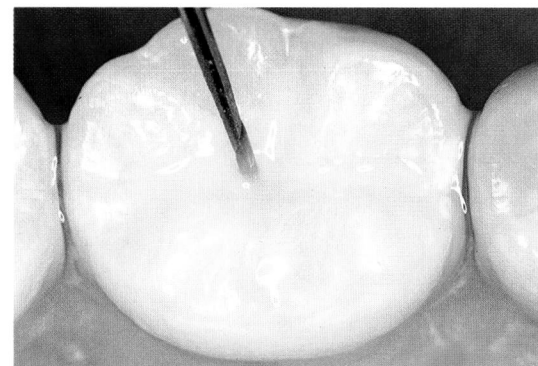

Fig. 12-5 Poly(acrylic acid) solution applied and raked into fissure with a sharp explorer.

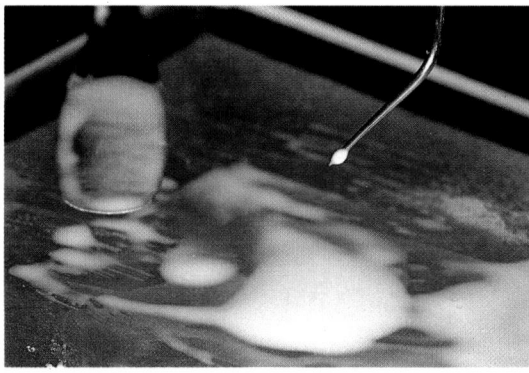

Fig. 12-6 Ideal mix of Type III cement for fissure sealing. A small bead of the cement is picked up on an explorer and transferred to the fissure.

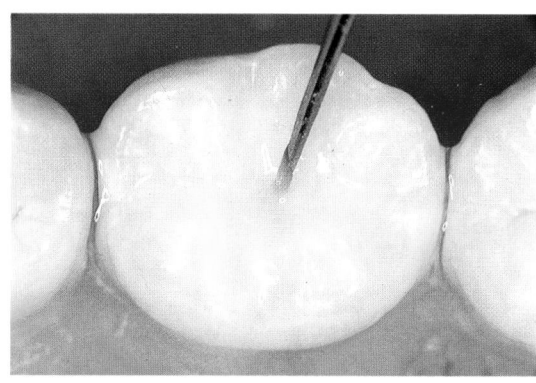

Fig. 12-7 Cement raked into fissure.

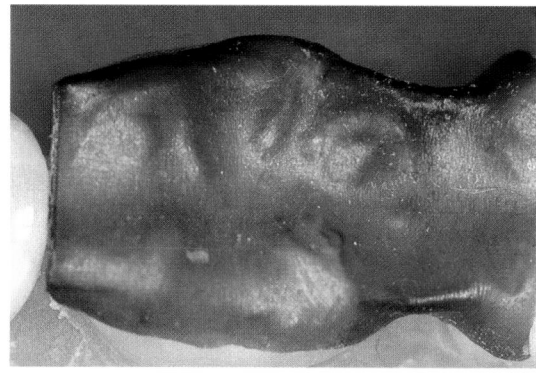

Fig. 12-8 Thin sheet wax applied over surface to protect the cement during setting.

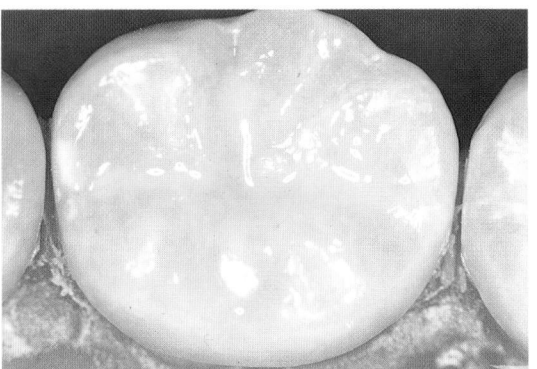

Fig. 12-9 Glass-ionomer cement after trimming excess, and application of another coat of varnish. A light-cured bonding resin may also be used.

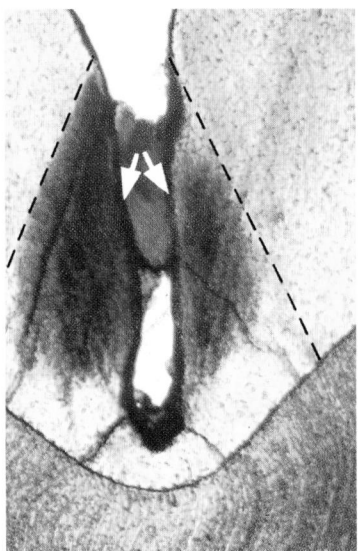

Fig. 12-10 Ground section of a carious enamel fissure viewed in transmitted light after imbibition with water (original magnification ×60). Note the lesions form bilaterally on the walls of the fissure *(arrows)* and advance to the enamel/dentine junction, giving the lesion the shape of a triangle with its base on the enamel/dentine junction *(dotted lines)*. Reprinted with permission from Kidd (1984).

jected into the fissures. In the case of hand-mixed materials, these can also be placed in a Hawe Centrix syringe* and injected into the fissures. However, it is still recommended that an explorer be used to rake the liquid cement into the fissure. This procedure, together with hydraulic pressure from the protective wax matrix, will ensure close adaptation to the walls of the fissure.

Treatment of fissure caries

The diagnosis of caries in fissures remains an area of great controversy, since the white spot lesion forms bilaterally on the walls of the fissure and is not easily visible (Mortimer, 1964). Kidd (1983) has shown that as the lesion advances to the enamel/dentine junction, it forms a triangle with the enamel/dentine junction as its base (Fig. 12-10). Unfortunately, a fissure that looks caries-free may histologically show signs of early lesion formation, and a so-called sticky fissure may be caries-free even though a sharp explorer can enter a patent fissure and bind on the walls, producing a tactile sensation of carious dentine. For this reason, diagnosis of early fissure caries should depend more upon visual examination rather than tactile exploration. Aids to achieving an accurate diagnosis are as follows:

1. Use magnifying loops.
2. Use fibre-optic lighting.
3. Clean and dry the teeth.
4. Use accurate bite-wing radiographs.

*Centrix Inc., Stratford, Conn.

5. Where explorers are used, do not exert pressure; rather, use them as a diagnostic tool to assess the width of the fissure orifice.

Clinicians are not only reporting strange caries patterns under occlusal fissures but are also becoming increasingly aware of the danger of missing occlusal caries (Stean, 1982; Vellender, 1982: Usher, 1982; Albers, 1985). These reports can no longer be regarded as anecdotal; they reveal a definite pattern of change in the disease. Fluoride-enriched enamel is hard and firm, but bacterial access is still gained through cracks and open fissures. This can result in a mushroom caries effect in the dentine, where, on opening the tooth, a large cavity is observed (Fig. 12-11). Clearly good bite-wing radiographs are essential in detecting dentine caries. The Backer-Dirk's holder is a useful tool to ensure reproducibility in serial radiographs (Fig. 12-12).

Even with all these modern aids and techniques the trained epidemiologist is only 70% to 80% reliable; examiner variability can make the choice of examiner as important as the choice of the test substance (Shaw and Murray, 1975). A "wait-and-see" policy can therefore be even more devastating than early mechanical intervention. The practising clinician should recognize that *caries is mainly ravaging dentine, not enamel,* and that pit and fissure caries is more rapid in its progress than approximal lesions, cavitation occurring after less than one year up to the age of 13 years (Backer-Dirks, 1961).

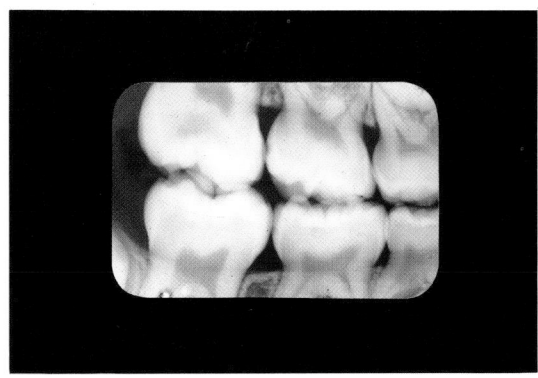

Fig. 12-11a Radiograph of intact enamel showing extensive caries in the dentine in teeth 16 and 46. Courtesy of F.J. Hill, M.D.S., D. Orth., R.C.S.

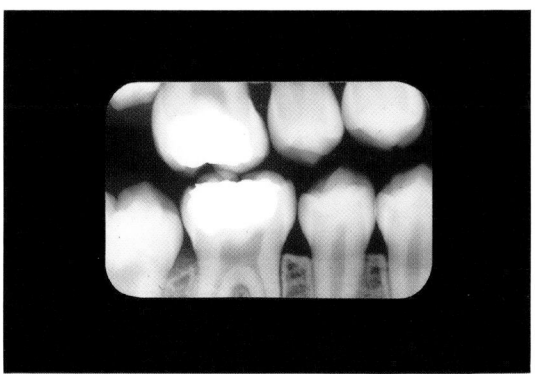

Fig. 12-11b Lesions after restoration with amalgam alloy.

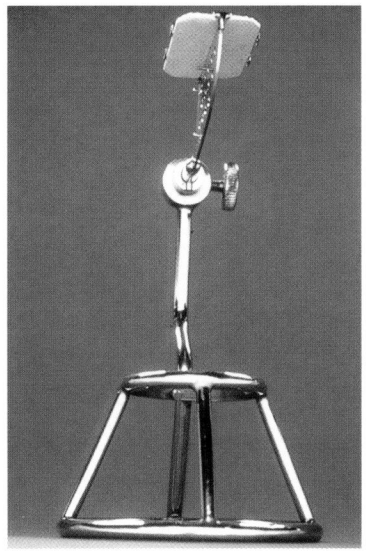

Fig. 12-12 The Backer-Dirks holder to aid in production of reproducible bite-wing radiographs. Reprinted with permission from Kidd (1984).

185

Guidelines for treating fissure caries

The following recommendations are made from experience in treating early carious lesions with glass-ionomer cements over the past 15 years:

1. Where radiological evidence shows caries, mechanical preparation is essential.
2. Where no radiological evidence is available and the fissure appears intact and the orifice is not patent, then no treatment is advised except for considering fissure sealing with a light-cured composite resin sealant.
3. Where no radiological evidence is available and the fissure is patent, fissure sealing should be mandatory, particularly where the patient's oral hygiene is poor or there is existing occlusal caries.
4. Where no radiological evidence is available and the fissure is stained and difficult to clean or the tooth enamel is discoloured, investigation of the fissure should be made using a fissure cleaning and widening procedure (Fig. 12-13).

Although procedure no. 4 remains controversial, it involves such minimal intervention that cases treated where no caries is detected can be justified on the grounds that it totally eliminates the risk factor of ignoring a carious fissure that could produce the devastating results shown in Fig. 12-11.

How do we diagnose the fissure that is difficult to clean? First, any explorer that can just enter a fissure will indicate that the fissure is patent with an opening of at least 80 μm, about the diameter of an explorer tip (McLean and von Fraunhofer, 1971). Where the explorer enters to a depth of 1 mm or more, it is likely that the fissure opening is at least 160 μm (Fig. 12-14).

Fissure widening and filling procedures

A fissure filling does not involve preparing an occlusal cavity but is merely a procedure where the fissure is widened and, where present, the carious dentine is removed using slow-speed handpieces. Fissure widening can be a painless procedure—for a child an experience no more traumatic than polishing the teeth. The procedure is as follows:

1. Using a very fine diamond point,* running at 150,000 rpm under water spray, enter the fissure and slightly widen it with a gentle rocking movement so that the base can be explored (Fig. 12-15). Use fibre-optic lighting and magnifying loops.
2. If dentine caries is not detected, no further widening or deepening of the fissure is necessary. Where caries is present the diamond point will usually drop into the softened dentine.
3. Where caries is detected, it should be removed with a slow-running handpiece and a small round bur (Fig. 12-16). Only a near-exposure of the pulp should be lined with calcium hydroxide. Do not extend the cavity into the enamel beyond the necessary access to remove all the carious dentine. The remaining fissures should be left intact except for slight widening (Fig. 12-16).
4. Isolate the tooth or teeth with cotton rolls and swab the fissures with a solution of 25% poly(acrylic acid) for ten seconds. This will clean the surface and partially remove the smear layer but will not open any cut dentinal tubules.
5. Clean off any debris or acid with air/

*D2 or D14 diamond point: Intensiv, Viganello, Switzerland.

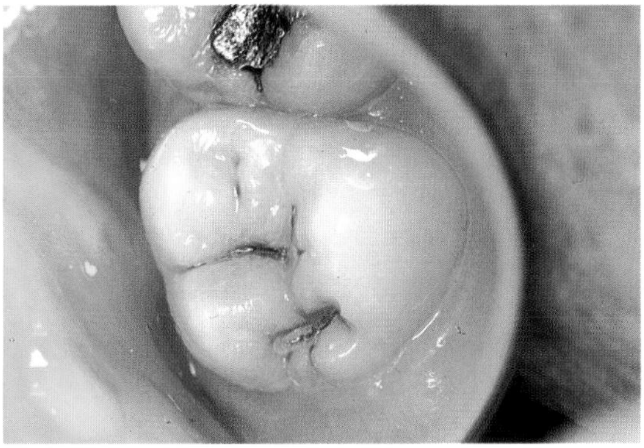

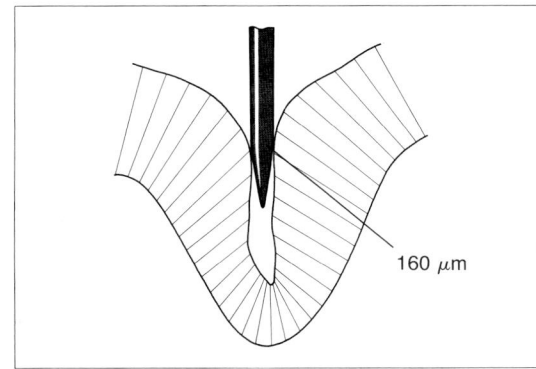

Fig. 12-13 Maxillary molar with stained fissures that are difficult to clean. A fissure cleaning and widening operation is advised.

Fig. 12-14 A patent molar fissure where the orifice is at least 160 μm wide.

160 μm

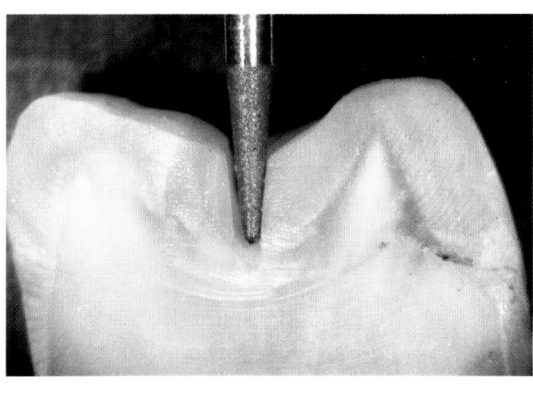

Fig. 12-15a Section through a molar showing use of diamond point for fissure widening and cleaning. The diamond point will normally drop into any soft dentine caries.

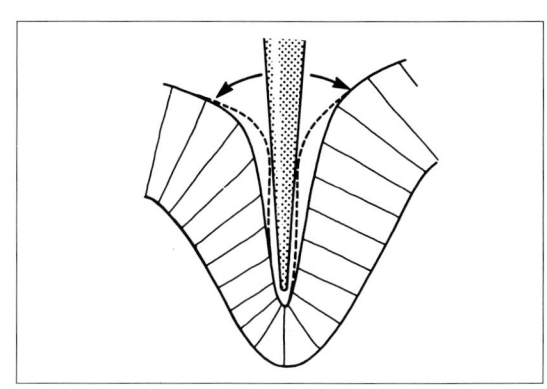

Fig. 12-15b The use of a diamond point for fissure widening.

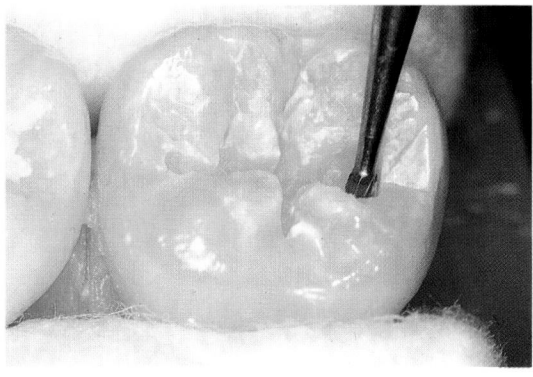

Fig. 12-16 Carious dentine removed with a slow-running round bur. Do not extend access beyond that necessary to remove the carious dentine.

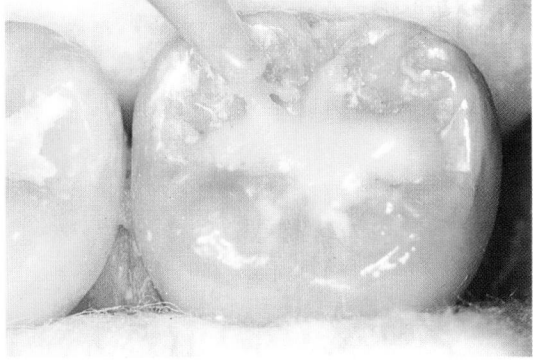

Fig. 12-17a Type II glass-ionomer cement injected into fissures.

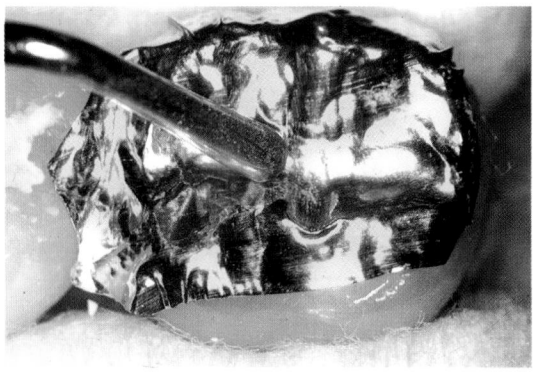

Fig. 12-17b Type II glass-ionomer cement injected into fissures and covered with Burlew's dry foil.

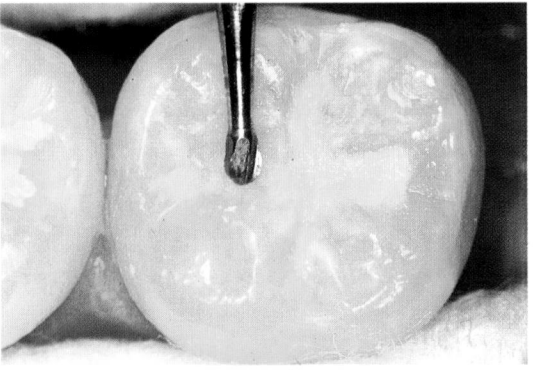

Fig. 12-18a Excess glass-ionomer cement removed with a small round bur.

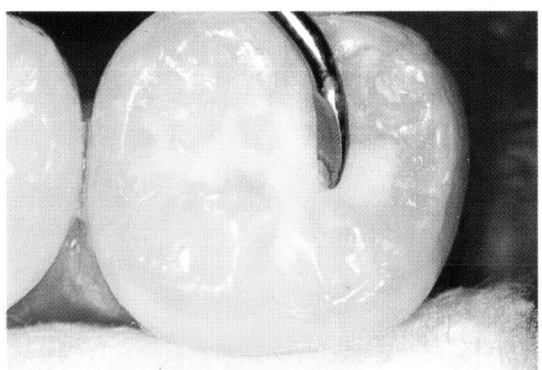

Fig. 12-18b Excess glass-ionomer cement removed with sharp excavator.

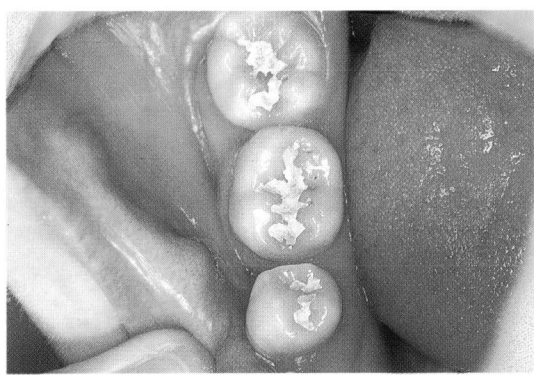

Fig. 12-19 Where more extensive caries is present and the cavity has to be extended, more abrasion-resistant material (Ketac-Silver) has been used.

water spray and dry the tooth with warm air for a few seconds only. Do not dehydrate.

6. Inject a mix of Type II glass-ionomer filling cement into the fissure (Fig. 12-17a) and cover with Burlew's dry foil,* which should be lightly burnished to position (Fig. 12-17b). Alternatively, apply Kerr's green occlusal indicator wax as recommended for the fissure sealing procedure (see Fig. 12-8).

7. After the requisite setting time specified by the manufacturer, the filling should be trimmed under water spray with fine round diamond stones or carbide burs (Fig. 12-18a). A sharp excavator also is useful in removing excess without damaging fine edges (Fig. 12-18b).

8. Immediately after trimming, the set cement should be coated with varnish or a light-curing bonding resin. The quicker the protective coating is applied, the better the final result.

Where occlusal caries is more extensive and the cavity has been widened, Type II glass-ionomer cements are more prone to erosion/abrasion (McLean, 1980). In these cases a silver-cermet cement such as Ketac-Silver* may be used to improve long-term abrasion resistance (Fig. 12-19). Ketac-Silver is better for maintaining centric occlusal contacts.

Glass-ionomer cements have been used as fissure fillings for the last 14 years and their long-term clinical success has been well established. Because of their anticariogenic properties and adhesion to tooth structure they offer a more attractive solution to the restoration of carious fissures than silver amalgam alloys.

The following recommendation was made in the findings of the British Dental Journal's Workshop on Alternatives to Amalgam Alloys (1984): "There is sufficient evidence to consider that modern glass-ionomer and composite materials could be used as an alternative to silver amalgam alloys for the restoration of simple fissures."

---

*Dentsply International Inc., Weybridge, England, and York, Pa.

*ESPE GmbH, Seefeld/Oberbay, West Germany, and Valley Stream, N.Y.

Figs. 12-20a and b Diagrams of breakdown of siloxane bonds in filler produced by hydroxyl ion and stress corrosion attack.

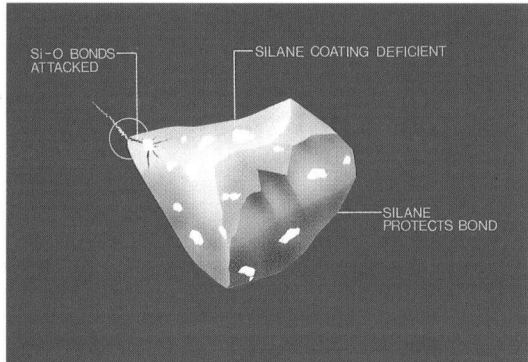

Fig. 12-20a Filler is more easily attacked when silane coating is deficient. Barium glasses are more prone to hydroxyl ion attack.

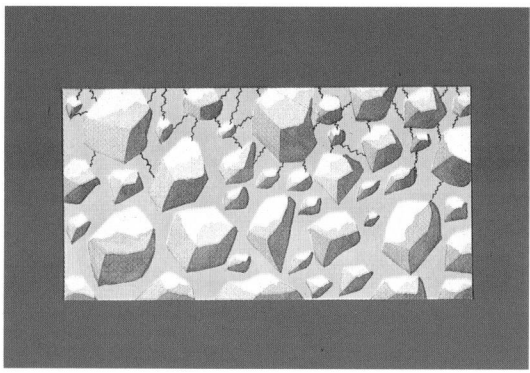

Fig. 12-20b Disintegration of surface produced by cracks.

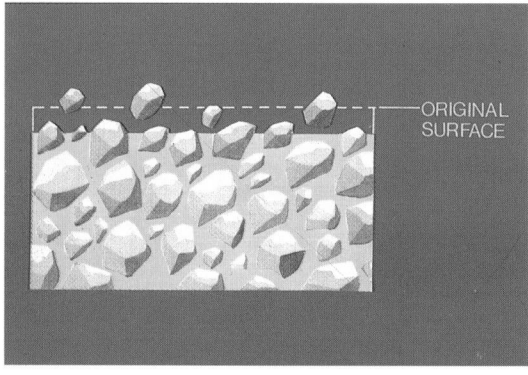

Fig. 12-21 Diagram of loss of filler produced by loss of polymer matrix.

The approximal lesion

New concepts in restorative dentistry concentrate more on preserving the integrity of the tooth rather than filling a cavity. The use of materials possessing both cariostatic properties and long-term adhesion is changing the approach to the treatment of the early Class II lesion.

Dental amalgam alloys, although serving the profession well for many decades, do not adhere to tooth structure and must be regarded as a metallic filling or plug inserted in the tooth, whose placement and possible replacement necessitates the loss of sound tooth material. Amalgam alloy fillings fail more through microleakage and secondary caries than through mechanical failure (Mjör, 1985). Although replacement with other materials giving long-term success in conventional cavities has not yet been achieved, this should not obscure the replacement of amalgam alloy fillings when new approaches to treating carious lesions are adopted.

The major problems with replacing amalgam alloys with composite resin filling materials in conventional Class II restorations involve two main factors: *(1)* lack of permanent adhesion to dentine, and *(2)* surface wear, often resulting in microleakage and postoperative sensitivity. Bond failure could be caused by the high shrinkage of the resin matrix setting up stresses at the tooth interface. Also, cuspal distortion may occur, which may cause pain (Causton et al., 1985).

Surface wear of composite resins results from two main causes, chemical degradation and wear of the polymer matrix due to friction. Long-term hydrolytic breakdown at the filler/matrix interface may result from hydroxy-ion and stress corrosion attack (Söderholm, 1983) (Fig. 12-20). This is increased with the use of radiopaque barium glasses which are more prone to hydroxy-ion attack (Fig.

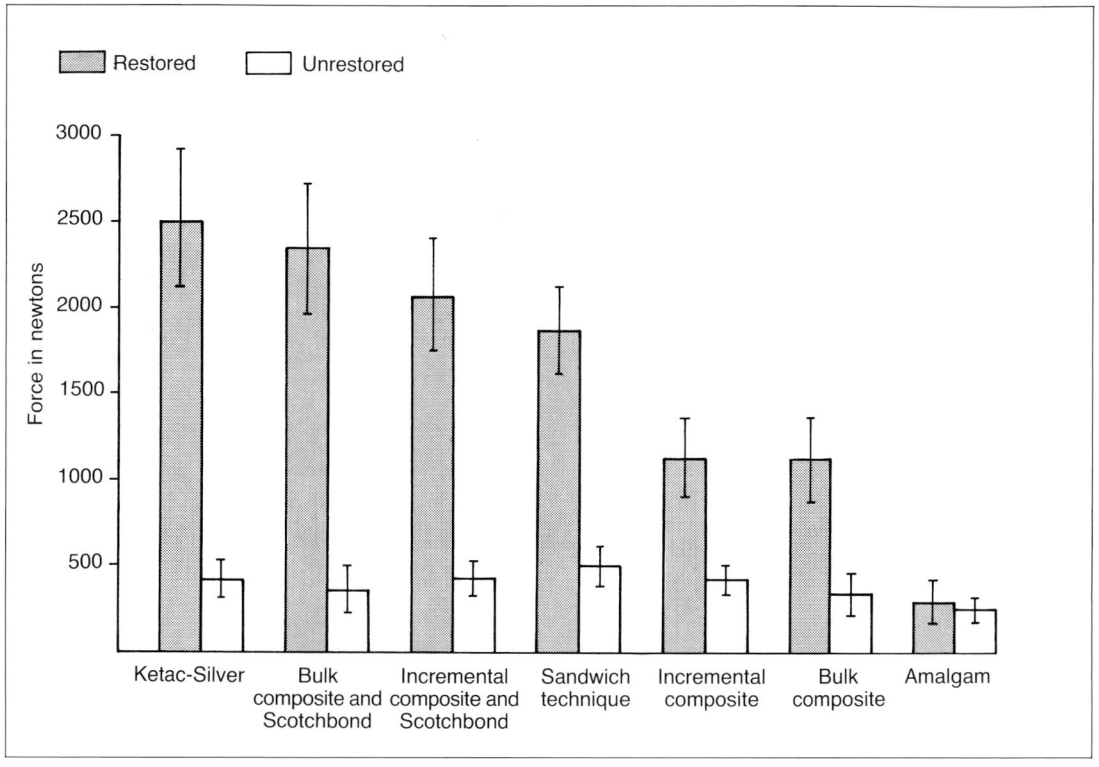

Fig. 12-22 Effect of adhesive restoratives on the strength of a lingual cusp in MOD restorations. Restored teeth were filled with amalgam, composite resins, and Ketac-Silver. Unrestored teeth with MOD cavities cut were used as controls. Modified from McCullock and Smith (1986).

12-20a). Surface wear due to loss of the polymer matrix is caused by frictional wear, adhesive failure of the filler, or cohesive failure through the polymer matrix (Fig. 12-21). Shear of the filler is more rare, since the polymer matrix is the weak link. Surface wear may flatten contact areas, eliminate centric occlusal contacts, and result in a steady deterioration of occlusal stability. By contrast, amalgam alloy, because of its low coefficient of friction, has a very slow rate of clinical wear. It is hardly surprising that amalgam alloy is still the most widely used material in the standard Class II preparation.

Traditionally, access to dentine caries in the approximal region has involved an occlusal approach in which the marginal ridge is destroyed and access is gained to the carious lesion via a comparatively large opening. The retention of marginal ridges where caries has undermined the dentine has been deprecated on the grounds that unsupported enamel will break. Most students have been taught to extend their preparations buccolingually until all unsupported enamel has been removed. This recommendation has remained ingrained in teaching and is correct when nonadhesive materials such as amalgam alloy are used. However, evidence is mounting that amalgam alloys can leave a tooth as weakened as an unfilled cavity. Studies on the fracture strength of posterior teeth in which mesial-occlusal-distal (MOD) cavities had been prepared showed that the use of adhesive materials such as acid-etched composite resins or glass-ionomer cements can increase fracture resistance by 81% to 362% when compared with the unrestored cavity (MacKenzie, 1981, 1986; McCullock and Smith, 1986) (Fig. 12-22).

Restoration of the Class II lesion using new technology and materials takes advantage of this improvement in adhesion. Glass-ionomer cements are used as dentine replacements and the enamel cap is preserved. To achieve success with this new approach it is essential to make an accurate diagnosis of the approximal lesion. The decision whether to treat it conservatively and use preventive measures assisting remineralisation, or to remove the caries with instrumentation, is one of fine judgement, which will now be discussed.

Diagnosis of the early approximal lesion

Ranking systems have been used in epidemiological studies that divide the enamel and dentine into inner and outer zones so that a more sensitive indication of the caries process is possible (Kidd, 1984). This system is illustrated in Fig. 12-23. Although a bite-wing radiograph will not reveal the full extent of a lesion, it gives some indication of zoning. Histologically, a lesion will always be larger than its radiological appearance. Approximal caries is usually a slow disease process that may take up to four years to progress through the enamel (Backer-Dirks, 1961; Berman and Slack, 1973a, 1973b, 1973c; Marthaler and Wiesner, 1973; Zamir et al., 1976; Granath et al., 1980). However, the clinician should bear in mind that there are always exceptions to the rule and treatment of patients should not be ruled by statistics, which sometimes are skewed.

How do we interpret the radiograph-

ic appearance of the carious lesion? Clearly, where no lesion in the enamel is apparent, no treatment is required (Fig. 12-23,a). Where radiolucency is confined to the enamel, preventive measures should be instituted (Fig. 12-23,b). However, in Figs. 12-23,c and 12-23,d the decisions are less clear-cut and need good judgement, whereas in Fig. 12-23,e there could be no question of not treating the lesion by operative procedures.

Lesions that reach the amelodentinal junction (Fig. 12-23,c) or are spreading laterally in dentine (Fig. 12-23,d) need more consideration. It could be argued that a lesion just entering the dentine should be left and remineralizing procedure adopted. However, the radiological appearance will not reflect the true histological state. The lesion in Fig. 12-23,c is the most difficult to treat and requires close monitoring with bite-wing radiographs if it is to be controlled. In these cases, a year can make a big difference since the caries has penetrated dentine where it can range far and wide. For this reason, if the patient cannot be examined regularly it is better to treat the lesion with the internal cavity approach to be described shortly.

Where caries in the dentine is visible on a radiograph, often the enamel is cavitated and has reached a point of no return. Monitoring of these lesions with bite-wing radiographs teeters on the brink of disaster because failure to diagnose correctly can result in either pulp exposure or fracture of marginal ridges—with all its attendant problems in the fu-

Fig. 12-23 Suggested ranking system for the diagnosis of dental caries. *(a)* No enamel lesion. *(b)* Lesion confined to outer half of enamel. *(c)* Lesion penetrating amelodentinal junction. *(d)* Lesion spreading laterally in dentine. *(e)* Lesion penetrating dentine, with the possibility of pulpal involvement.

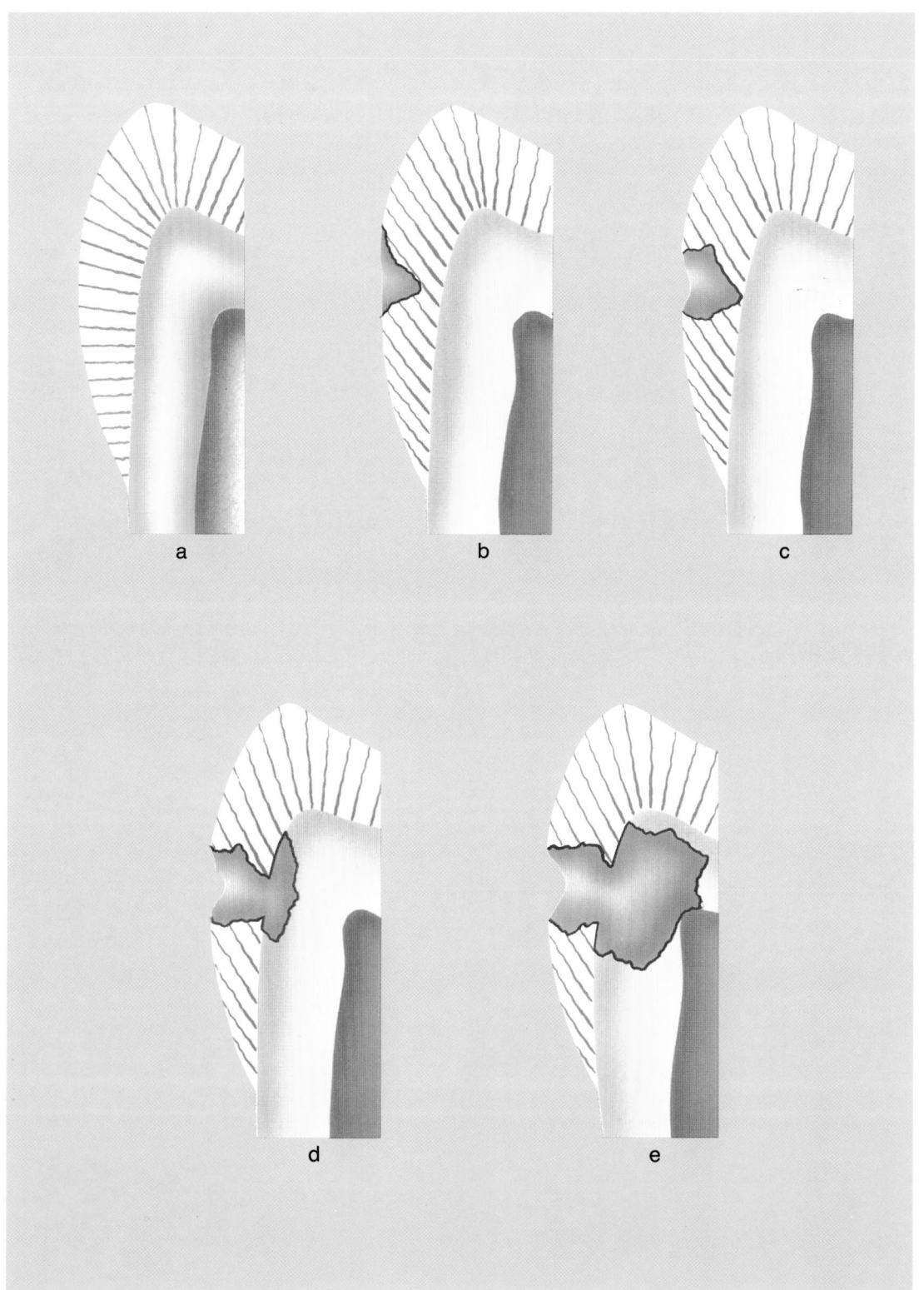

ture. The following recommendations can be made for treating the early carious lesion:

1. When enamel is sound on bite-wing radiograph, do not treat (Fig. 12-23,a).
2. When radiolucency is confined to the enamel, institute preventive measures and attempt to remineralize (Fig. 12-23,b).
3. When radiolucency is confined to the enamel but just reaches the amelodentinal junction, monitor closely with bite-wing radiographs and, if lesion is progressing, restore via internal cavity preparation (Fig. 12-23,c).
4. When radiolucency has entered the dentine and the patient has a high caries rate, treat immediately via internal cavity preparation. Where caries incidence is low, monitor with bite-wing radiographs. If the patient is not available for regular inspection, treat immediately (Fig. 12-23,d).
5. When radiolucency in dentine is close to the pulp, treat immediately; where possible use an internal occlusal cavity approach. Always line with calcium hydroxide (Fig. 12-23,e).

In all cases preventive measures should be introduced. An improvement in oral hygiene can often make a dramatic change and tilt the balance toward remineralization (see Fig. 12-2).

References

Albers, H.F. (1985) Tooth-Coloured Restoratives. 7th ed. Cotati, Calif.: Alto Books.

Backer-Dirks, O. (1961) Longitudinal dental caries study in children 9–15 years of age. Arch. Oral Biol. 6: (Special Suppl.) 94–108.

Berman, D.S., and Slack, D.L. (1973a) Dental caries in English school children: A longitudinal study. Br. Dent. J. 133:529–538.

Berman, D.S., and Slack, G.L. (1973b) Caries progression and activity in an approximal tooth surfaces: A longitudinal study. Br. Dent. J. 134:51–57.

Berman, D.S., and Slack, G.L. (1973c) Susceptibility of tooth surfaces to carious attack: A longitudinal study. Br. Dent. J. 134:135–139.

British Dental Association/Department of Health and Social Security Working Party (1986) Fissure sealants: Report of the joint BDA/DHSS Working Party. Br. Dent. J. 161:343.

Causton, B.E., Miller, B., and Sefton, J. (1985) The deformation of cusps by bonded posterior composite resins: An in vitro study. Br. Dent. J. 159:397–403.

Granath, L., Kahlmeter, A., Matsson, L., and Schröder, V. (1980) Progression of proximal enamel caries in early teens related to caries activity. Acta Odontol. Scand. 38:247–251.

Handelman, S.L., Leverett, P.M., Espeland, M.A., and Curzon, J.A. (1986) Clinical radiographic evaluation of sealed carious and sound tooth surfaces. J. Am. Dent. Assoc. 113:741–754.

Kidd, E.A.M. (1983) The histopathology of enamel caries in young and old permanent teeth. Br. Dent. J. 155: 196–198.

Kidd, E.A.M. (1984) The diagnosis and management of the "early" carious lesion in permanent teeth. Dental Update March: 69–81.

Levine, R.S. (1976) The action of fluoride in caries prevention: A review of current concepts. Br. Dent. J. 140: 9–14.

McCullock, A.L., and Smith, B.G.N. (1986) In vitro studies of cusp reinforcement with adhesive restorative material. Br. Dent. J. 149:368–373.

MacKenzie, D.F. (1981) Reinforcing posterior teeth using adhesive restorative materials. M.Sc. Thesis, University of London.

MacKenzie, D.F. (1986) The reinforcing effect of mesio-occluso-distal acid etch composite restorations on weakened posterior teeth. Br. Dent. J. 161:410–416.

McLean, J.W. (1980) Aesthetics in restorative dentistry: The challenge for the future. Br. Dent. J. 149: 368–373.

McLean, J.W., and von Fraunhofer, J.A. (1971) The estimation of cement film thickness by an in vivo technique. Br. Dent. J. 131:107–111.

McLean, J.W., and Wilson, A.D. (1974) Fissure sealing and filling with an adhesive glass ionomer cement. Br. Dent. J. 136:269–276.

Mjör, I.A. (1985) Frequency of secondary caries at various anatomical locations. Oper. Dent. 10:88–92.

Marthaler, T.M., and Wiesner, P.K. (1973) Rapidity of penetration of radiolucent areas through mesial enamel of the first permanent molars. Helv. Odontol. Acta 17:19–26.

Mortimer, K.V. (1964) Some histological features of fissure caries in enamel. In J.L. Hardwick, J.-P. Dustin, and H.R. Meld (eds.) Advances in Fluorine Research and Dental Caries Prevention. Vol. 2. Proceedings of the 10th Congress of the European Organization for Research on Fluorine and Dental Caries Prevention. Oxford, England: ORCA, and New York: Pergamon Press.

Mount, G. (1984) Glass-ionomer cements: Clinical considerations. chapt. 20A In J.W. Clark (ed.) Clinical Dentistry. Philadelphia: Harper & Row.

Shaw, L., and Murray, J.J. (1975) Inter-examiner and intra-examiner reproducibility in clinical and radiographic diagnosis. Int. Dent. J. 25:280–288.

Söderholm, K.J. (1983) Leaking of fillers in dental composites. J. Dent. Res. 62:126–130.

Stean, M.S. (1982) Is there a change in the carious process? Br. Dent. J. 152:301.

Usher, P.J. (1982) Is there a change in the carious process? (letter) Br. Dent. J. 152:399.

Vellender, B. (1982) Is there a change in the carious process? (letter) Br. Dent. J. 152:399.

Zamir, T., Fisher, D., and Sharrar, Y. (1976) A longitudinal radiographic study of the rate of spread of human approximal dental caries. Arch. Oral Biol. 21:523–526.

Chapter 13

Designs of Microcavities for Approximal Lesions

The introduction of glass-ionomer cements has made possible a number of new approaches to treating approximal caries, particularly in cases where the marginal ridge is still intact. McLean (1980) first suggested the use of glass-ionomer cements in low-stress-bearing micropreparations in which the approximal caries was removed either via a buccal or lingual approach or, when accessible, below the marginal ridge. Knight (1984) and Hunt (1984) used an occlusal approach in which entry was made internally through the fossa, preserving the marginal ridge and removing caries through a tunnel preparation. McLean (1986) and Albers (1985) also found this approach viable, and many clinicians are now adopting the principle of nondestruction of marginal ridges in their treatment of approximal caries.

For the purposes of classification, Class II preparations may fall under the following headings:

Occlusal approach

Approximal Class II cavity (Fig. 13-1)
Approximal Class II microcavity (Fig. 13-2)
Tunnel or internal fossa cavity (Fig. 13-3)

Approximal approach

Approximal microcavity (Fig. 13-4)
Buccolingual approximal cavity (Fig. 13-5)

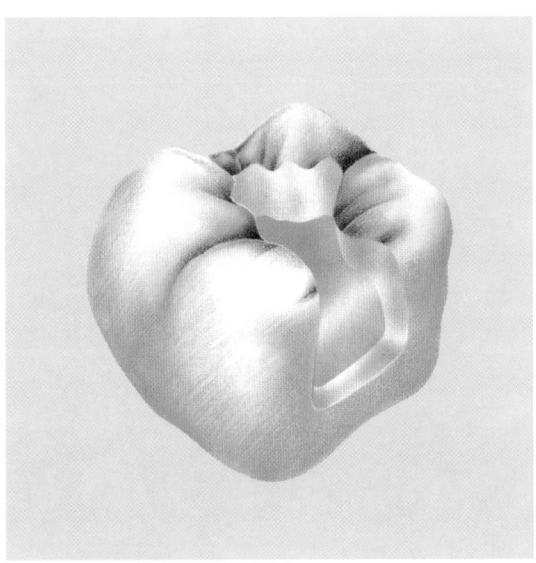

Fig. 13-1 Standard Black's Class II cavity, occlusal approach.

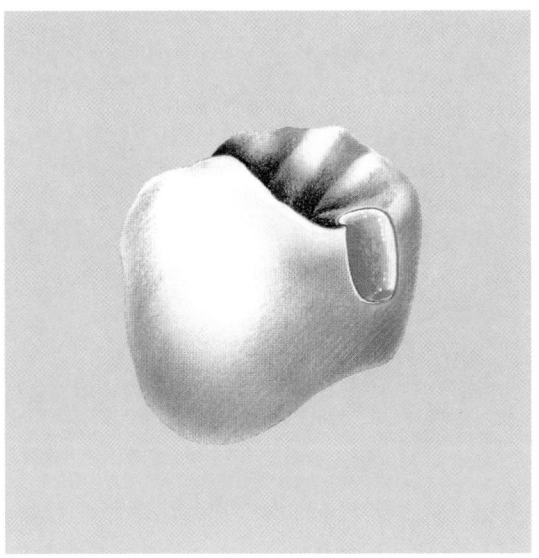

Fig. 13-2 Approximal Class II microcavity, occlusal approach.

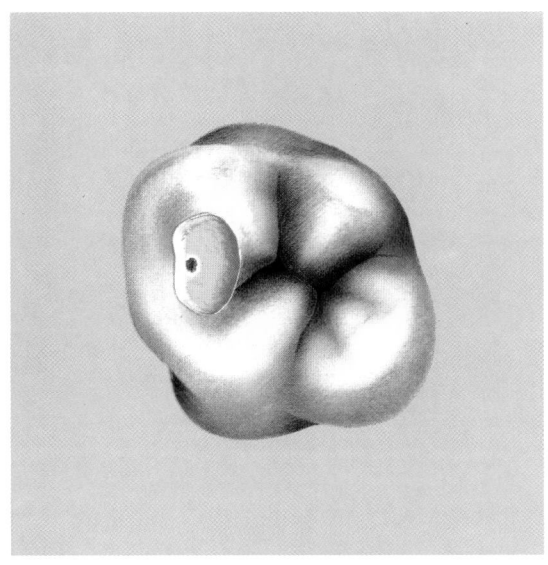

Fig. 13-3 Internal occlusal fossa cavity, occlusal approach.

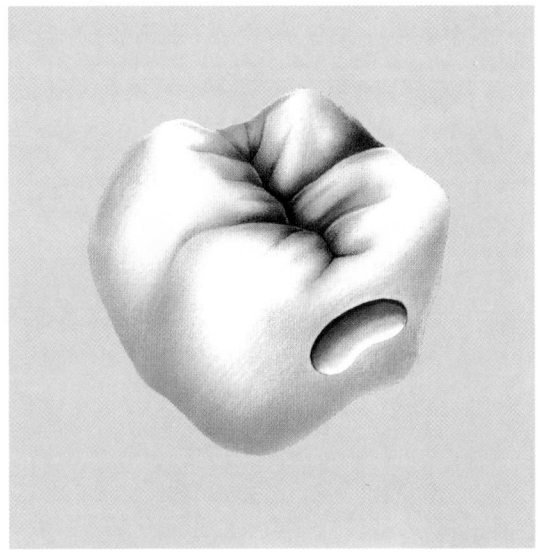

Fig. 13-4 Approximal microcavity, approximal approach.

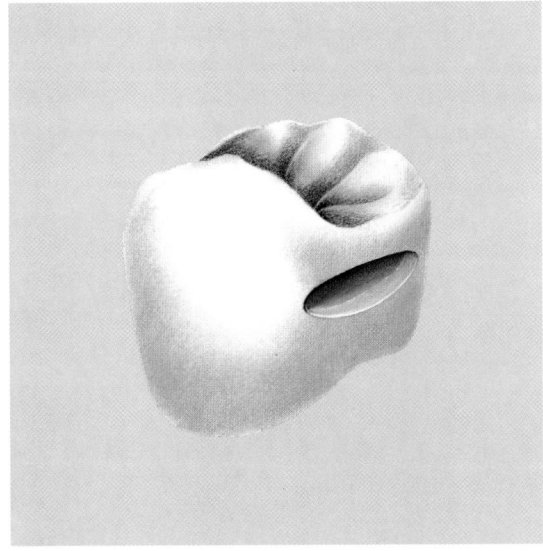

Fig. 13-5 Buccolingual approximal cavity, buccal or lingual approach.

Application of materials

The flexural strength of glass-ionomer cements is low, ranging from 9 to 30 MPa for filling materials and 4 to 15 MPa for luting agents. In addition, they are brittle materials subject to chipping and greater wear than either composite resins or amalgams. However, the silver-cermet ionomer cements show considerable improvement in wear resistance, probably because of the lubricating effect of the fine silver particles bonded to the glass surface. For this reason, silver-cermet materials such as Ketac-Silver* are to be preferred over standard Type II glass-ionomer cements for the restoration of occlusal areas where centric holding stops are present. In addition, Ketac-Silver is less liable to wear on approximal microcavities where dental floss is used. Even the cermet-type glass-ionomer cements, however, cannot replace dental amalgams in the standard Class II preparation because the flexural or shear strengths required to resist fracture in proximal boxes and isthmuses are too high for this range of brittle cements (Table 13-1). Amalgam alloys and posterior composite resins are more than four times stronger than glass-ionomer cements and will continue to be the materials of choice for load-bearing areas. For this reason the use of glass-ionomers for the restoration of Class II cavities will not be discussed except as they are used as linings under posterior composite resins.

Table 13-1 Comparison of flexural strengths

Material	Breaking stress (MPa)
Amalgam alloy	140
Composite resin	
Conventional	110–135
Posterior	120–150
Microfil	60–80
Glass-ionomer Type II cement	9–30
Silver-cermet-ionomer cement	32–40
Gold alloy yield strength	350–500

Occlusal approach to an approximal Class II microcavity

Indications for use

When early caries in the dentine and marginal ridge cracks are detected when transilluminated under fibre-optic lighting, then an occlusal approach through the marginal ridge may be the entry point of choice. A lateral marginal ridge approach is also indicated where access can be gained below the marginal ridge and the contact areas are located at least 2 mm below the crest of the ridge (Fig. 13-6).

*ESPE GmbH, Seefeld/Oberbay, West Germany, and Valley Stream, N.Y.

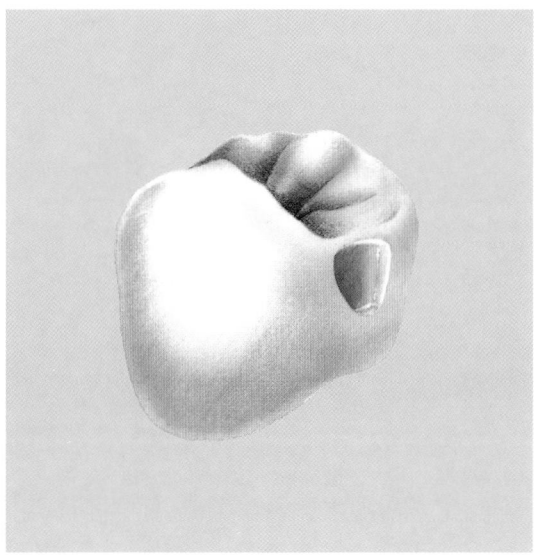

Fig. 13-6 Approximal Class II microcavity using lateral marginal ridge approach.

Procedure

1. A small round diamond stone* is used to enter the approximal side of the marginal ridge. Entry to the carious lesion is made with the aid of magnifying loops and fibre-optic lighting. The orifice of the cavity should be large enough to allow good visibility and provide clear access to the carious dentine (Fig. 13-7).

2. The cavity should be extended cervically only as far as the lesion, and the cervical floor should be rounded. All caries is removed with a slow-running round carbide bur. Very slight undercuts in the dentine will then increase the resistance form of the restoration. Essentially the cavity should be a miniature proximal box cavity. It should not extend beyond the periphery of the lesion (see Fig. 13-2).

3. If a lesion is present in the adjoining tooth, access can be gained through the proximal box. A microcavity prepared in this tooth will allow preservation of the marginal ridge (Fig. 13-8).

4. Prior to restoration, the cavity should be cleaned with a solution of 25% poly(acrylic acid) for ten seconds, then washed thoroughly (Fig. 13-9).

Matrix technique

A thin, soft metal matrix band* is inserted, contoured, and wedged firmly into position. It is important that the soft metal matrix is contoured very accurately to provide a contact area and not a contact point; light burnishing should leave it in close contact with the adjoining tooth (Fig. 13-10). A separator† can also be used to improve separation (Fig. 13-10).

*Rocky Mountain Orthodontic Band, Rocky Mountain Dental Co., Denver, Colo.; 0 Tofflemire Orthodontic Band, HO Dental Co., Goleta, Calif.
†McKean Separator, Rocky Mountain Dental Co., Denver, Colo.

*HiDi521, Dentsply International Inc., Weybridge, England and York, Pa.

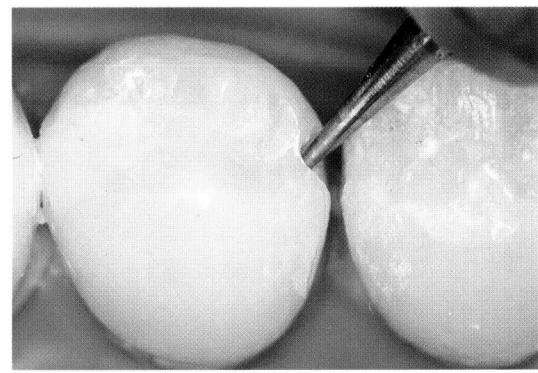

Fig. 13-7a Access gained to approximal lesion using small round diamond bur.

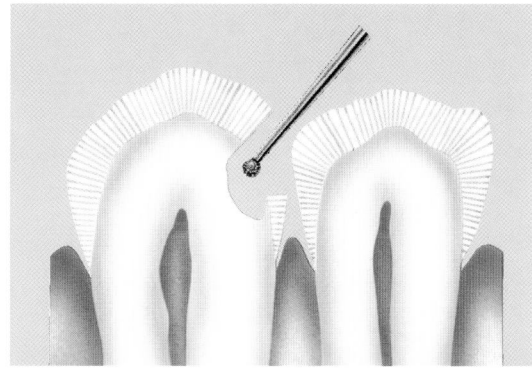

Fig. 13-7b Marginal ridge approach.

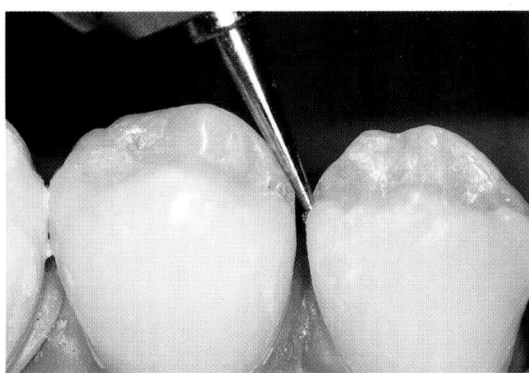

Fig. 13-8 Where caries is present in adjoining tooth, access is easily gained via cavity opening in the Class II microcavity.

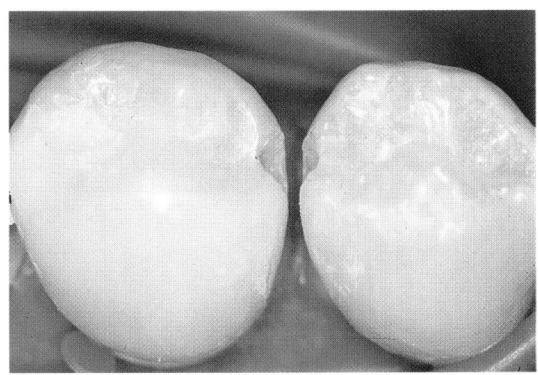

Fig. 13-9 Completed Class II microcavities after surface conditioning with 25% polyacrylic acid.

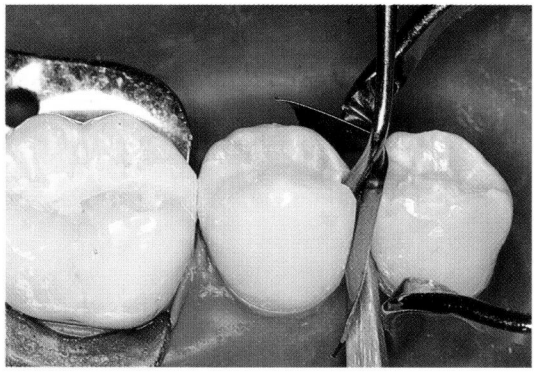

Fig. 13-10 Soft-metal matrix band inserted and wedged firmly. Band is burnished toward contact area. A separator is used to open contact area.

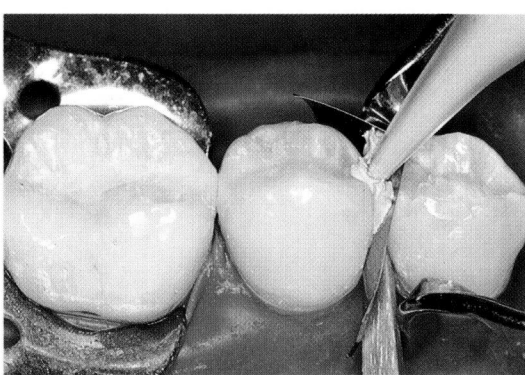

Fig. 13-11 Silver-cermet cement injected into cavity.

Insertion of silver-cermet cement

Unless there is a near exposure of the pulp, calcium hydroxide linings are not required.

After mixing, the silver-cermet cement capsule is inserted into the applicator and syringed into the cavity (Fig. 13-11). Where access is difficult the mix can be transferred to a Centrix syringe* with a finer tip. It is important to syringe the material into the base of the cavity to avoid trapping air, and excess material should be left on the surface. The band may now be burnished over the marginal ridge, taking care to burnish toward the contact area (Fig. 13-12).

Finishing

After five minutes of setting, excess material can be removed with a no. 5 fluted carbide bur (Fig. 13-13) or a similarly shaped fine-diamond stone, running under water spray. Approximal excess may also be removed with a sharp curved scalpel blade. The surface may then be lightly burnished. Do not trim in dry conditions since this may cause crazing of the cement.

After the silver-cermet cement restoration is completed, the adjacent tooth is ready for filling. At this stage, do not remove the matrix band but simply remove the wedge and reinsert it on the opposite side of the band (Fig. 13-14). It is now a simple procedure to inject silver-cermet cement into the adjacent cavity and reburnish the soft matrix band over the

*Centrix Inc., Stratford, Conn.

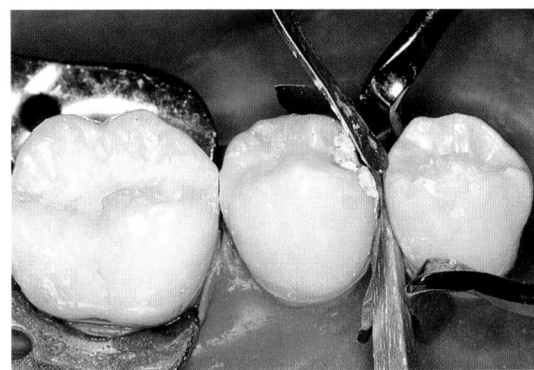

Fig. 13-12 Matrix band burnished over cermet cement to develop contact area.

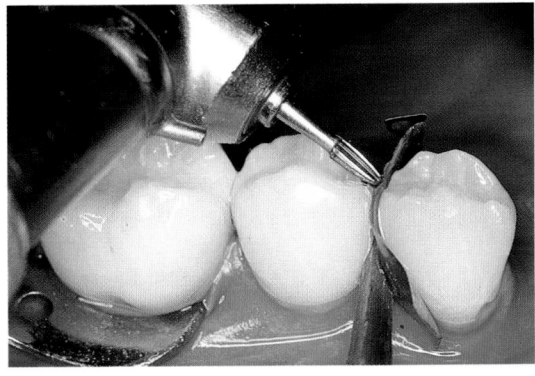

Fig. 13-13 Fluted carbide bur used under water spray to remove excess silver-cermet cement. Sharp knife may be used to remove approximal excess.

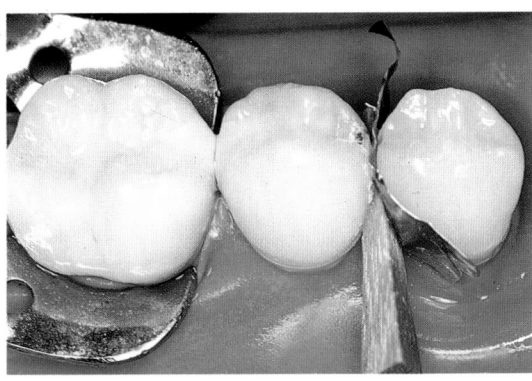

Fig. 13-14 Wooden wedge removed and applied to opposite side of band prior to filling adjoining cavity.

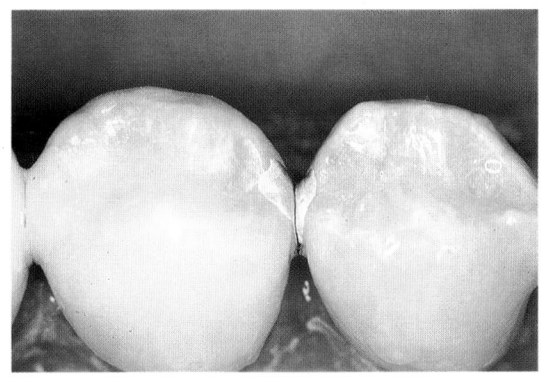

Fig. 13-15 Completed restorations after finishing. Apply a coat of light-cured bonding agent as an added protection against moisture contamination.

marginal ridge. Trim and burnish and apply a coat of protective varnish to both restorations (Fig. 13-15).

Occlusal adjustment

The silver-cermet cement should be trimmed using slow speeds not exceeding 30,000 rpm. A copious water supply is essential. This material is a water-based system and will not withstand prolonged drying. Early strength of silver-cermet cement is higher than glass-ionomer cements but is still not adequate to resist the full force of the patient's bite. Heavy occlusal pressure by the patient can cause minute cracks to develop in the cement that may not be observed during occlusal adjustment. The patient should be instructed to exert very light pressure, as when adjusting amalgam alloy restorations. Failure to observe this procedure may be the cause of fracture of the restoration at a later date.

Occlusal approach to an internal occlusal fossa cavity

Knight (1984) and Hunt (1984) first described a method of removing approximal caries through an access channel cut in the occlusal fossa. This preparation has been described as a "tunnel cavity." For the beginner, however, this can be misleading—working through a tunnel can prove difficult, with the operator often leaving caries undermining the enamel. For this reason, the beginner should regard this preparation as an occlusal internal fossa cavity closely resembing an occlusal cavity, except in its extent. Access to the approximal caries should be extended buccolingually be-

cause the internal fossa preparation concentrates on the removal of carious dentine and *the preservation of the enamel marginal ridge.* This requries more skill from the operator but is made easier providing the occlusal access channel is large enough to clearly see all the caries. This will not weaken the tooth if the clinician stays within the 2-mm peripheral ring of marginal ridge enamel (Fig. 13-16).

Indications for use and procedure

The internal fossa preparation is particularly useful for treating the type of lesion previously discussed and shown in Figs. 12-23c and d. Access through the fossa should be predetermined by using Kerr's green occlusal indicator wax* to mark out the centric holding stops (Fig. 13-17). Where possible these areas should be avoided, *but not at the expense of access to the lesion.* This is a common mistake and results in the clinician working through a tunnel with "tunnel vision." If occlusal centric holding stops are involved, Ketac-Silver is recommended because of its better resistance to abrasion. The internal fossa preparation is not suitable for restoring teeth where the marginal ridge is cracked or undermined to the extent that less than 2 mm of enamel is remaining either occlusally or approximally (Fig. 13-18).

Accurate bite-wing radiographs must be available and the lesion clearly identified (Fig. 13-19). Transillumination of the teeth using fibre-optic lighting is a further aid to diagnosis. Generally, the enamel lesion is at least 2.5 mm below the marginal ridge, and the cavitation in the enamel rarely exceeds more than 1 mm in diameter (Fig. 13-20). A periodontal

*Kwik-Wax, Kerr Mfg. Co., Div. of Sybron Corp., Romulus, Mich.

Figs. 13-16a and b Ideal occlusal access for the internal fossa preparation.

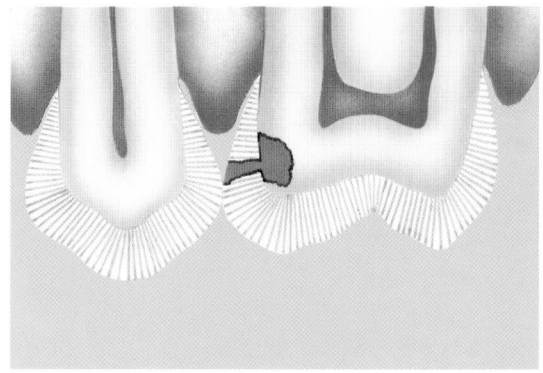

Fig. 13-16a Carious lesion prior to cavity preparation.

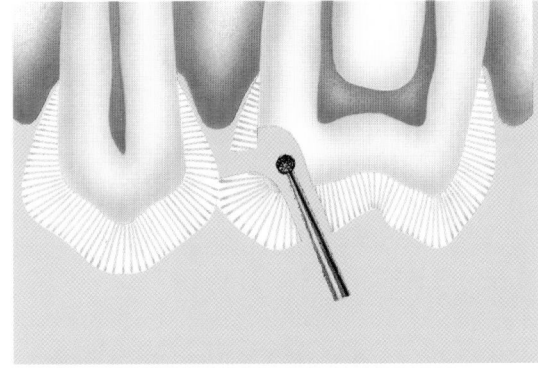

Fig. 13-16b Occlusal access gained through mesial fossa.

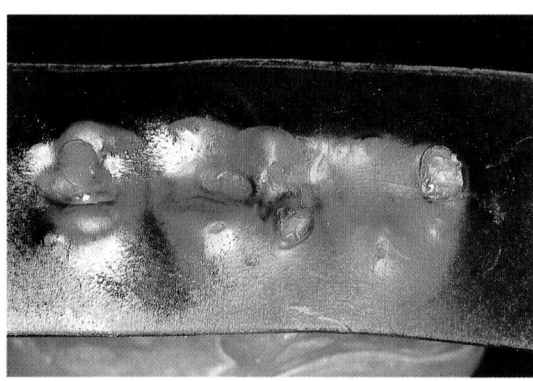

Fig. 13-17 Kerr's green occlusal indicator wax used to establish area of centric holding stops.

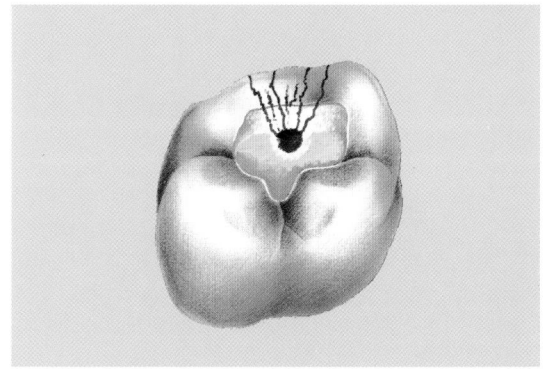

Fig. 13-18 A lesion unsuitable for the internal fossa preparation. Initial lesion and subsequent cavitation has undermined the marginal ridge, and cracks are now developing due to lack of dentinal support undermined by caries.

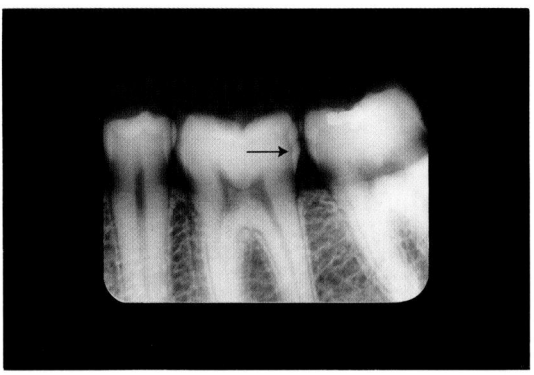

Fig. 13-19 Radiograph of approximal lesion in tooth 36 suitable for the internal occlusal fossa preparation.

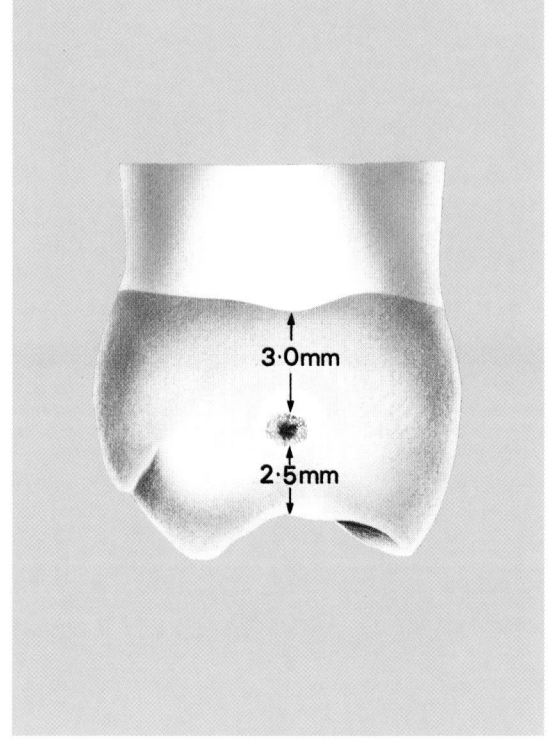

Fig. 13-20 *(right)* Diagram of proximal surface of a molar showing ideal lesion for treatment with the internal occlusal fossa preparation. At least 2 mm of supporting enamel must be left on the marginal ridge.

probe may be used to measure and determine the depth of the lesion. It is essential to leave a section of marginal ridge of at least 2 mm × 2 mm if long-term resistance to fracture is to be achieved.

Cavity preparation

The initial approach to the lesion should be made through the occlusal fossa, avoiding where possible occlusal centric holding stops, and must not involve the marginal ridge. Speeds of up to 150,000 rpm are preferred to those of air turbines.

1. Using a small round diamond stone, entry is made in the occlusal fossa leaving at least 2 mm of marginal ridge *intact* (Fig. 13-21). Entry to the soft caries is made by directing the diamond stone very slightly diagonally.

2. Widen the access channel bucco-lingually until all the soft caries is visible. Magnification and fibre-optic lighting are essential tools for this type of microcavity preparation. At this stage, make certain that the marginal ridge is intact and transilluminate it for detection of micro-cracks (Fig. 13-22). This procedure also aids in the detection of caries, which is then removed using round carbide burs in a slow-speed handpiece. Do not attempt to cut into the enamel lesion but use the slow-running round bur as a tactile instrument for detecting soft caries in the dentine. Hunt (1984) has suggested using a caries-detection solution such as basic fuchsin in propylene glycol for detection of bacteria in the dentine. However, Handelman et al. (1986) have shown that, provided the surface seal is intact on a restoration, such as in a fissure filling, bacterial growth does not

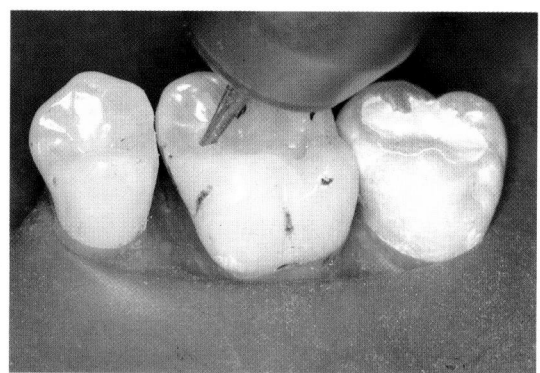

Fig. 13-21 Entry made in occlusal fossa with a small round diamond.

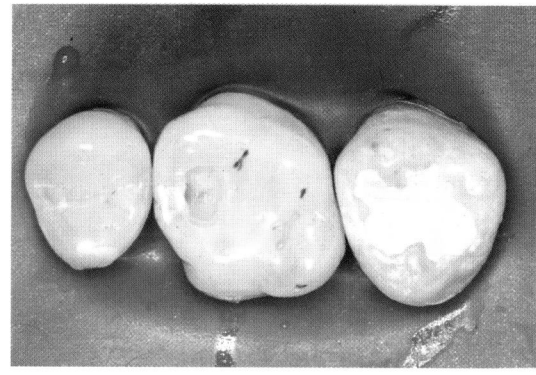

Fig. 13-22 Widen the access channel buccolingually to make certain all caries is removed. Enamel ridge should be illuminated with fibre-optic light and examined for cracks.

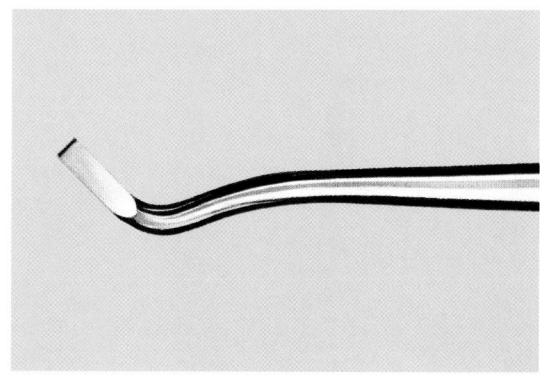

Fig. 13-23a Double-bladed chisel used to smooth the enamel walls where cavitation is present.

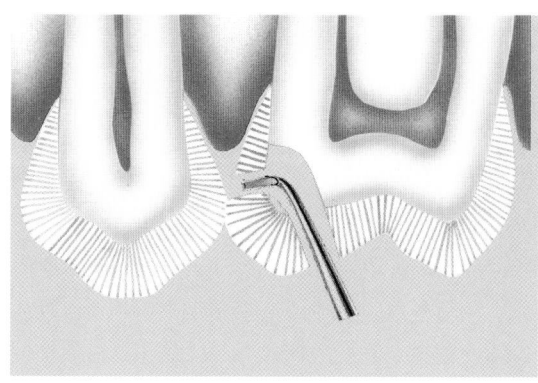

Fig. 13-23b The use of a double-bladed chisel.

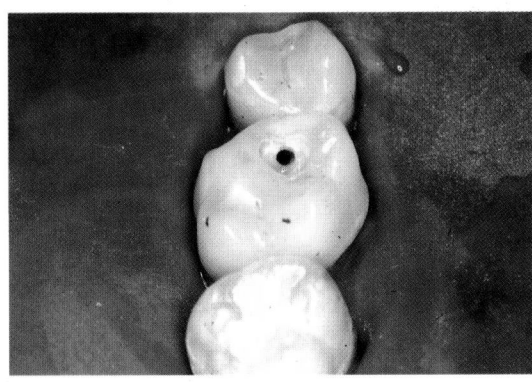

Fig. 13-24 Completed internal occlusal fossa preparation after smoothing cavosurface margins with fine diamonds.

proceed. For this reason, the operator should not cut sound dentine that may show the presence of small amounts of bacteria if pulpal involvement is likely.

3. The proximal enamel lesion is usually very small and slightly porous (the white spot lesion). Cutting into this lesion with rotary instruments is strongly deprecated, since Kidd and Joyston-Bechel (1986) have shown that a white spot lesion, even when exposed to fluoride toothpaste, becomes more resistant to further demineralisation. The leaching of fluoride from the glass-ionomer cement will also contribute to this effect. Instrumentation is only necessary when the enamel is cavitated and a definite hole is located. For these cases a specially designed double-bladed chisel is now available* (Fig. 13-23), which may be used to remove any weak or porous enamel at the margins of the cavitation. Do not attempt to break through intact enamel even when a white spot lesion is present. In these cases extension for prevention is strongly deprecated.

After gently smoothing the edges of the enamel cavitation, fine diamonds should be used to smooth the occlusal enamel exits (Fig. 13-24). At this stage a

confirmatory bite-wing radiograph may be taken to check accuracy and completeness of caries removal—but once experience has been gained with this technique a confirming radiograph is rarely necessary.

When preparing an internal occlusal fossa cavity the clinicians should appreciate that the main objective is to remove infected dentine, not enamel. Preservation of the enamel cap and approximal enamel is the key to success.

Insertion of glass-ionomer cement

Any Type II glass-ionomer cement may be used for restoring the occlusal fossa internal preparation, but improved wear characteristics and strong radio-opacity can be obtained by using a silver-cermet cement such as Ketac-Silver, as previously explained.

1. If an enamel access channel has been made, insert a thin metal matrix band lightly lubricated with silicone oil into the contact area and wedge it tightly so that a close fit can be seen through the access channel (Fig. 13-25). If necessary, place wedges of compound to seal the band to the tooth.

2. Cleanse the cavity for ten seconds with a solution of 25% poly(acrylic acid)

*MC1 Chisel, Cottrell Ltd., London, and Parker, Colo.

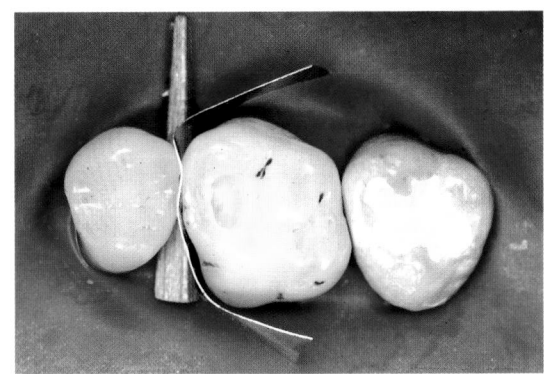

Fig. 13-25 Matrix band wedged tightly to occlude the approximal cavitation.

and wash and dry. Line with calcium hydroxide if there is a near-exposure, but place it only over the pulp chamber to avoid loss of bonding sites for the glassionomer cement.

3. Mix the silver-cermet cement in a high-energy automatic mixer for ten seconds, and then insert it into the applicator and inject through the occlusal access channel (Fig. 13-26). Where the channel is narrow, use a Centrix syringe, as previously described.

4. The cement may be forced into position using a slightly damp pledget of cotton-wool and then covering with Burlew's dry foil.* Light burnishing will ensure an accurate occlusal fit.

5. After five minutes of setting, the silver-cermet cement may be safely trimmed with round diamond stones or tungsten carbide burs. Sintered diamond stones are also very useful tools for fine finishing. It is essential to use constant water spray when trimming and never to allow the cement to dry out. Gentle scraping with sharp excavators will also remove small amounts of excess cement peripherally. Apply a light-cured bonding agent if the silver-cermet cement is to be the main restoration.

6. If aesthetics is of prime importance, a posterior composite resin may be used to seal the occlusal surface of the restoration.

After setting, the silver-cermet cement is removed to a depth of not more than 2 mm and the enamel and cement are etched for 30 seconds with a 37% phosphoric acid gel (Fig. 13-27). After washing and thoroughly drying, a bonding agent is applied and light cured. The faster the bonding agent is applied the better, since it will seal and preserve an uncontaminated surface (Fig. 13-28). A bulk composite is then inserted by standard techique and light cured for at least 40 seconds (Fig. 13-29). Trimming and polishing may be done using fine diamond stones and round burs for the refinement of grooves (Fig. 13-30). The grooves and fissures are polished with Shofu rubber abrasive points* and the restoration finished with rubber polishing cups and a slurry of 30 μm aluminum oxide (Fig. 13-31).

Clinical cases illustrating the use of silver-cermet cement and silver-cermet cement composite resin laminate restorations are shown in Figs. 13-32 to 13-34.

*Dentsply International Inc., Weybridge, England, and York, Pa.

*Shofu Dental Corp., Kyoto, Japan, and Menlo Park, Calif.

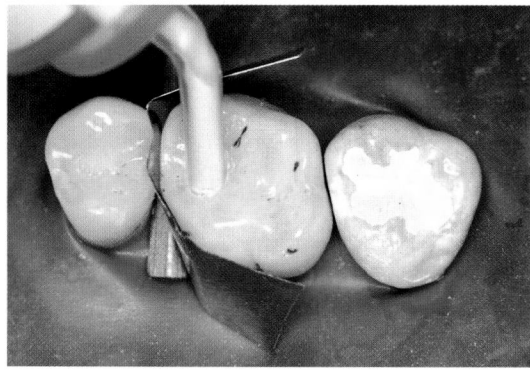

Fig. 13-26a Silver-cermet cement injected into occlusal fossa preparation.

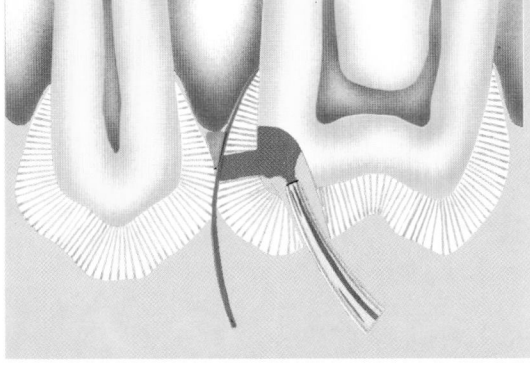

Fig. 13-26b Injection of silver-cermet cement.

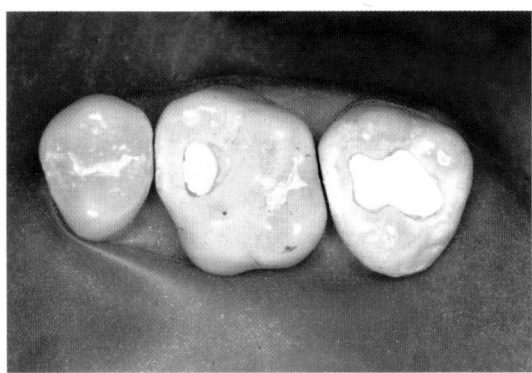

Fig. 13-27a Silver-cermet cement removed to a depth of 2 mm and etched for 30 seconds.

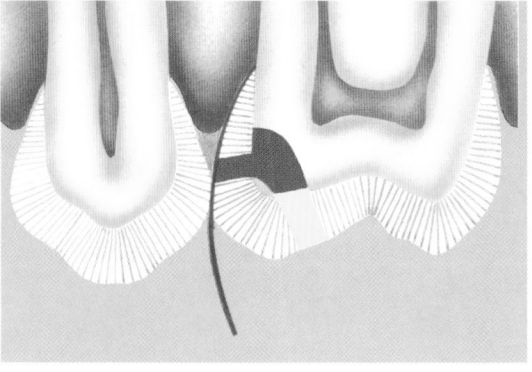

Fig. 13-27b Diagram of correct amount of occlusal space for composite resin restoration.

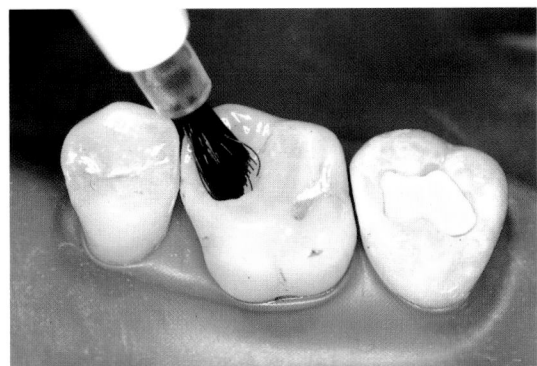

Fig. 13-28 Bonding agent applied to enamel and silver-cermet cement surface.

Fig. 13-29 Occlusin* bulk composite resin applied and light cured.

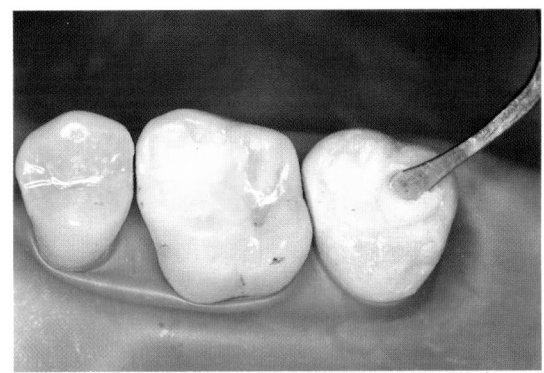

*ICI Dental, Macclesfield, Cheshire, England.

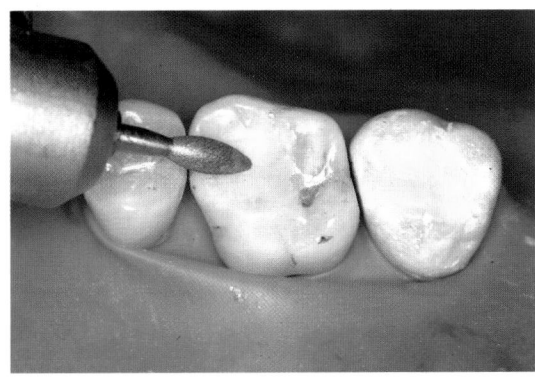

Fig. 13-30a Fine-plated diamond used to trim excess.

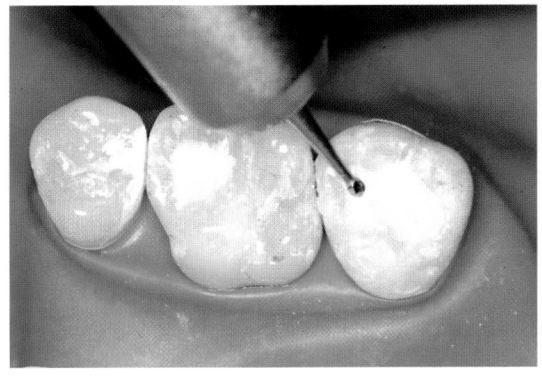

Fig. 13-30b Round bur for the refinement of the grooves.

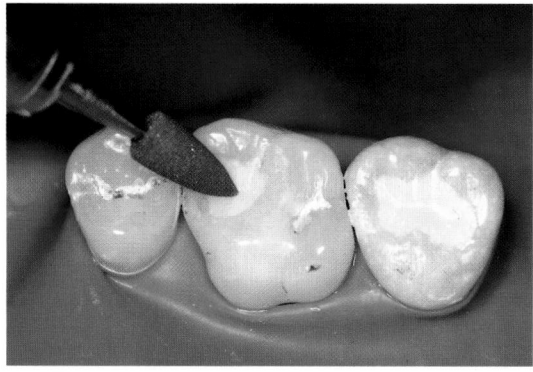

Fig. 13-31a Grooves and fissures polished with polishing points.

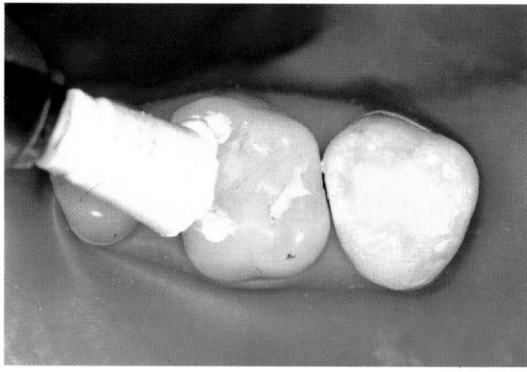

Fig. 13-31b Grooves and fissures polished with rubber cups and a slurry of 30-μm aluminium oxide.

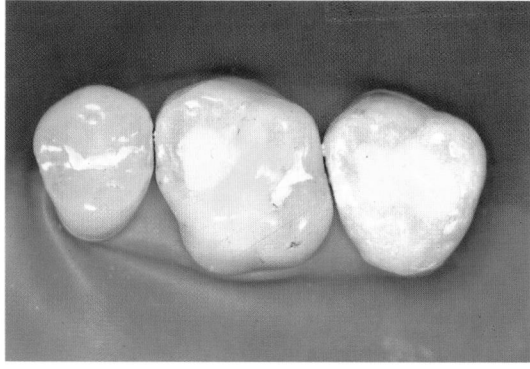

Fig. 13-31c Completed restorations in maxillary molars.

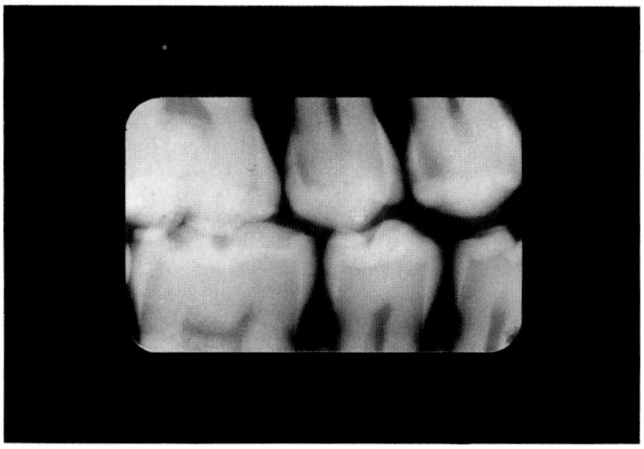

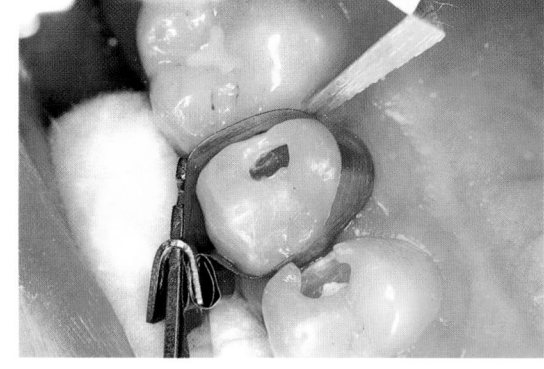

Fig. 13-32a Bite-wing radiograph of carious lesions in teeth 14 and 15. The lesion in tooth 14 is more extensive and not suitable for internal occlusal fossa preparation.

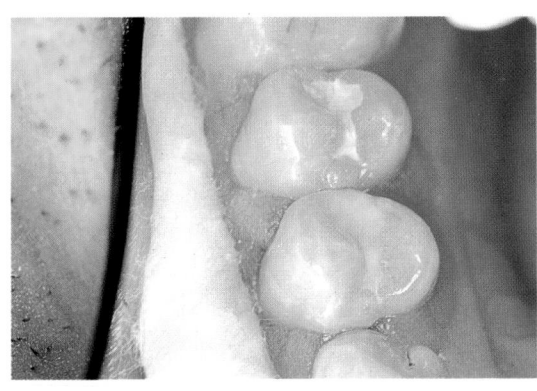

Fig. 13-32b Internal occlusal fossa preparation in tooth 15. Patient aged 18 years is an epileptic and being treated with phenytoin sodium. High caries rate and hypertrophic gingival condition make him an ideal candidate for treatment with glass-ionomer cement. Carious lesion in tooth 14 unsuitable for treatment due to undermining of marginal ridge by more extensive caries.

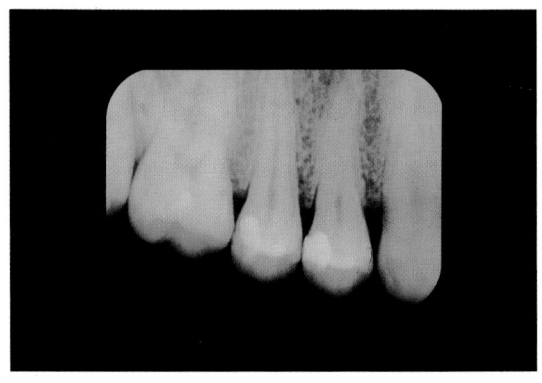

Fig. 13-33a Completed silver-cermet cement restoration in tooth 15 and Ketac-Silver/Occlusin Class II laminate restoration in tooth 14.

Fig. 13-33b Radiograph of completed restorations in teeth 14 and 15.

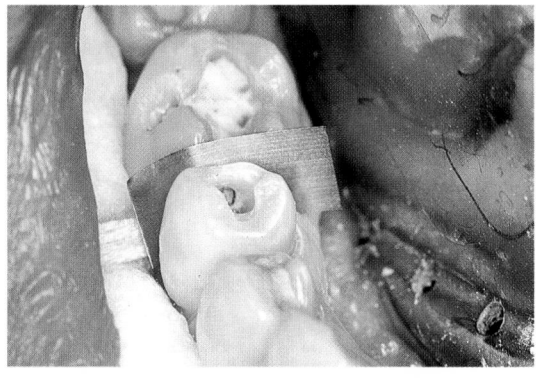

Fig. 13-34a Large distal cavity preparation in tooth 45. Note white spot lesion left intact and marginal ridge enamel still strong enough to use an internal occlusal fossa preparation.

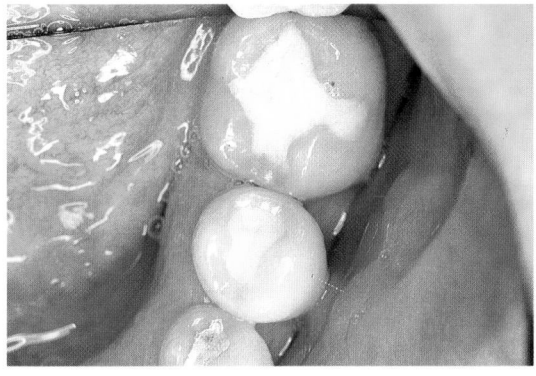

Fig. 13-34b Completed restoration in tooth 45 using Ketac-Silver/Occlusin laminate. Experimental Occlusin restoration in tooth 46.

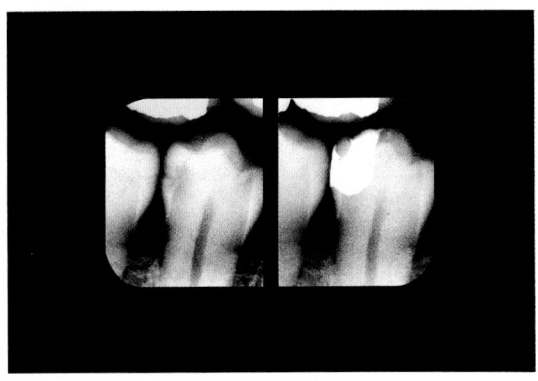

Fig. 13-34c Radiographs of tooth 45 before and after treatment.

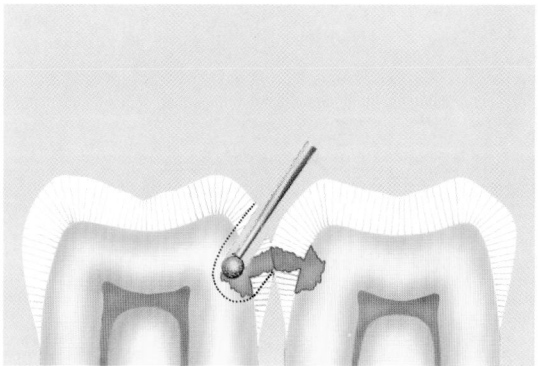

Fig. 13-35 An ideal approximal cavity where access can be gained directly into the carious lesion, or mechanical separation has allowed direct access.

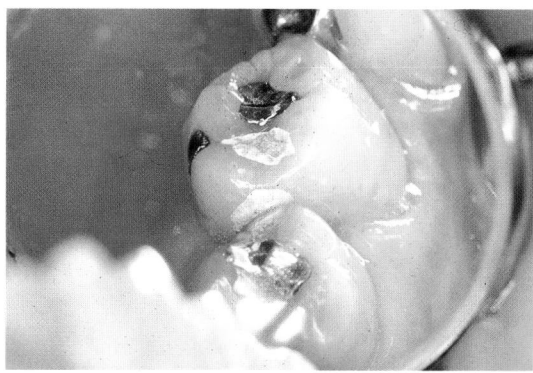

Fig. 13-36 Approximal lesion in tooth 17 restored with silver-cermet cement. Access was easily gained directly into the carious lesion.

Advantages of the occlusal fossa internal preparation

1. Marginal ridge of enamel is left intact; strength of cusps is preserved.
2. Original contact area and embrasure space are maintained.
3. The potential for proximal microleakage is greatly reduced when compared with a Class II amalgam alloy, since the cavity does not involve either proximal or cervical enamel or cause damage to the gingiva.
4. Fluoride release of glass-ionomer provides an artificial dentine barrier to further diffusion of bacteria and possible demineralization, and may assist in remineralization of the white spot lesion.
5. Adjoining tooth is not damaged during preparation.
6. More aesthetic results than for standard Class II restorations.

Disadvantages of the occlusal fossa internal preparation

1. Requires greater skill in preparation and the use of microcutting techniques.
2. May undermine the marginal ridge if badly prepared, causing fracture of the enamel at a later date.
3. Inadequate access channels may not reveal all the dentine caries, particularly in molar teeth.

Approximal approach to an approximal microcavity

Where access is available or mechanical separation of the teeth has been used, the simplest treatment for an approximal lesion is a cavity cut directly through the cavitation in the enamel. The enamel lesion should only be opened sufficiently to gain access to the carious dentine and no attempt should be made to widen the cavity into so-called easy cleansable areas (Fig. 13-35). Glass-ionomer cements give some caries protection so that a microcavity preparation is highly suitable for these materials (Fig. 13-36).

Even though the approximal microrestoration is not subject to much wear, some patients can cause loss of margins when using dental floss. For this reason we often use the glass-ionomer cement/composite resin laminate, which provides a better surface for movement of dental floss and thereby preserves marginal integrity. Where aesthetics is of no importance, silver-cermet cement should be used as illustrated in Fig. 13-36.

Buccolingual approach to an approximal cavity

The treatment of approximal caries using a buccolingual approach requires great skill and should not be attempted unless access can be gained to the lesion easily (McLean, 1980). Generally, the mesial lesion is easier to restore than the distal one (Fig. 13-37); access becomes increasingly difficult the further posteriorly the operator goes.

Premolars are the most suitable for this technique. In particular, the mesial aspects of first premolars can provide easy access (Fig. 13-38). The buccolingual approach should really be compared with a Class III preparation, where enamel is removed only to gain access to the carious dentine.

Procedure

Apply a thin matrix band to the adjoining tooth and using a round diamond stone (HiDi no. 520)* enter the enamel either

*DeTrey, Dentsply International, Inc., Weybridge, England, and York, Pa.

buccally or lingually over the carious lesion (Fig. 13-38). Accurate bite-wing radiographs and fibre-optic lighting will assist in pinpointing the location. Once the enamel has been penetrated, use a no. 2 round bur running at slow speed to remove the carious dentine, and finish the cavity edges with a fine diamond stone. Wash and dry the cavity and release the matrix band but do not remove it. Condition the surface with poly(acrylic acid), as described previously, and line with a Type III glass-ionomer cement (Fig. 13-39). The cement is acid etched, and a composite resin material injected. For these cases, a Centrix syringe is ideal (Fig. 13-40). Fold the matrix band over the composite resin and lightly burnish to position. Trimming can be done with sharp curved scalpels or fluted tungsten carbide burs.

A radio-opaque glass-ionomer cement is preferred for this technique because it allows marginal inaccuracy to be detected easily.

Choice of cavity preparation design

The decision as to what type of cavity preparation design to use when restoring teeth with glass-ionomer cement is fairly complex and depends upon the extent of the dentine caries and the integrity of the enamel marginal ridges. However, certain recommendations can be made:

1. Whenever access is available, prepare an approximal microcavity directly through the cavitated enamel (see Fig. 13-4).
2. Where access is easy, prepare a buccal or lingual approximal cavity similar

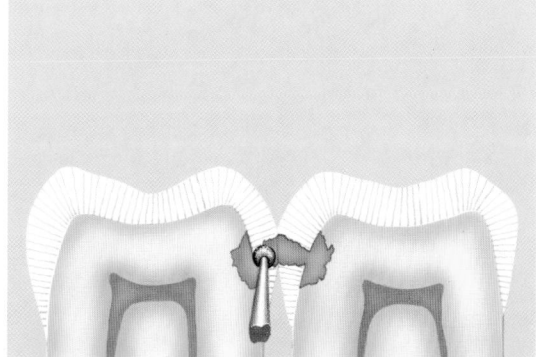

Fig. 13-37 Buccolingual approach into the approximal carious lesion.

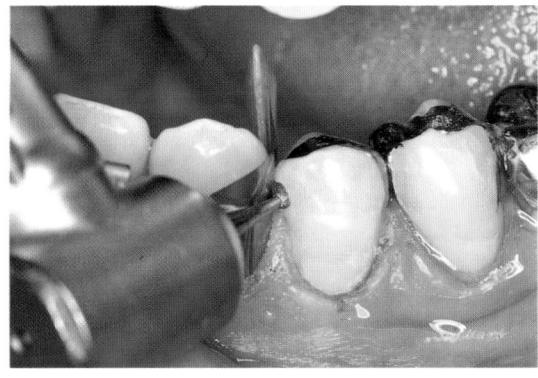

Fig. 13-38 Entrance to carious lesion in tooth 34 made buccally with a small round diamond using matrix band to protect adjoining tooth.

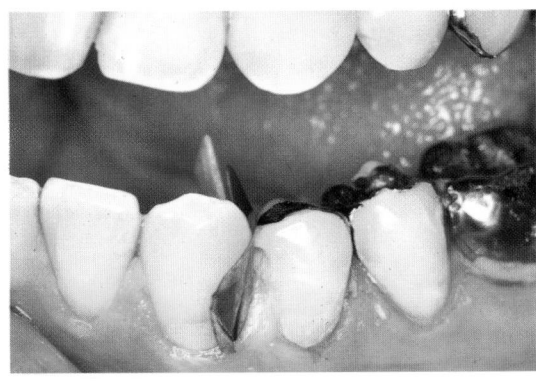

Fig. 13-39 Matrix band released and Type III glass-ionomer cement lining applied prior to filling cavity with composite resin in a syringe.

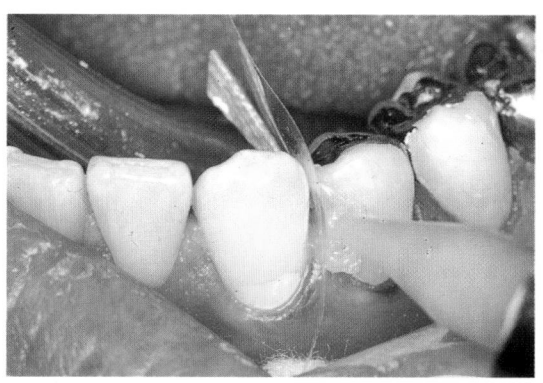

Fig. 13-40 Composite resin injected into cavity in tooth 34 using buccal approximal approach.

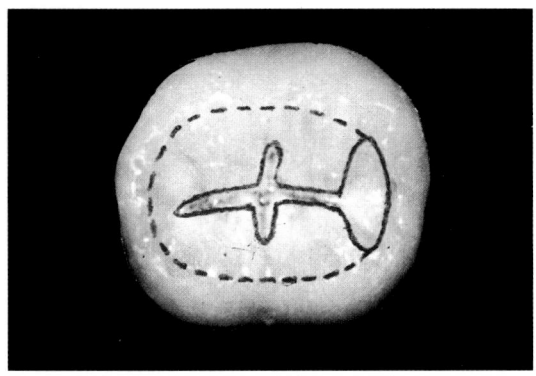

Fig. 13-41a Outline of a typical internal occlusal preparation for a Class II carious lesion. Dotted line indicates maximum size of preparation where extensive dentinal caries is present.

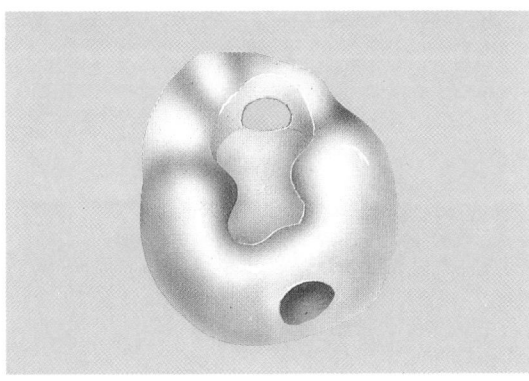

Fig. 13-41b Occlusal view of an internal occlusal preparation for Class II carious lesions where dentinal caries is extensive.

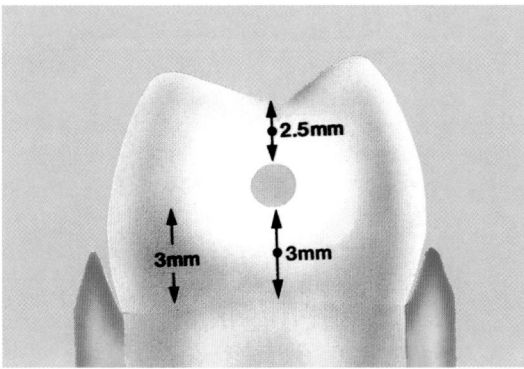

Fig. 13-41c Proximal view of enamel lesion that is generally quite small, leaving a large supporting shell of enamel.

to a Class III lesion (see Fig. 13-5). This type of cavity should not be attempted where dentine caries is extensive or the lesion is not completely visible. Premolars are most suited to this method.

3. Where the caries is confined to the amelodentine junction or entering the dentine, use the internal fossa or tunnel preparation (see Fig. 13-3).

4. Where the marginal ridge is cracked, missing, or severly undermined, prepare an approximal Class II microcavity using an occlusal approach (see Fig. 13-2).

5. Where the marginal ridges are still in-

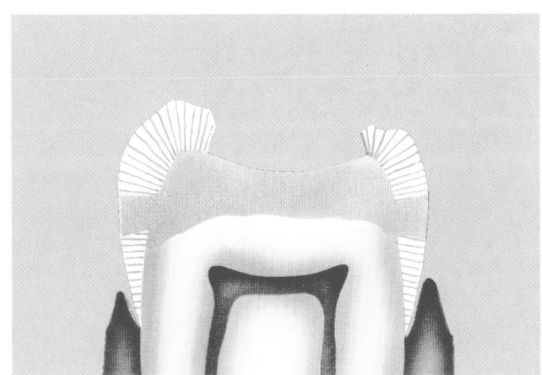

Fig. 13-42a Internal occlusal preparation for a bonded posterior composite resin/glass-ionomer cement laminate in a large Class II carious lesion.

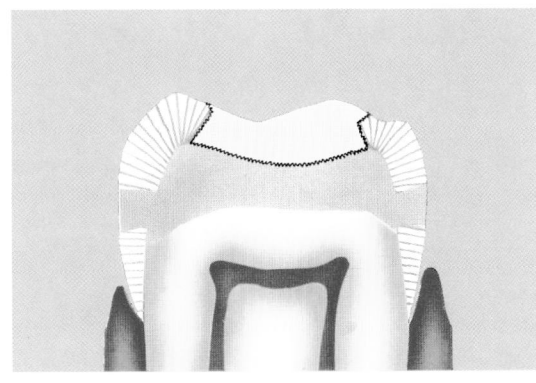

Fig. 13-42b A section through a bonded posterior composite resin/glass-ionomer cement laminate after completion.

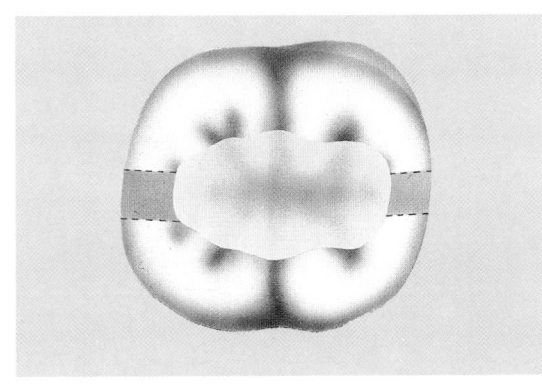

Fig. 13-42c An occlusal view of a bonded posterior composite resin/glass-ionomer cement laminate. The glass-ionomer cement is indicated by the dotted line. For improved strength and abrasion resistance, silver-cermet cement is preferred where aesthetics is not critical.

tact and the peripheral enamel shell is judged to be strong, it is still possible to prepare an occlusal cavity using an internal occlusal fossa approach to the lesion. Providing the operator stays within 2 mm of the peripheral enamel, an extensive occlusal cavity can be prepared to enable all the dentine caries to be removed. The approximal enamel lesions may then be cleaned with chisels (Fig. 13-41). A bonded posterior composite resin will further strengthen the enamel walls (Fig. 13-42).

References

Albers, H.F. (1985) Tooth-Coloured Restoratives. 7th ed. Cotati, Calif: Alto Books.

Handleman, S.L., Leverett, D.H., Espeland, M.A., and Curzon, J.A. (1986) Clinical radiographic evaluation of sealed carious and sound tooth surfaces. J. Am. Dent. Assoc. 113:751–754.

Hunt, P.R. (1984) A modified Class II cavity preparation for glass ionomer restorative materials. Quintessence Int. 15:1011–1015.

Kidd, E.A.M., and Joyston-Bechal, S. (1986) Susceptibility of natural carious lesions in enamel to an artificial caries like attack in vitro. Br. Dent. J. 160:345–347.

Knight, G.M. (1984) The use of adhesive materials in the conservative restoration of selected posterior teeth. Aust. Dent. J. 229:324–331.

McLean, J.W. (1980) Aesthetics in restorative dentistry: The challenge for the future. Br. Dent. J. 149:368–372.

McLean, J.W. (1986) New concepts in cosmetic dentistry using glass-ionomer cements and composites. J. Calif. Dent. Assoc. 21:20–27.

Chapter 14

Restoration of Primary Teeth

Croll and Phillips (1986) have used glass-ionomer/silver-cermet cements for the restoration of primary teeth, and after a two-year clinical trial described the following applications:

1. Class I and II restorations in primary molars, especially when the cement is in contact with adjacent molars
2. Restoration of lingual surfaces (not involving the incisal edge) of primary maxillary incisors damaged by "nursing bottle decay" or other dental caries
3. Restoration of distal surfaces of primary canine teeth
4. Bonded base covering dentine and local areas of calcium hydroxide liner under silver amalgam restorations in primary molars and young permanent posterior teeth
5. As a chemically bonded base under certain composite resin restorations (a 37% phosphoric acid etch for 30 seconds is used to attach the composite)
6. Repair of stainless steel crown surfaces that are worn through because of masticatory abrasion
7. Class V restorations for primary teeth where aesthetics is not important
8. Final restoration of primary molar or canine teeth after a pulpotomy procedure in which the teeth are expected to exfoliate within two years
9. Replacement of amalgam restorations where fracture has occurred
10. Bonded interior restorations awaiting results of direct or indirect calcium hydroxide capping of primary or permanent molars

Croll and Phillips (1986) stated that fractures occurred in some Class II silver-cermet restorations and advocated their use in bulk to overcome this problem. They also advised that restored marginal ridges should be left slightly out of occlusion and that the basic principles of "retention form" must be observed for best results. Mechanical retention will enhance the success of an adhesively bonded glass-ionomer cement restoration.

Fluoride release

The use of glass-ionomer cements in primary teeth is of particular value in preventing recurrent caries and protecting adjoining enamel surfaces in permanent teeth. Fluoride release from these cements over two years is often sufficient to prevent early approximal lesions from developing at a later date.

Clinical procedure for the Class II restoration

Clinical procedures for restoring the Class II carious lesion are illustrated in Figs. 14-1 to 14-21. (Clinical technique by Dr. T. P. Croll.)

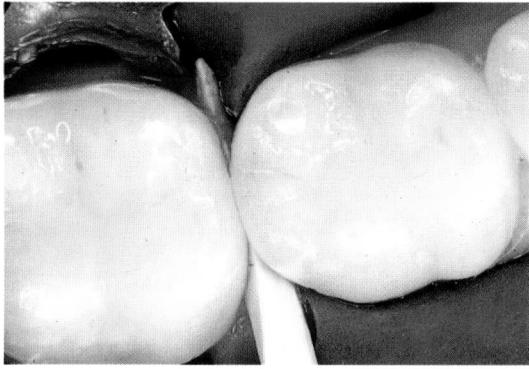

Fig. 14-1 Rubber dam placed using the "slit-dam" technique (Croll, 1985a). A wooden wedge is inserted to protect the gingiva.

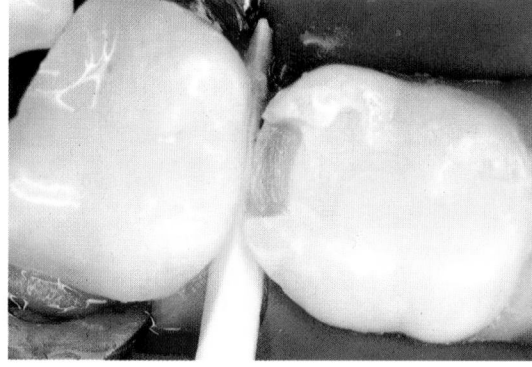

Fig. 14-2 The disto-occlusal preparation is made wider than a traditional amalgam preparation to allow for a larger bulk of silver-cermet material.

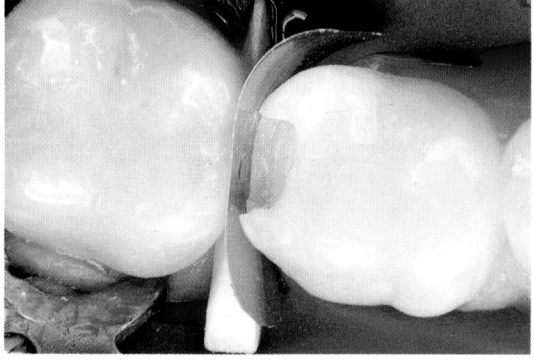

Fig. 14-3 A custom-contoured metal matrix segment is positioned and firmly wedged into place (Croll, 1985b).

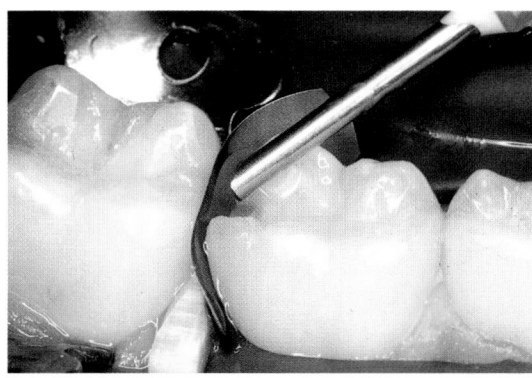

Fig. 14-4 Diluted poly(acrylic acid) is applied to the cavity preparation for five to ten seconds using a 5-cc storage syringe and an 18-gauge blunted needle.

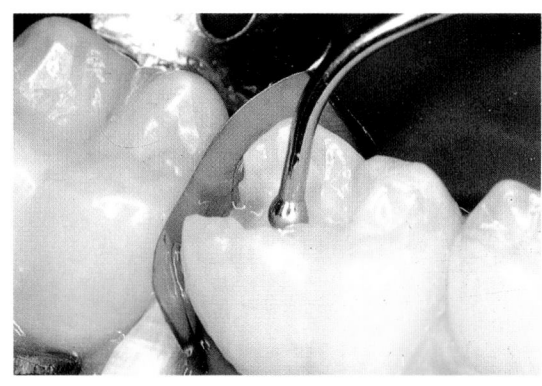

Fig. 14-5 The poly(acrylic acid) is agitated throughout the preparation for five to ten seconds. Such treatment removes the "smear layer," enhancing bonding of material to tooth structure. Had dentinal penetration been deeper, a limited amount of calcium hydroxide liner would have been placed.

Fig. 14-6 After five to ten seconds, the poly(acrylic acid) is washed from the preparation and the silver-cermet cement capsule activated and mixed according to the manufacturer's instructions. The material is immediately injected into the tip of a Centrix syringe.*

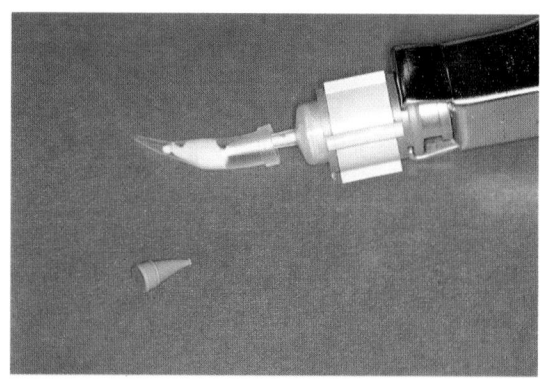

*Centrix Inc., Stratford, Conn.

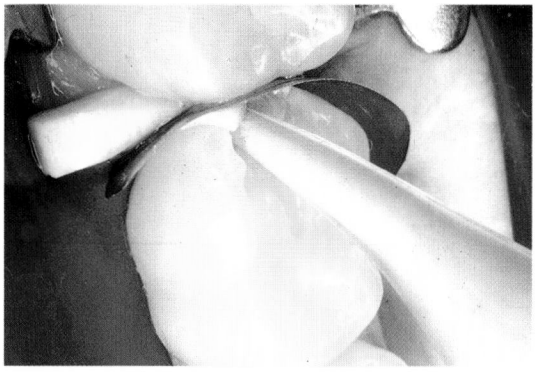

Fig. 14-7 The Centrix syringe tip can be cut to any desired tip diameter, according to the size of the cavity. The silver-cermet cement is then expressed deep into the confines of the preparation. Slow, careful injection avoids entrapment of air bubbles.

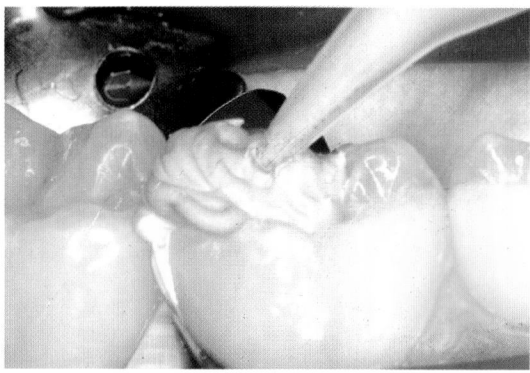

Fig. 14-8 The entire preparation is slowly over-filled with the silver-cermet cement.

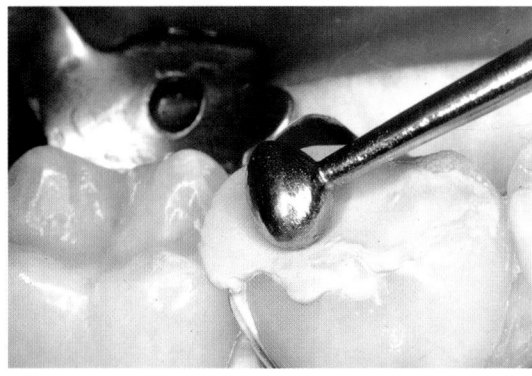

Fig. 14-9 A large burnisher, wiped with water or isopropyl alcohol to avoid sticking, compresses the cement.

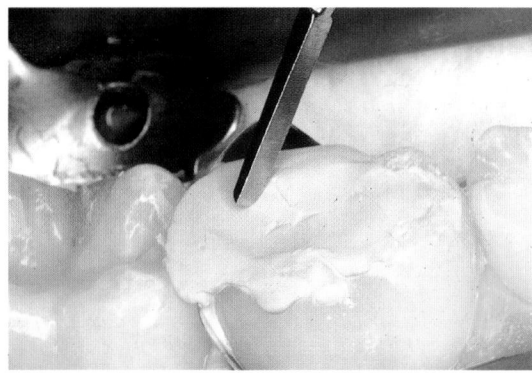

Fig. 14-10 The overfilled restoration is tested with a binangle chisel to see if the surface indents. After about five to seven minutes it is usually hard enough to commence finishing procedures.

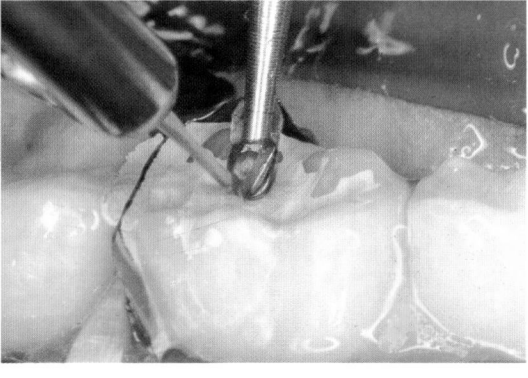

Fig. 14-11 Under copious water spray, bulk excess cement is removed to avoid dehydration of the surface.

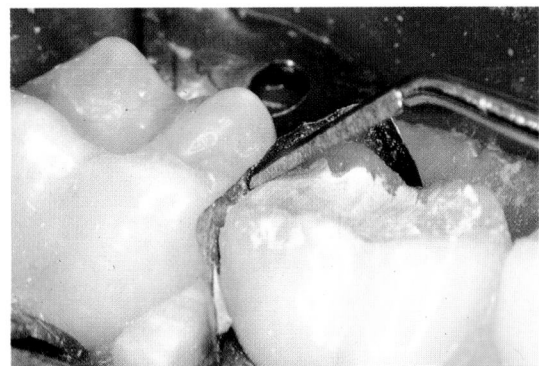

Fig. 14-12 A sharp binangle chisel trims and shapes the marginal ridge region, with the matrix segment retained in place.

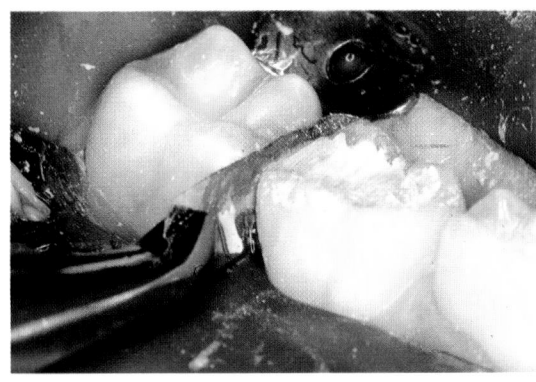

Fig. 14-13 The wooden wedge and matrix are slid buccally for removal.

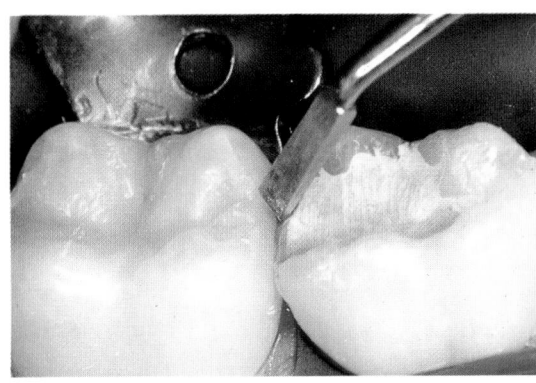

Fig. 14-14 The binangle chisel carves and refines the marginal ridge once more. To avoid fracture in Class II silver-cermet restorations, the marginal ridge is carved slightly out of occlusion and a spoon excavator completes final contours.

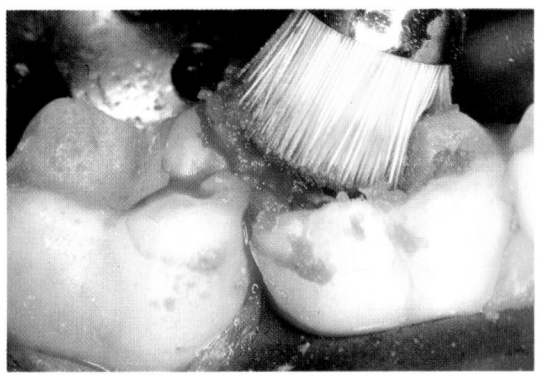

Fig. 14-15 Moist fluoridated prophylaxis paste and a brush are used to smooth the cement.

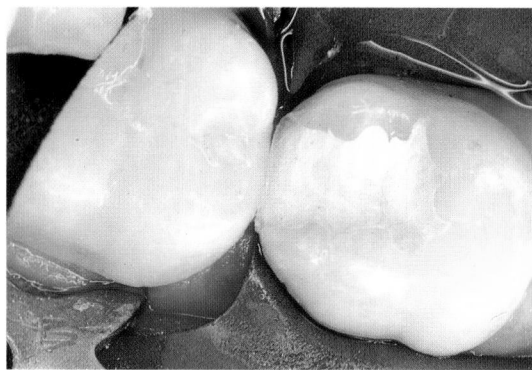

Fig. 14-16 After final polishing, the restoration is seen. Note that a fine feathered edge of marginal cement "flash" remains. The cement should not be finished to the cavosurface margin for at least 24 hours. Practically, final marginal polishing of primary-tooth silver-cermet restorations can wait until the six-month re-evaluation visit.

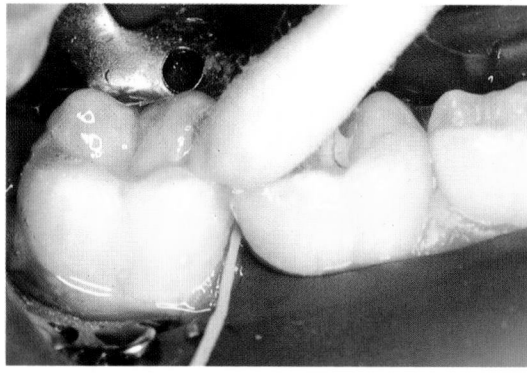

Fig. 14-17 The entire quadrant is treated with a topical fluoride solution as a preventive service to the patient.

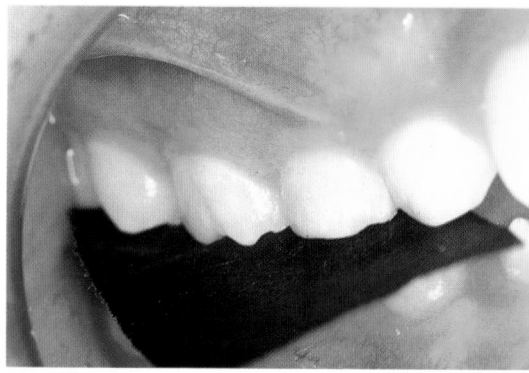

Fig. 14-18 Articulating paper is used to reveal areas of traumatic occlusal contact.

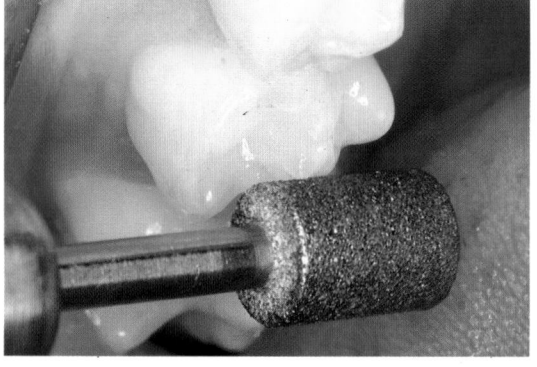

Fig. 14-19 Opposing cusp tips of primary teeth can be blunted to eliminate traumatic occlusal loading on the silver-cermet cement. No significant occlusal alterations result from such trimming of primary teeth.

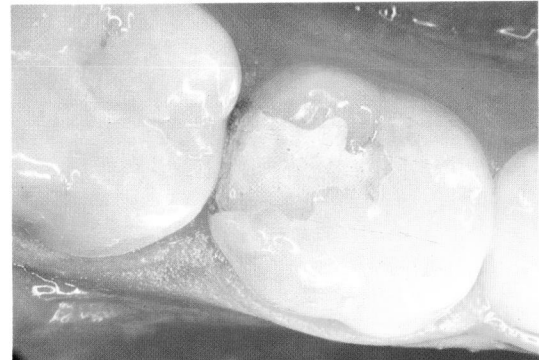

Fig. 14-20 The restoration is shown six months postoperatively after marginal finishing and polishing with prophylaxis paste.

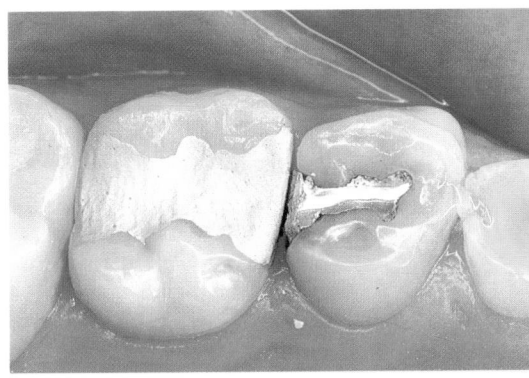

Fig. 14-21 An MOD silver-cermet restoration is seen six months after placement. Note the absence of marginal black stain, which occurred in the early batches of the material due to production of silver oxides.

References

Croll, T.P. (1985a) Primary canine full coronal restoration: New considerations. Quintessence Int. 16:143–150.

Croll, T.P. (1985b) Alternative methods for use of the rubber dam. Quintessence Int. 16:387–392.

Croll, T.P., and Phillips, R.W. (1986) Glass ionomer-silver cermet restorations for primary teeth. Quintessence Int. 17:607–615.

Chapter 15

Glass-Ionomer Luting Cements

The ideal properties of a luting cement have been described by McLean (1979) and Wilson et al. (1977). They may be summarized as follows:

1. Low viscosity and film thickness
2. Long working time with rapid set at mouth temperature
3. Good resistance to aqueous or acid attack
4. High compression and tensile strength
5. Resistance to plastic deformation
6. Adhesion to tooth structure and restoration
7. Cariostatic properties
8. Biological compatibility with the pulp
9. Translucency
10. Radio-opacity

Type I luting cements

The first experimental glass-ionomer cement made for luting purposes was based on a standard mix of calcium aluminosilicate glass powder and a polyacid liquid. The liquid contained a copolymer of acrylic and itaconic acids (Wilson et al., 1977). After the introduction of tartaric acid as a hardener in 1973, further improvements were sought.

The first commercial luting cement was marketed in 1978 using this principle.* However, one of the problems with using these high-viscosity liquids is judging correct consistency; there is a tendency to use a too low powder/liquid ratio, which may result in a weaker cement. In addition, increased film thickness and solubility in saliva during the early stages of setting were noted (Prosser et al., 1984).

To overcome these problems the water-hardening glass-ionomer cements were investigated and recourse was made to a system developed at the Laboratory of the Government Chemist in 1969 by Wilson and Kent and tested clinically by McLean. Early clinical trials in 1978 with a water-hardening glass-ionomer cement, ASPA Va, revealed that excellent working properties could be obtained while meeting most of the above requirements (McLean et al., 1984). Two forms of water-hardening cement based on the use of tartaric acid are possible (Wilson et al., 1977). The acid can either be dissolved in water or blended with the glass-polyacid powder. In the case of ASPA Va (see chapter 2), a powder blend was prepared by mixing 2.5 parts G-200 glass (ground to less than 15 μm), one part solid copolymer PA-2 (prepared by

*Fuji Ionomer I, G. C. International Corp., Tokyo, and Scottsdale, Ariz.

freeze-drying L-2 solution),* and 0.1 part tartaric acid. The results of these early clinical trials indicated that water-hardening glass-ionomer cements offered considerable promise for future commercial exploitation. The following were advantages of this system:

1. Development of very low viscosity in the early mixing stages with easy seating of the restoration
2. Rapid set at mouth temperature
3. Easy dispensing and mixing technique
4. Excellent shelf life

The first commercial water-hardening luting cement, Ketac-Cem† was produced and clinically tested in 1979. The powder is a blend of a copolymer of acrylic and maleic acids with an aluminosilicate glass. The liquid is a 10% solution of tartaric acid.

Physical and mechanical properties

Ketac-Cem possesses excellent physicomechanical properties, which may be summarised as follows:

1. Low viscosity producing a film thickness of c. 20μm
2. Long working time (five minutes; Fig. 15-1)
3. Rapid set four to five minutes
4. Low solubility (1% after seven-minute set)

5. Cariostatic properties due to leaching of fluoride
6. High compressive strength

The properties of water-hardening cements are given in Table 15-1, where they are compared with those of a conventional material.

According to Reisbick (1981), the main disadvantages of these luting cements were lack of radio-opacity, adherence to dry gingiva, and difficulty of removal from the teeth. In addition, their biological compatibility still remains questionable. However, since Reisbick made his comments, radio-opaque versions have appeared.

Biological compatibility

The biological compatibility of the glass-ionomer cements has been reviewed in chapter 8. It is now generally recognized that glass-ionomer cement restorative and lining materials are only mildly irritant to pulpal tissue. In the case of water-based luting materials, however, examples of postoperative sensitivity have been reported that can no longer be regarded as anecdotal. A number of theories have been advanced to explain this phenomenon.

1. A low pH is recorded in the early stages of setting and does not rise as rapidly as zinc phosphate cements (Smith and Ruse, 1986).
2. Because of the exceptionally low viscosity and film thickness of the mixed cement, hydrostatic pressure may be exerted through the dentinal tubules. Full crowns and near-parallel restorations increase the potential for a rise in hydrostatic pressure.

---

*PA-2 is a homopolymer of acrylic acid. L-2 is an aqueous solution of PA-2.
†ESPE GmbH, Seefeld/Oberbay, West Germany, and Valley Stream, N.Y.

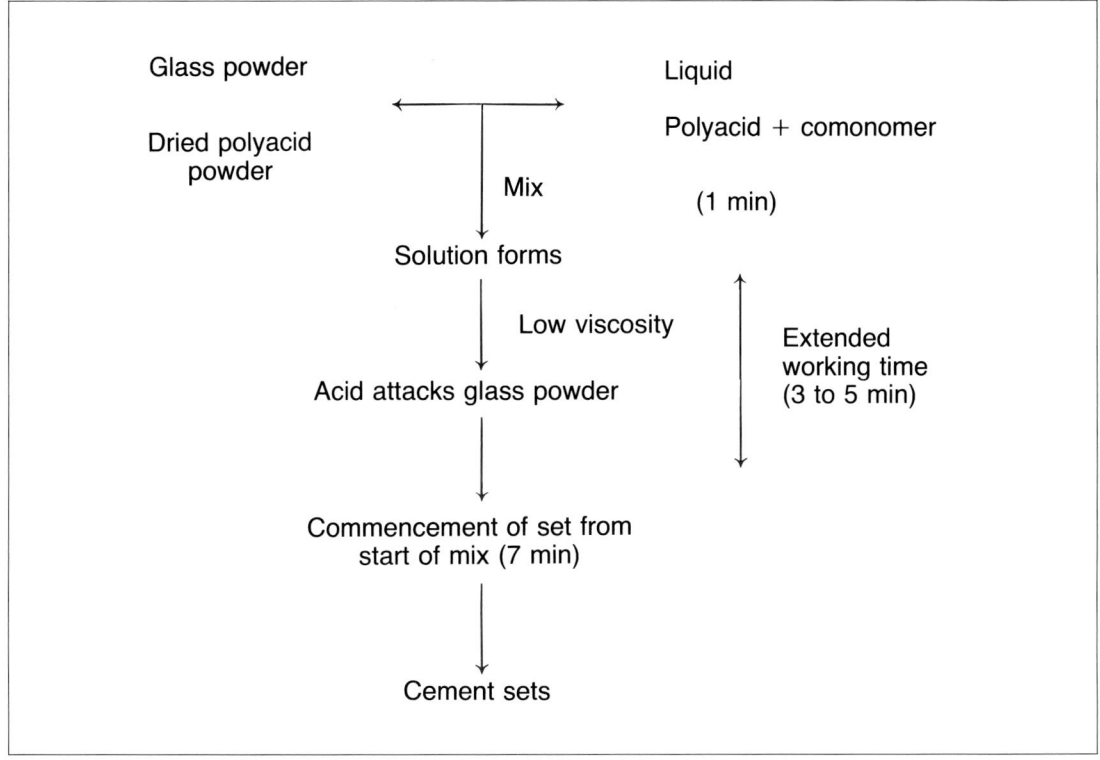

Fig. 15-1 Working time of water-based glass-ionomer cements is extended by the freeze-dried poly-acid powder forming a solution with the liquid prior to any reaction with the glass powder.

Table 15-1 Comparison of properties of conventional and water-hardening cements*

		Water-hardening	
	ASPA IVa†	ASPA Va†	Ketac-Cem‡
Powder/liquid ratio (g/ml)	1.7	3.6	3.4
Consistency disc diam (mm)	29	31	38
Film thickness (μm)	24	22	20
Working time at 23°C (min)	2.5	4.2	5.7
Setting time at 37°C (min)	4.5	5.0	4.5
Compressive strength (MPa)	128	124	105
Water-leachable material (%)	0.9	0.7	0.4
Early vulnerability to water (%)	—	1.8	1.0

*Based on data obtained from McLean et al. (1984).
†Laboratory of the Government Chemist, London.
‡ESPE GmbH, Seefeld/Oberbay., West Germany, and Valley Stream, N.Y.

3. When heavy pressure is exerted during seating of the restoration, the low film thickness may result in the restoration contacting the tooth. A rebound of the restoration may then cause voids in the cement film, which could result in subsequent microleakage and bacterial penetration of the dentine.

4. Too thin a mix can result in washout of cement if the margins are exposed to saliva. Also, evaporation of water from the liquid could increase tartaric acid concentration.

A recent paper by Heys and coworkers (1987) compared pulpal histological responses after crown cementation with zinc phosphate cement, polycarboxylate cement, and a glass-ionomer luting agent, and showed no statistical differences between any of the materials.

The causes of postoperative sensitivity would appear, therefore, to be more related to technique rather than to the chemistry of the glass-ionomer cements. Thin mixes would appear to be the major problem; for this reason, great care should be taken to ensure correct dosage of powder and liquid. Low powder/liquid ratios may also account for the postoperative sensitivity experienced when using glass-ionomer luting cements in which the polyacid is incorporated into the liquid. In the latter case it is very easy to make too thin a mix because of the high-viscosity liquid. It is possible that the introduction of capsulated luting agents could alleviate this problem. It is also inadvisable to remove the smear layer where large tracts of dentine have been exposed.

Surface preparation of tooth and metal surfaces

Preparation of tooth

Prepared surfaces of teeth are always covered with a layer of grinding debris probably composed of particles whose sizes range from less than 1 μm to more than 15 μm (Eick et al., 1970). This debris, the so-called smear layer, can consist of both organic and inorganic material. In addition, the surface can be contaminated with saliva, blood, or remnants of the temporary filling. Grinding debris will invariably contain microorganisms that may remain during cementation (Brännström and Nyborg, 1974). Further, Jendresen and Glantz (1980) have shown that pellicle (biofilm) forms on all surfaces in the mouth and is substantially complete within two hours, converting clean, high-energy surfaces into low-energy, less-easily-wettable substrates.

The cleaning of tooth surfaces does present a considerable problem. There is little doubt that if the dentine is etched with a weakly acidic complexing agent such as a 50% solution of citric acid, all grinding debris can be removed. But such a procedure will undoubtedly open the dentinal tubules and damage the pulp, where large areas of dentine are involved. In addition, Brännström and Johnson (1974) have shown that etching with 37% phosphoric acid can open and widen the tubular apertures of the dentine, thus exposing the pulp to maximum onslaught of the cementing material. Another relevant factor is surface roughness. Even the most carefully finished preparation is rough when considered at microscopic level. For optimum bonding by physicochemical means, adhesion is improved when the substrate surfaces are smooth (Fig. 15-2), as Aboush and

Jenkins (1986) have shown. Surfaces left unfinished after coarse grinding with diamond stones can result in trapping air in re-entrant angles, reducing the area for adhesion (Fig. 15-3).

When preparing a tooth surface for physicochemical adhesion, the clinician must take all the above factors into account. Essentially, the tooth surface should be finished to a macroscopically smooth surface and the contaminated dentine treated with a surface conditioner prior to cementation. Ideally the conditioner should partially remove the smear layer, leaving the tubules still blocked, or react with the smear layer to form bonding sites for the cement (see chapter 6).

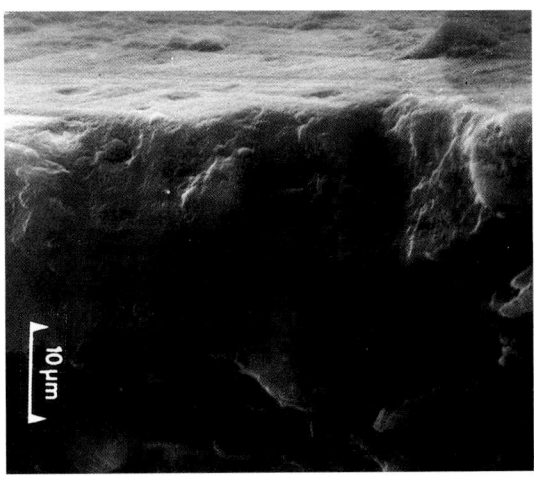

Fig. 15-2 Molecular bonding to dentine surfaces is improved when surface is finished with 40-μm diamonds. Tooth has been fractured to show the very light smearing of the surface.

Tooth-surface finishing instruments

After gross cutting of the tooth preparation, surface roughness should be reduced by using fine diamond stones under copious water spray. Two types of diamond stones are available (Fig. 15-4): sintered diamonds* and microdiamond-plated stones (manufactured by most major diamond stone suppliers). Forty-micrometer diamonds are recommended. Sintered diamonds or microdiamond-plated stones produce a macroscopically smooth surface that can then be surface conditioned (see Fig. 15-2).

Surface conditioning

After finishing with fine diamonds and washing with air-water spray, the dentine surface is still grooved and contaminated

*Hi-Di, Dentsply International Inc., Weybridge, England, and York, Pa.

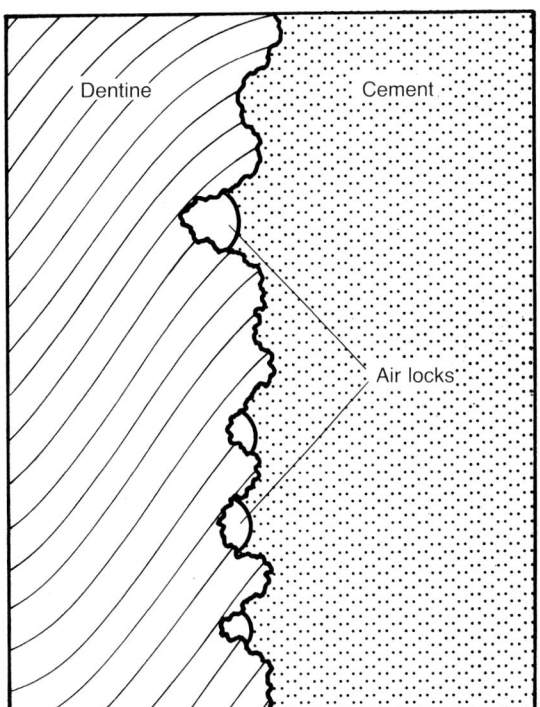

Fig. 15-3 Loss of adhesion due to rough surfaces producing reentrant angles. Good adhesion of the cement is prevented by air entrapment.

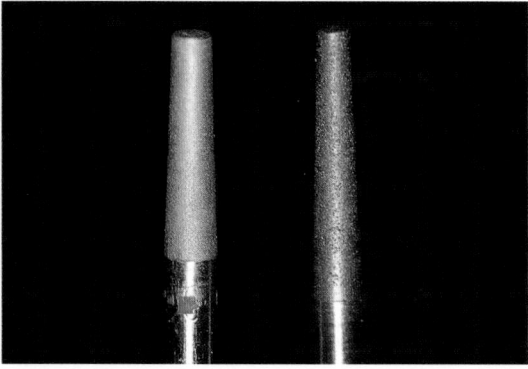

Fig. 15-4 Sintered diamond stone *(right)* and a microfine plated diamond stone *(left)*.

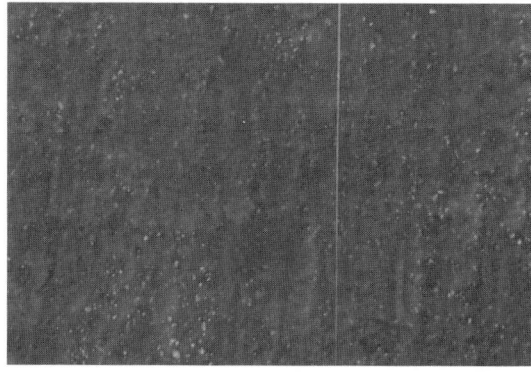

Fig. 15-5 Electron micrograph of the so-called smear layer in dentine produced by grinding with fine diamonds (original magnification ×200).

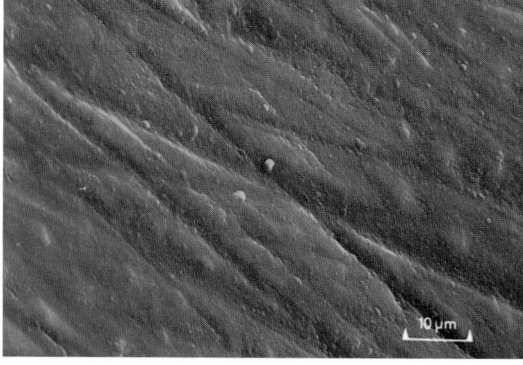

Fig. 15-6 Electron micrograph of dentine surface treated with tannic acid. Note the smooth surfaces are only interrupted by blisters where the dentinal tubules are present.

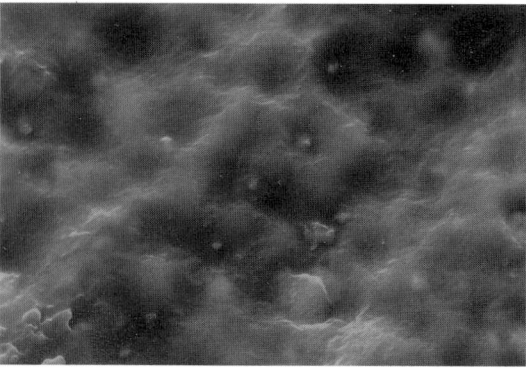

Fig. 15-7 Smear layer partially removed when dentine is treated with a 25% poly(acrylic acid) solution for ten seconds.

with grinding debris—the smear layer (Fig. 15-5). The dentinal tubules remain blocked and can only just be observed. The strength of the bond between the glass-ionomer cement and this surface is only 3.1 MPa (Powis et al., 1982). Treatment of the dentine with a 25% tannic acid solution, a tanning agent for collagen, yielded a smooth striated surface with small blisters indicating the location of tubules (Fig. 15-6). Collagen reacts with tannic acid and the smooth topography is attributed either to the smear layer caused by grinding or the formation of a layer of reaction products. The bond strength of the glass-ionomer cement to this surface was high (6.3 MPa). Results obtained with poly(acrylic acid) solution were similar (Powis et al., 1982), except that 25% poly(acrylic acid) will partially remove the smear layer (Fig. 15-7).

Powis et al. (1982) concluded that the bond strengths of glass-ionomer cements to tooth material can be enhanced greatly by the use of a suitable conditioner for the pretreatment of enamel or dentine. Solutions of 25% tannic acid, poly(acrylic acid), or a fluoride-containing surface-active substance (dodicin) were found to be most effective. The adhesive bond strength of the glass-ionomer cement to enamel or dentine could be made to approach the true tensile strength of the cement. *In the case of a full-veneer crown preparation where large areas of dentine are exposed, a 25% tannic acid solution applied for 30 seconds and lightly dried is preferred.*

Preparation of metal surfaces

Improved bonding of glass-ionomer cements to metal may be achieved when some surface oxides are present. In the case of metals used for porcelain bonding, no further treatment of the metal surface is required, since these alloys are designed specifically to provide oxide surfaces for porcelain attachment. In the case of the gold alloys used for crown and inlay construction, tin-plating of the nonfit surface can be beneficial (Hötz et al., 1977; McLean, 1977). A maximum coating of 2 μm is required and should be lightly oxidized at 500°C for one minute. A tin-oxide surface will provide the means for chemical bonding to the carboxyl groups in the glass-ionomer cement. When tin-plating inlays, the nonfit surfaces should be coated with wax or varnish prior to plating and oxidizing (Fig. 15-8). The Vita Ceramiplater,* used for plating foils in the aluminous porcelain crown technique, is a suitable machine for this purpose because it is designed to limit the tin-plate thickness to around 2 μm, which does not interfere with bonding (Fig. 15-9). Bond strengths of Aspa IVa glass-ionomer cement to a gold casting alloy gave figures of 0.05 MPa for unplated gold against 4.3 MPa for tin-plated and oxidized gold (Hötz et al., 1977). The inlay cemented with water-hardening glass-ionomer luting cement is illustrated in Fig. 15-10.

*Vita Zahnfabrik, Bad Säckingen, West Germany.

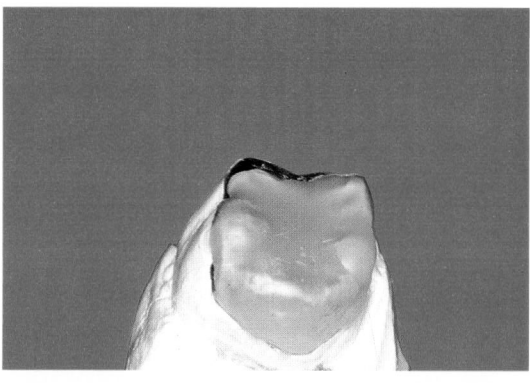

Fig. 15-8 Nonfit surface of gold inlay coated with wax to prevent plating of the polished surface.

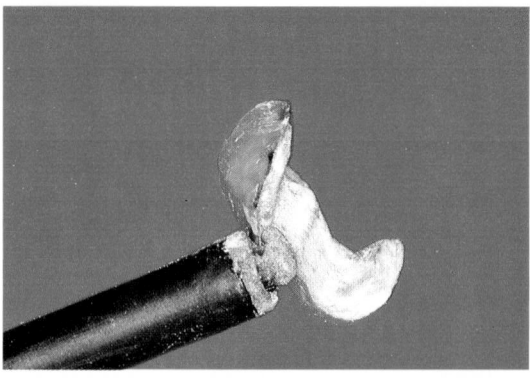

Fig. 15-9a Inlay attached to Ceramiplater clip and coated with tin.

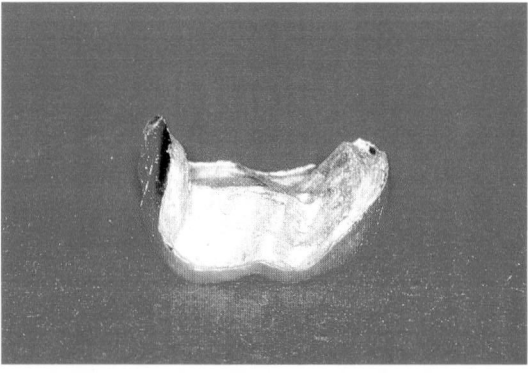

Fig. 15-9b Wax burned off and tin lightly oxidized at 500°C.

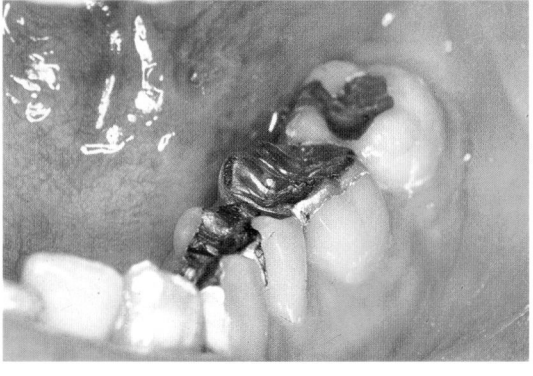

Fig. 15-10 Inlay in tooth 36 cemented with water-hardening glass-ionomer luting cement.

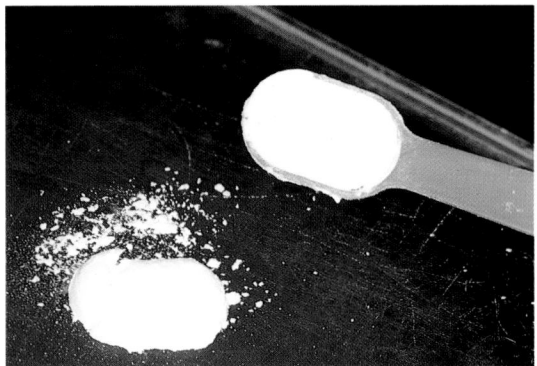

Fig. 15-11a Ketac-Cem luting powder dispensed from measuring scoop.

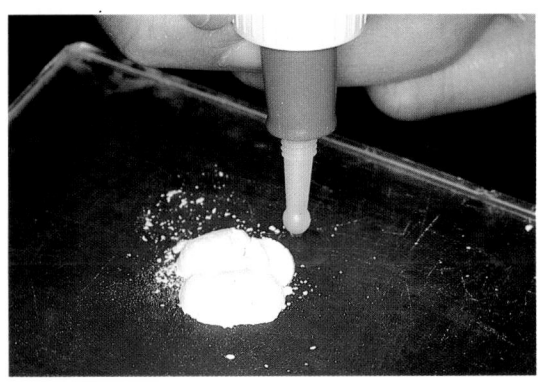

Fig. 15-11b Tartaric acid solution dispensed by inverting bottle to prevent drops of liquid from running down side of dispenser.

Clinical procedures for glass-ionomer luting cements

The principles for mixing a water-hardening glass-ionomer cement will be given using the first such commercially-developed material, Ketac-Cem.

Dispensing and mixing

The procedure for mixing Ketac-Cem luting cement should be followed closely, since failure to achieve a mix in which the optimum powder/liquid ratio is used can result in thin mixes that may cause pulpal sensitivity.

1. Shake the cement powder bottle prior to filling the measuring scoop. The scoop should be firmly filled but not compacted and the powder levelled to the rim with a spatula (Fig. 15-11a). Average weight of the powder should be in the region of 0.35 g.
2. Dispense the powder onto a clean glass slab that has been chilled and wiped dry. According to the mix required, each scoop of powder requires two drops of liquid, which gives a powder/liquid ratio of approximately 3.5 g/ml.
3. Invert the liquid bottle and dispense the tartaric acid solution drop by drop onto the slab according to the number of measures of powder. Generally two scoops are needed for each crown (Fig. 15-11b).

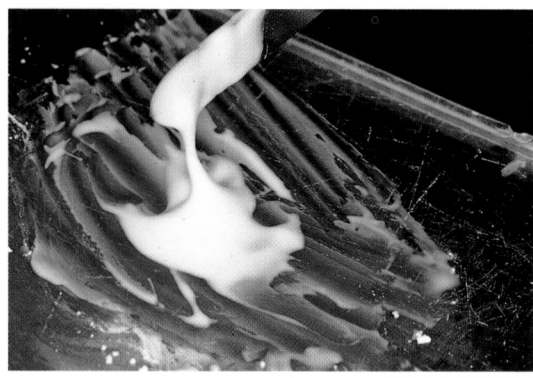

Fig. 15-12 Ideal mix of Ketac-Cem cement showing creamy consistency. Do not mix cement too thinly since this can produce postoperative sensitivity due to hydraulic pressure.

4. Incorporate the powder into the liquid as quickly as possible using a tantalum or stainless steel spatula. At first the mix will be watery. Do not be tempted to add more powder, because as the liquid dissolves the polyacid powder the mix will thicken and become creamy. The viscosity of the mix should allow it to run off the spatula (Fig. 15-12).

Cementation

1. Clean the surface of the dentine as previously described with a 25% tannic acid solution. Tannic acid is best applied for 30 seconds. If a zinc oxide temporary cement is still present remove it, using rubber cups and pumice flour mixed in water, prior to surface conditioning. Wash off all debris with a continuous blast of air/water spray and lightly dry the tooth with absorbent cotton (Fig. 15-13).

Tooth surfaces should be clean, but not dehydrated, when the cement is applied. Overdrying may also contribute to postoperative sensitivity. Unless there is a problem in maintaining a dry field, a rubber dam is not required because its use may result in dehydration of the dentine if the tooth is left exposed to the atmosphere for too long.

2. Apply the cement to the restoration and tooth with a small, stiff brush. The mixed cement is easily picked up on the brush, and the inlay or crown surface is lightly coated, with care taken to wet out all surfaces thoroughly (Fig. 15-14). It has been found that brushing a light coat of cement into the crown promotes a better fit than completely filling the crown with cement (Ishikiriama et al., 1981). Brush a light coat of cement onto the tooth surface and make certain that the cement is worked into all the line angles of the preparation (Fig. 15-15).

3. Seat the restoration on the tooth with firm pressure with a ball-ended burnisher. For complete porcelain veneer crowns, only finger pressure is required (Fig. 15-16). Do not ask the patient to bite on a wooden spatula or similar device to ensure seating. Not only can this procedure weaken a porcelain crown by introducing microcracks, but it may also cause excessive hydrostatic pressure, as discussed previously. With gold inlays, undesirable stresses can be placed on dentine walls. Restorations should have a free sliding fit, and the use of die spacers in construction is recommended (Eames, 1981). The seating of the castings may also be improved by vibration.

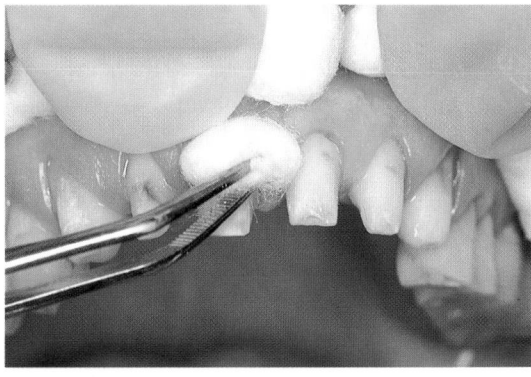

Fig. 15-13 After surface conditioning with 25% tannic acid the tooth should be lightly dried with absorbent cotton wool. Do not dehydrate under air spray because this may decrease wettability and cause pulpal damage.

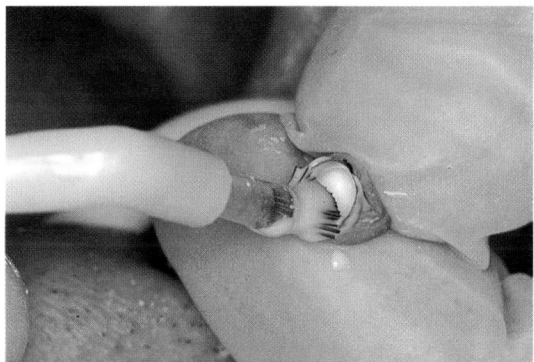

Fig. 15-14 Crown lightly coated with cement, taking care to wet out the internal line and point angles.

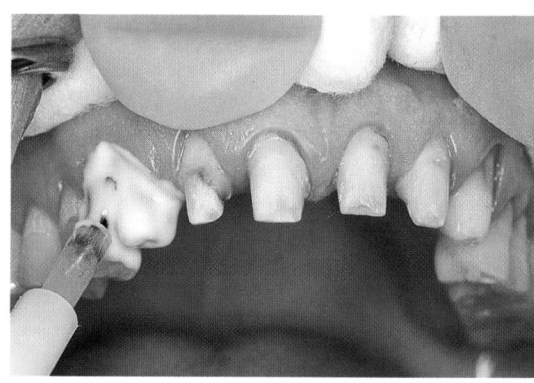

Fig. 15-15 Tooth surface lightly coated with cement.

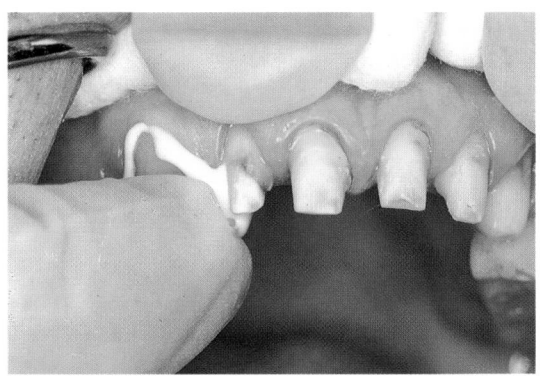

Fig. 15-16 Crown seated with finger pressure.

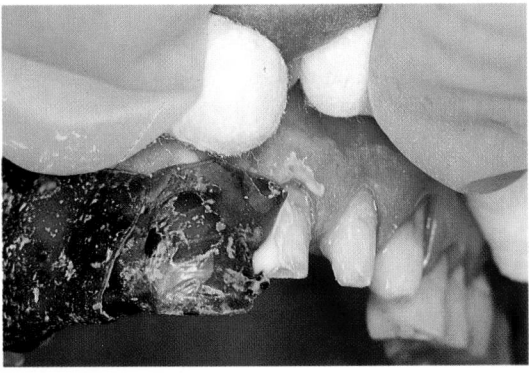

Fig. 15-17 Restoration and cement protected with occlusal indicator wax during setting.

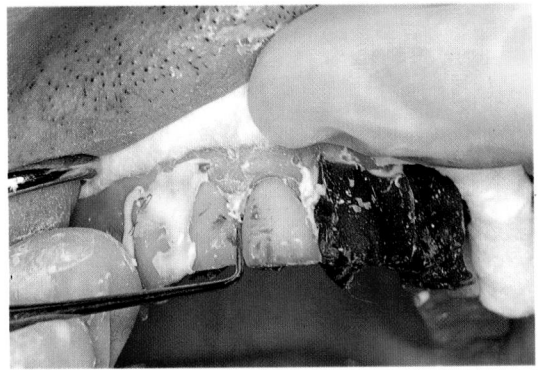

Fig. 15-18 After setting, excess cement carefully removed with an explorer or ultrasonic scaler.

Figs. 15-19a and b Anterior view of crowns cemented on maxillary teeth.

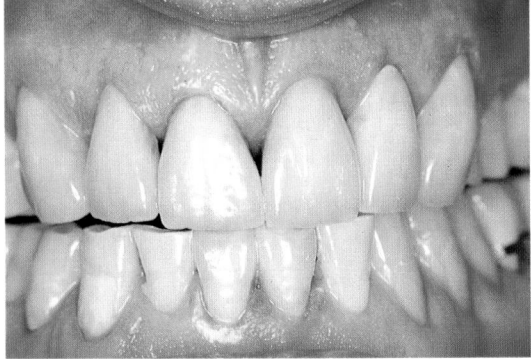

Fig. 15-19a

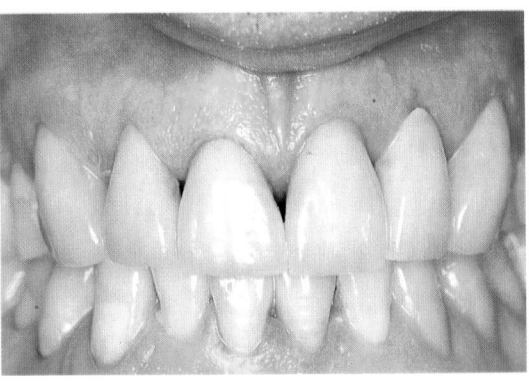

Fig. 15-19b

4. Immediately after seating, cover the entire restoration gingival margin with a soft wax (Kerr's green occlusal indicator wax*) so that all margins are tightly adapted. The wax will prevent any gingival seepage during setting and is an excellent way of stopping ingress of saliva (Fig. 15-17).

5. Allow the cement to set for five minutes. Timing should start only after the restoration is seated and covered with wax. At the end of five minutes the wax is peeled off and the cement removed from the margins with a sharp explorer or an ultrasonic scaler (Fig. 15-18). The margins may then be varnished as an added protection.

The crowns cemented in the mouth are shown in Fig. 15-19.

Cementation of post crowns

Glass-ionomer cements are ideally suited for cementation of posts because of their low viscosity and excellent wettability.

1. Clean all temporary cement or debris out of the root canal with mechanical and water irrigation. A root canal file is a useful instrument for this purpose. Dry the canal with paper points and then wash out with a 50% citric acid solution. The stronger acid will remove all debris and is probably better than poly(acrylic acids) for root canals. Wash and dry the canal again with paper points (Fig. 15-20). Cast gold posts may be tin-plated and oxidized to improve bonding to the cement.

2. After mixing the cement, brush it onto the post to form a thin film (Fig. 15-21). Brush some cement into the canal

orifice and ream it into the root canal with a spiral root filler (Fig. 15-22a) and spread it with an engineer's twist drill. A hand-held drill will ensure that the cement is wetting all surfaces of the canal, thus avoiding the risk of air entrapment (Fig. 15-22b). After spreading the cement, add a little more to the post hole with a spiral filler.

3. Insert the post into the canal and seat to position with steady pressure. Do not hammer or tap the post into position, since this can cause cracking of the dentine and possible root splitting (Fig. 15-23). The low viscosity of the water-hardening glass-ionomer cements allows easy seating without the risk of post "rebound" because of rapidly stiffening pastes. The crown cemented on tooth 12 is shown in Fig. 15-24.

Retention of castings with glass-ionomer cement

The retentive ability of glass-ionomer cements is good—in one in vitro study the glass-ionomer cement required an average of 65.2% more tensile force to unseat the inlays than was required to unseat those luted with zinc phosphate cement. Similarly, an improvement (27.7%) was noted for the glass-ionomer cement over the zinc silicophosphate cement (McComb, 1982).

---

*Kwik-Wax, Kerr Mfg. Co., Div. of Sybron Corp., Romulus, Mich.

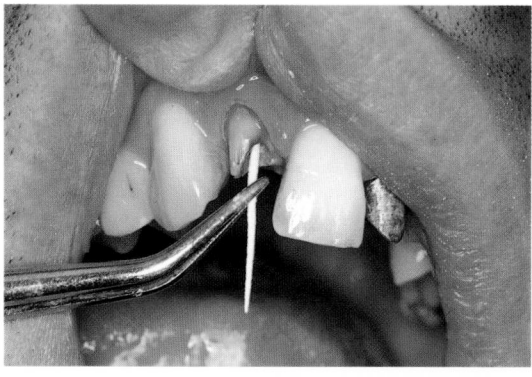

Fig. 15-20 Paper points used to thoroughly dry canal after surface conditioning.

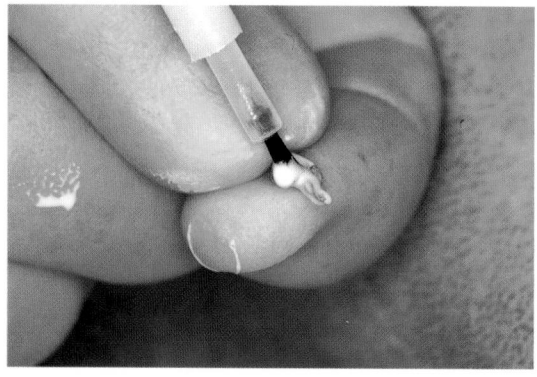

Fig. 15-21 Post lightly coated with cement.

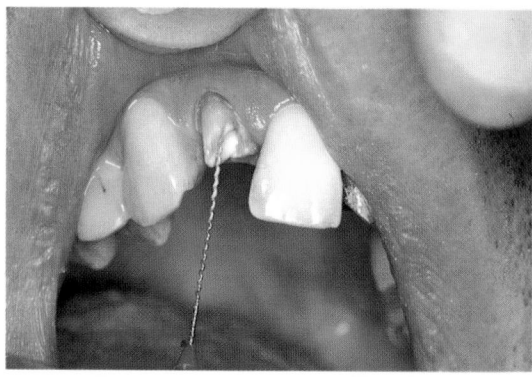

Fig. 15-22a Cement has been spun into the canal with a spiral filler.

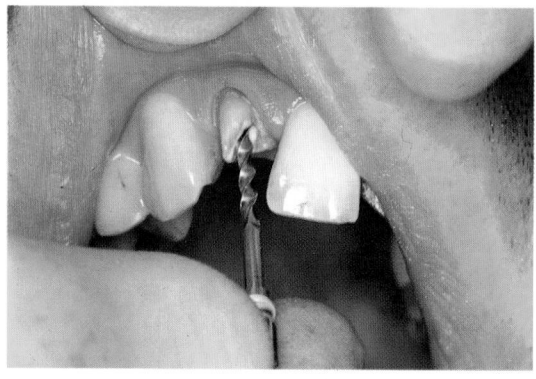

Fig. 15-22b An engineer's twist drill may be used to spread cement evenly over the canal walls.

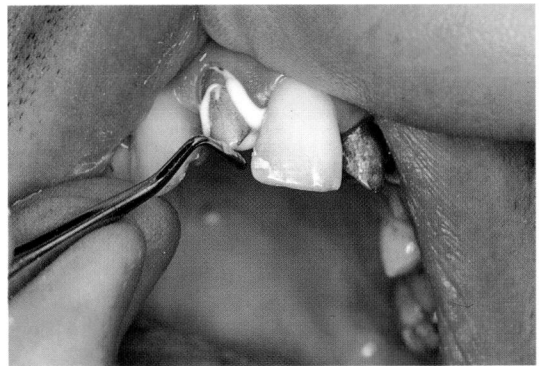

Fig. 15-23 Post and core seated with firm finger pressure. Do not tap or hammer the post to position since there is a high risk of causing microcracks in the dentine.

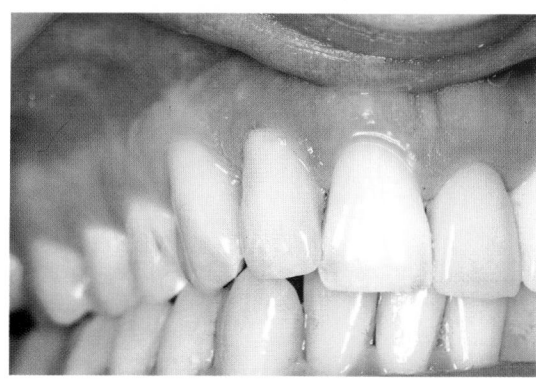

Fig. 15-24 Completed crown on tooth 12.

Anticariogenic effect of glass-ionomer luting cements

The ability of the glass-ionomer cements to leach fluoride and provide some anticariogenic effect is well known. A recent study on secondary caries formation in vitro around glass-ionomer restorations by Hicks and coworkers (1986) showed that glass-ionomer cements provided protection against a carieslike attack at the enamel/restoration interface, as evidenced by the absence of cavity wall lesions. The lesions in surface enamel adjacent to the glass-ionomer cements were reduced significantly, when compared with control lesions.

Kidd and McLean (1979) investigated the cavity sealing ability of cemented cast gold restorations assessed in vitro by an acidified gel artificial caries technique. Where glass-ionomer cement was used as the luting agent it was observed that the area of positive birefringence of the outer lesion was at some distance from the cavity wall (Fig. 15-25). In the case of restorations cemented with zinc phosphate cement, the outer wall lesion adjoined the cavity wall (Fig. 15-26). These authors suggested that the fluoride in the glass-ionomer cement was responsible for the diminution of the extent of the outer lesion in Fig. 15-25.

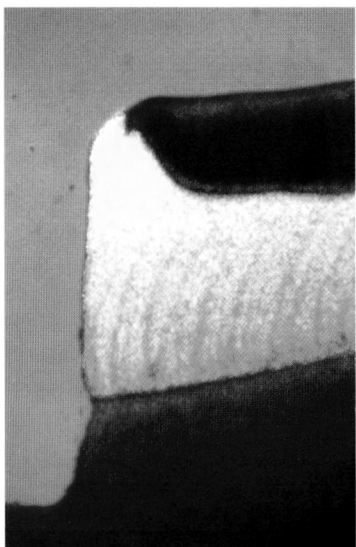

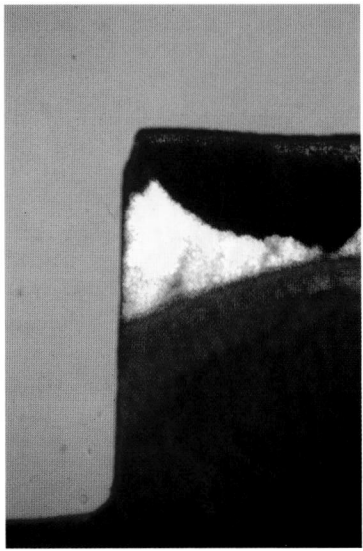

Fig. 15-25 Section of cavity wall of an inlay cemented with Ketac-Cem. Outer lesion is at some distance from the cavity wall due to action of fluoride leached from the cement. The fluorapatite crystals are more resistant to acid attack. Reprinted with permission from Kidd and McLean (1979).

Fig. 15-26 Section of cavity wall of an inlay cemented with zinc phosphate cement. Outer lesion adjoins the cavity wall where no fluoride is present. Reprinted with permission from Kidd and McLean (1979).

References

Aboush, Y.E.Y., and Jenkins, C.B.G. (1986) An evaluation of the bonding of a glass-ionomer restorative to dentine. Br. Dent. J. 161:79–184.

Brännströmm, M., and Nyborg, H. (1974) Bacterial growth and pulpal changes under inlays cemented with zinc phosphate cement and epoxylite CBA 9080^p. J. Prosthet. Dent. 31:556.

Brännströmm, M., and Johnson, G. (1974) Effects of various conditioners and cleaning agents on prepared dentin surfaces: A scanning electron microscopic investigation. J. Prosthet. Dent. 31:42.

Eames, W.B. (1981) The casting misfit: How to cope. J. Prosthet. Dent. 45:283–285.

Eick, J.D., Wilks, R.A., Anderson, C.H., and Sorensen, S.E. (1970) Scanning electron microscopy of cut tooth surfaces and identification of debris by use of electron microprobe. J. Dent. Res. 49:1359–1368.

Heys, R.J., Fitzgerald, M., Heys, D.R., and Charbeneau, G.T. (1987) An evaluation of a glass ionomer luting agent: Pulpal histological response. J. Am. Dent. Assoc. 114:607–611.

Hicks, M.J., Flaitz, C.M., and Silverstone, L.M. (1986) Secondary caries formations in vitro around glass ionomer cements. Quintessence Int. 17:527–532.

Hötz, P.R., McLean, J.W., Sced, I.R., and Wilson, A.D. (1977) The bonding of glass ionomer cements to metal and tooth substrates. Br. Dent. J. 142:41–47.

Ishikiriama, A., Oliviera, J. de F., Vieira, D. F., and Mondelli, J. (1981) Influence of some factors on the fit of cemented crowns. J. Prosthet. Dent. 45:400–404.

Jendresen, M.D., and Glantz, P.-O. (1980) Clinical adhesiveness of tooth surface. Acta Odontol. Scand. 38:379–383.

Kidd, E.A.M., and McLean, J.W. (1979) The cavity sealing ability of cemented cast gold restorations. Br. Dent. J. 147:39–41.

McComb, D. (1982) Retention of castings with glass ionomer cement. J. Prosthet. Dent. 48:285–288.

McLean, J.W. (1977) A new method of bonding dental cements and porcelains to metal surfaces. Oper. Dent. 2:130–142.

McLean, J.W. (1979) The Science and Art of Dental Ceramics. Vol. 1. Chicago: Quintessence Publ. Co., p. 325.

McLean, J.W., Wilson, A.D., and Prosser, H.J. (1984) Development and use of water-hardening glass-ionomer luting cements. J. Prosthet. Dent. 52:175–181.

Powis, D.R., Folleras, T., Merson, S.A., and Wilson, A.D. (1982) Improved adhesion of a glass-ionomer cement to dentine and enamel. J. Dent. Res. 61:1416–1422.

Prosser, H.J., Powis, D.R., Brant, P., and Wilson, A.D. (1984) The characterisation of glass-ionomer cements. 7. The physical properties of current materials. J. Dent. 12:231–240.

Reisbick, M.H. (1981) Working qualities of glass-ionomer cements. J. Prosthet. Dent. 52:182–189.

Smith, D.C., and Ruse, N.D. (1986) Acidity of glass-ionomer cements during setting and its relation to pulp sensitivity. J. Am. Dent. Assoc. 112:654–657.

Wilson, A.D., Crisp, S., Lewis, B.G., and McLean, J.W. (1977) Experimental luting agents based on the glass-ionomer cements. Br. Dent. J. 142:117–122.

Chapter 16

Posterior Restorations

Composite resin restorations in posterior teeth is still a matter of controversy, the two main criticisms being surface wear and lack of permanent adhesion to dentine (see chapters 6 and 11). Recently, the use of glass-ionomer cement bases to replace missing dentine has become popular. Although this technique was originally described by McLean and Wilson in 1977, manufacturers were slow to develop fast-setting glass-ionomer cements for this purpose. Only recently have Type III fast-setting glass-ionomer cements become available for bonding composite resins to dentine (see chapter 2).

Glass-ionomer cements have four main advantages when used for the attachment of posterior composite resins to dentine:

1. Minimal shrinkage with good adhesion and dimensional stability arise from their hydrophilic nature.
2. Adhesion is not affected when the cement is bulk packed. The volume of composite resin veneer required to complete the restoration is less, further reducing shrinkage problems.
3. Anticariogenic properties result from leaching of fluoride.
4. The cement can be acid etched to provide mechanical bonding sites for the composite resin.

The disadvantage of using a glass-ionomer cement/composite resin laminate system is that the strength of the bond between resin and cement or dentine and cement is still inadequate for use in high-stress-bearing areas. Generally failure will be a cohesive one in the cement at the resin or dentine interface.

Fortunately, in the posterior restoration, composite resin attachment to enamel is strong enough to give some protection to the glass-ionomer cement. The main purpose of the cement base is to prevent microleakage and postoperative sensitivity at the dentine interface.

At the present time, no long-term clinical studies have been done on the success of glass-ionomer cements as alternatives to "dentine-bonding agents," based, for example, on phosphonate esters. However, their increasing use is indicative of the clinician's success in reducing dentine sensitivity under posterior composite resins (Miller, 1986).

When using glass-ionomer cement bases it should be appreciated that certain combinations of glass-ionomer cement and posterior composite resin are better than others (Hinoura et al., 1987). These are difficult to quantify, but certain recommendations can be made:

1. Thicker layers of glass-ionomer cement ($>$0.5 mm) are better than a thin

wash lining. Thin linings may disintegrate when etched with acid.

2. Type II glass-ionomer cements are stronger and give improved bond strengths as compared with Type III lining cements.

3. Metal-reinforced glass-ionomer cements give the highest bond strengths (Hinoura et al., 1987) and are radio-opaque.

4. Although giving lower bond strengths, the fast-setting Type III glass-ionomer cements can be safely etched after much shorter time periods and, provided that very high strengths are not required, are the materials of choice. Most are radio-opaque.

5. Low-viscosity bonding resins, with their improved wettability, tend to produce higher bond strengths (Mount, 1986).

6. Reduction of the bulk of composite resin by using a glass-ionomer base will reduce polymerization contraction and improve the longevity of the bond. Veneer thicknesses should be in the range of 1.5 mm to 2 mm.

Clinical procedures

In order to illustrate the use of glass-ionomer cements for bonding composite resins to dentine, a typical Class II restoration, which would normally be restored with amalgam or gold, will be illustrated. In the case of the early approximal lesion, the microcavity techniques described in chapter 13 would be preferred. All posterior composite resins should be inserted under a rubber dam, and the use of magnification is strongly recommended.

Cavity preparation

After removal of the caries or old amalgam restoration, the cervical floor angles should be rounded. Where possible, all interproximal exit angles should be finished to a 90° angle (Fig. 16-1). Microdiamond stones are ideal for this procedure. The occlusal isthmus should not be widened more than is required for removal of the existing amalgam restoration. Any caries or soft dentine should be removed with slow-running round burs or sharp excavators. Some mechanical retention is beneficial, since the strength of the glass-ionomer cement or composite resin acid-etch bond may prove insufficient if sudden occlusal stresses occur—such as when eating very sticky foods.

Lining

Where a near-exposure of the pulp is observed, a very small bead of setting calcium hydroxide should be placed just over the pulp horn (Fig. 16-2). The cavity is then washed and dried and a 25% solution of poly(acrylic acid) applied for ten seconds to partially remove the smear layer. The tooth is again washed and dried and a creamy mix of lining cement is prepared and applied to all dentine surfaces with the applicator (Fig. 16-3). We prefer a Type III cement, such as Ketac-Bond,* for this purpose. *Do not apply a thin wash,* but rather make certain that a layer of at least 0.5 mm is inserted. Preferably, this layer should be thicker for best results. However, a space must be left occlusally for at least 1.5 mm of composite resin (Fig. 16-4). With practice, the cement can be applied to cover the dentine exactly, but in the event of any excess flowing over the enamel, it

*ESPE GmbH, Seefeld/Oberbay, West Germany, and Valley Stream, N.Y.

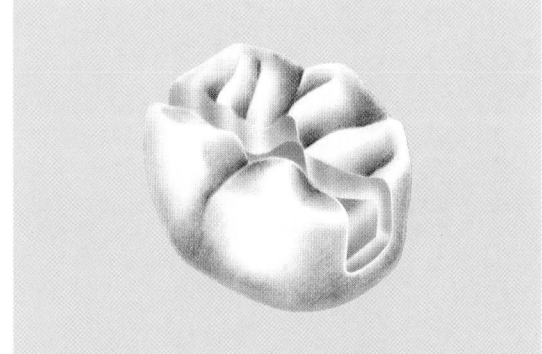

Fig. 16-1a An ideal preparation for a Class II composite resin restoration. All exit angles should be finished to a 90° angle and the cervical floor angles rounded.

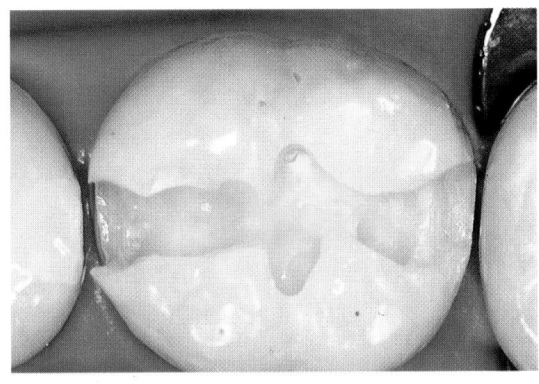

Fig. 16-1b MOD cavity in mandibular first molar prepared with rounded cervical margins and approximal exit angles finished to a 90° angle.

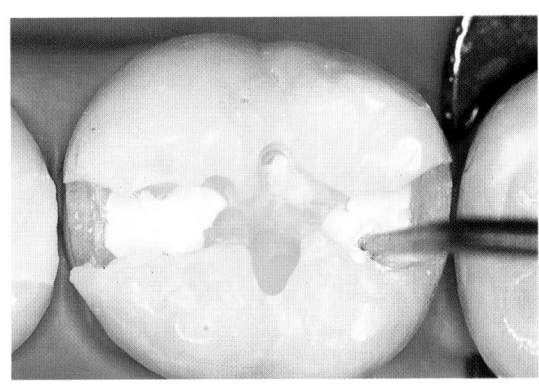

Fig. 16-2 Setting calcium hydroxide applied to deepest part of cavity.

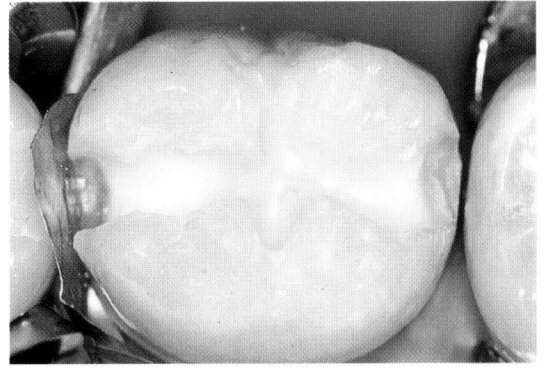

Fig. 16-3 After surface conditioning, fast-setting Ketac-Bond is applied to the dentine and built up to leave approximately 1.5 mm occlusal space for the composite resin filling. Matrix bands are inserted to protect adjoining teeth prior to acid etching.

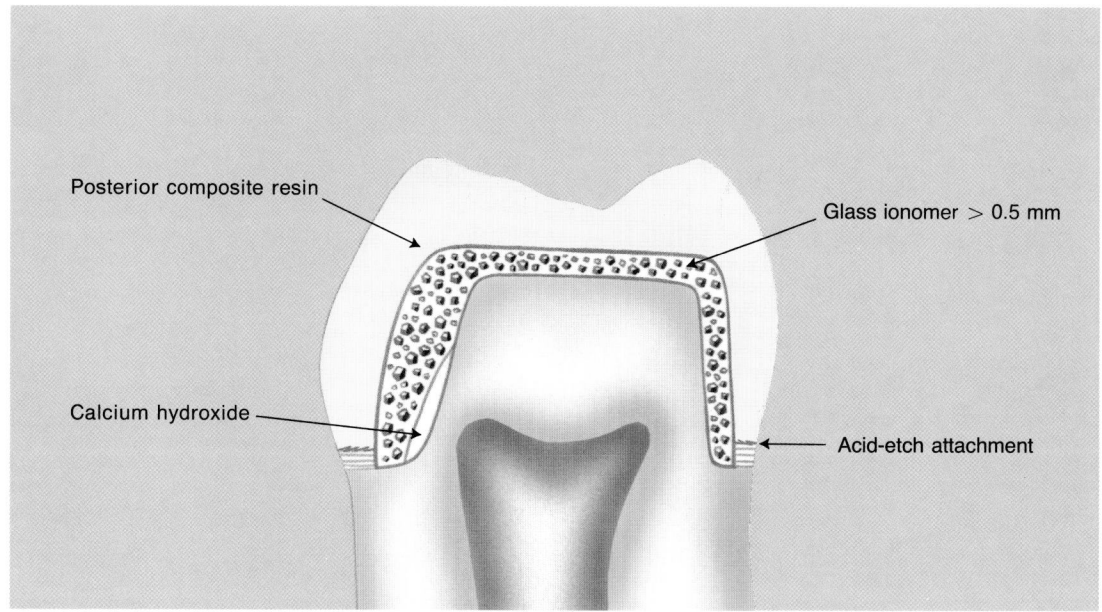

Fig. 16-4a   Ideal thicknesses of calcium hydroxide liner, glass-ionomer cement, and posterior composite resin.

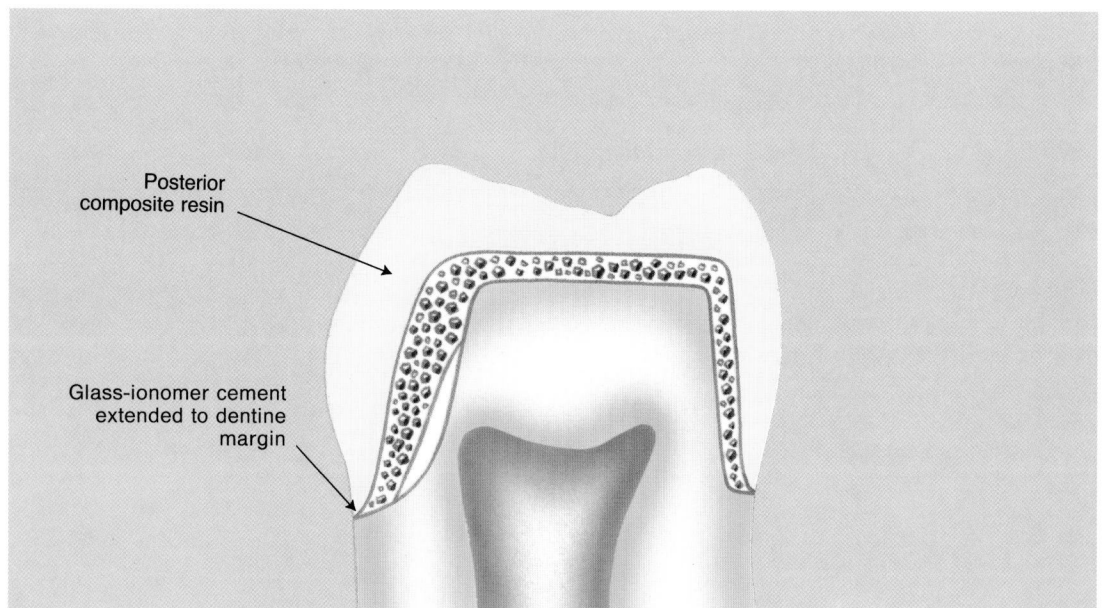

Fig. 16-4b   If cervical dentine is involved, the glass-ionomer cement must be extended to the margin.

should be removed with sharp excavators. Allow to set for two minutes and then check the surface with an explorer. When no indentation can be made without exerting heavy pressure, the cement should be ready for etching. This period generally does not exceed three minutes after insertion into the cavity. Prior to acid etching, it is essential to insert protective matrix bands to prevent damage to adjoining teeth (see Fig. 16-3).

Matrix application

The maintenance of tight contact areas is the most difficult procedure during insertion of a posterior composite resin restoration. In addition, because of their lack of body, composite resins cannot be packed against a band like amalgam alloys can. For this reason, precontoured matrix bands are preferred. These are supplied in both metal and plastic, but the latter are thicker and present even bigger problems in maintaining tight contacts. Plastic matrices allow light curing of the gingival margin using clear plastic wedges, but despite this advantage, the ease of contouring and sealing metal bands probably makes them the material of choice. It is also possible to insert clear plastic wedges after removal of the metal matrix band and recure the cervical area.

Matrix retainers are not always required for matrix band retention, and overtightening can cause cuspal distortion. Very thin matrix bands should be used. Alternatively, a number of sectional matrices are available.* The advantage of using sectional matrices or thin matrix bands is that very accurate adaptation can be achieved at the approximal walls.

*Nos. 1 or 2 Tofflemire, HO Dental Co., Goleta, Calif.; Sectional Matrices, Palodent, Portola Valley, Calif.; Contour Matrix Bands, Teledyne Getz, Elk Grove Village, Ill.

Wedging

After application of the matrix the cervical area should be firmly wedged and, if necessary, a separator* used to increase the opening (see Fig. 16-3). Make certain that the wedges do not alter the contour of the band and cause a concavity to develop in the embrasure space. When filling two proximal surfaces on the same tooth, Albers (1985) recommends that each box should be wedged, filled, and light cured prior to filling the other side. Before filling, burnish the metal band against the adjoining tooth. If magnification is used, a *contact area* should be observed, not a *contact point* (see Fig. 16-3).

Etching

A gel etchant (37% phosphoric acid) is preferred for ease of control, and should be applied for 30 seconds to both enamel and glass-ionomer cement base (Fig. 16-5). After washing for at least 15 seconds with air-water spray, the tooth must be thoroughly dried with oil-free warm air. If the etch patterns are correct, the enamel should appear frosted and the glass-ionomer cement surface like unglazed porcelain (Fig. 16-6). It is useful, at this stage, to rewedge the tooth from the lingual to increase the opening mesially. Prior to filling, the wedge may be replaced buccally and the McKean separator applied to the mesial aspect of the wedge.

Applying bonding resin

Etching and the application of the bonding resin is the most critical procedure;

*McKean, Rocky Mountain Dental Co., Denver, Colo.

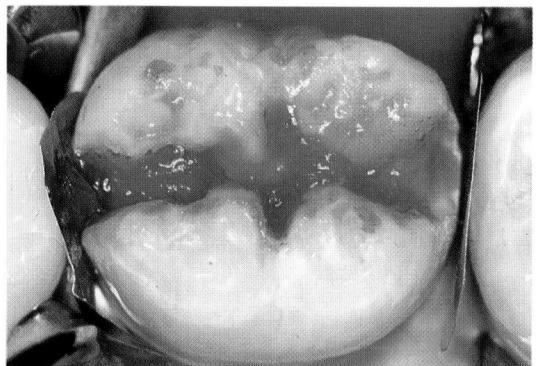

Fig. 16-5 Tofflemire contoured band applied to both ends of MOD cavity, one end wedged firmly. A McKean separator has been applied to increase the opening. The band should be burnished against the adjoining tooth to ensure a proper contact area, as opposed to a contact point. The glass-ionomer base and enamel may then be etched for 30 seconds with a 37% phosphoric acid gel prior to washing and drying.

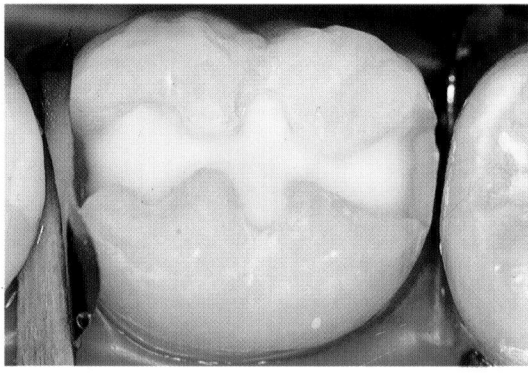

Fig. 16-6 Glass-ionomer cement base and enamel after etching showing frosted appearance. The distal matrix band is now removed to ensure a tight contact at the mesial aspect.

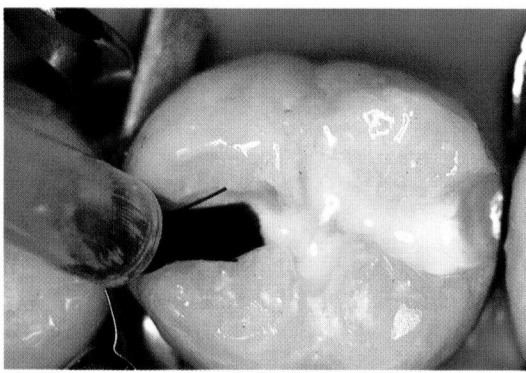

Fig. 16-7 After washing and drying, the bonding agent is applied and spread thinly over the surface with a stream of air.

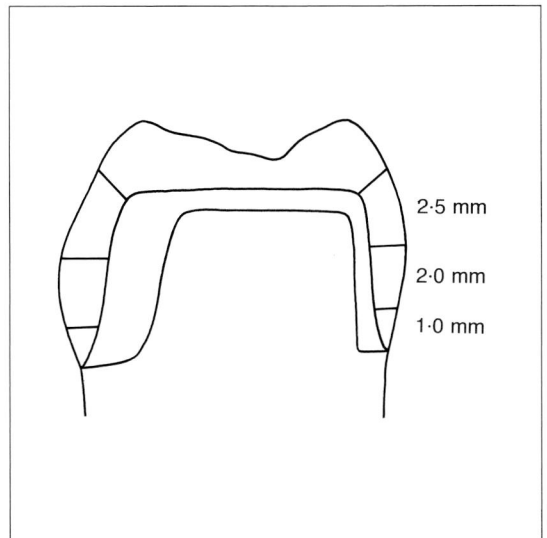

Fig. 16-8 Ideal method of reducing polymerization shrinkage in composite resins. The proximal box should be built up in layers.

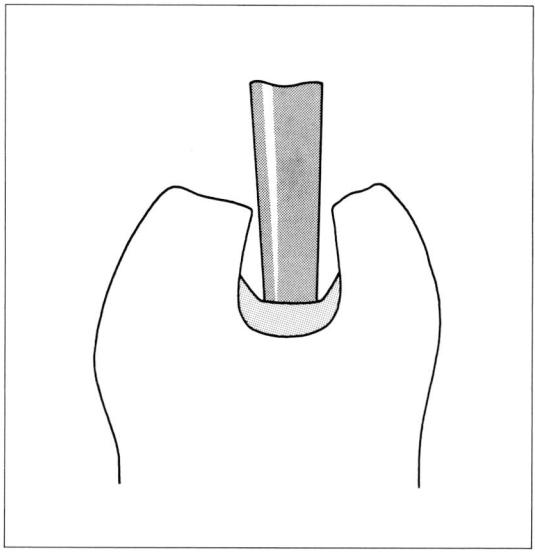

Fig. 16-9 Amalgam plugger used to condense composite resin.

long-term success hinges on the attainment of an uncontaminated bond area. For this reason, immediately after drying, the light-cured bonding resin should be applied and spread with a light blast of clean air (Fig. 16-7). Light cure immediately for 20 seconds to ensure attachment to the high-energy surface enamel.

Placement of composite resin

If the polymerization contraction of composite resin is to be controlled, then opposing cavosurfaces should not be filled and light cured at the same time. It is generally agreed that the cervical material should not exceed 1 mm in thickness prior to curing (Albers, 1985) and that each layer should be cured for at least 40 seconds for optimum results. The proximal box should then be built up in opposing layers (Fig. 16-8), with each layer of composite resin being covered with a very thin layer of bonding resin to prevent layering. Conventional amalgam pluggers are useful tools to condense the composite resin (Fig. 16-9). Composite syringes can aid in delivering the material accurately but are not essential, provided a layering technique is used. When the contact area is being filled it is essential to make sure that the band is in close opposition to the adjoining tooth. This can be achieved if the band is held firmly with a burnisher while the approximal walls are filled and light cured (Fig. 16-10). The mesial wedge is removed and transferred to the distal end prior to completing the restoration (Fig. 16-11). Rewedging or increasing pressure on the wedge at intervals is strongly recommended since loose contact is the most common cause of failure during placement of posterior composite resin restorations.

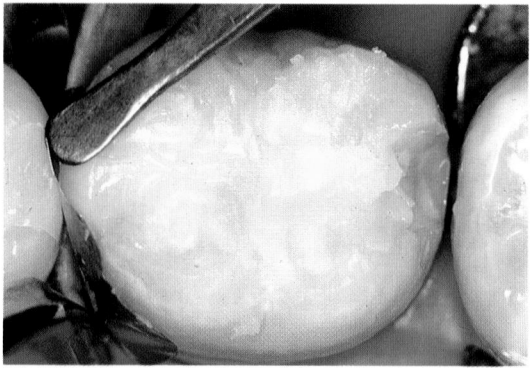

Fig. 16-10 Matrix band held tightly against contact area with a plastic instrument during light curing of composite resin.

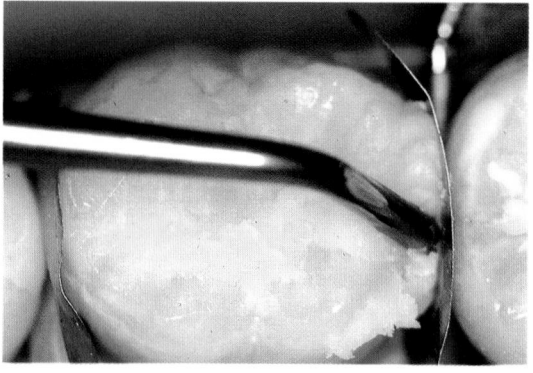

Fig. 16-11 Mesial wedge and McKean separator removed and new band inserted in distal box. Using this method increases the chances of maintaining tight contact areas. The composite resin is applied in layers to complete the MOD restoration. Prior to completion of the distal end of the restoration the mesial band may also be removed.

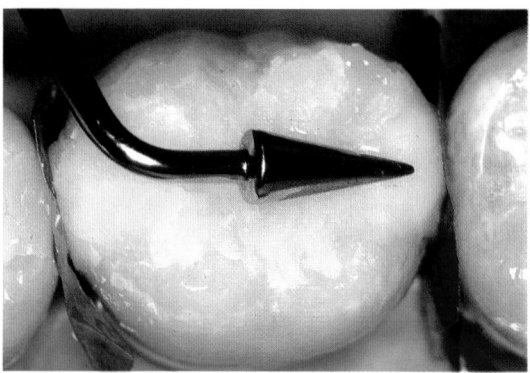

Fig. 16-12 Cone-shaped burnisher used to develop occlusion.

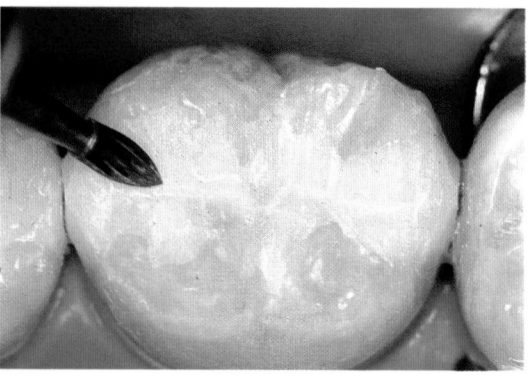

Fig. 16-13 Fluted tungsten burs used to refine the occlusal surface. By using magnification it is possible to avoid any damage to the enamel.

Provided magnification is used, it is possible to contour the marginal ridges and occlusal surfaces very accurately with cone-shaped burnishers (Fig. 16-12). Finishing procedures are then kept to the minimum. Many failures in posterior composite resins occur because of insufficient light curing. For this reason, it is strongly recommended that the final occlusal cure should be extended to 60 seconds prior to removal of the wedges and matrices and the cervical area recured using clear plastic wedges to increase light transmission.

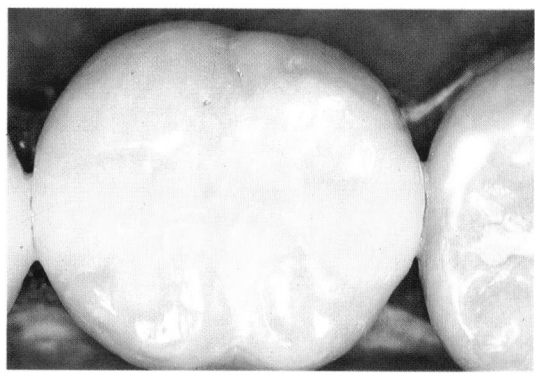

Fig. 16-14 Completed restoration in tooth 46 after polishing with rubber cups and a slurry of aluminium oxide.

Finishing

The use of fibre-optic lighting and magnification is essential when finishing composite resin restorations, since the colour contrast at the cavosurface margins is poor. If gross reduction is required, this is best done with fine-grit conventional diamonds. However, provided that contouring is accurate, it should be possible to finish the surface using light pressure and slow-running round tungsten carbide burs or flame-shaped fluted tungsten burs (Fig. 16-13). These burs will allow sufficient tactile sense to be transmitted to avoid damage to the enamel. In addition, if the operator is using magnification and a dry field, it is much easier to confine trimming to the composite resin restoration, and only the lightest touch is required at the cavosurface margins. Microdiamond burs are also useful but will grind enamel rather more easily without providing definite tactile sensation. Exposed proximal margins are best finished with flexible discs. Sharp no. 12 curved scalpel blades are also useful. After finishing, it is essential to check the contacts and any overhanging margins with dental floss.

Occlusion

After removal of the rubber dam the occlusion is checked. Ideally, occlusal stops should not be placed within the composite resin material but rather on the enamel. However, where amalgam restorations are replaced, existing centric holding stops may be present. Occlusal adjustment should therefore follow the procedure for adjusting gold occlusal surfaces, in which centric holding stops are maintained and heavy balancing contacts removed. Heavy occlusal contact on composite marginal ridges (ie., two-tooth contact) should be avoided because the flexural and shear strengths of these materials are still comparatively low. Posterior composite resins will last longer with a canine-protected occlusion rather than in group function where continuous grinding of occlusal surfaces may occur.

Polishing

Posterior composite resin restorations can be polished with impregnated rubber wheels or points. It is useful to use

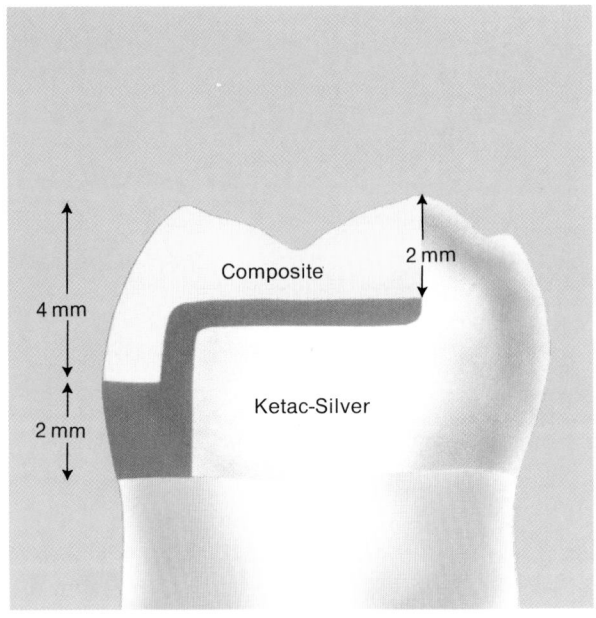

Fig. 16-15   Ideal thickness of Ketac-Silver and composite resin in the approximal box.

these polishers with a slurry of fine aluminium oxide. The completed restoration is shown in Fig. 16-14.

The posterior composite resin restoration involving large occlusal areas must still be regarded as experimental and is better confined to the premolars. Until the problems of hydrolytic instability and high shrinkage are solved, the long-term seal and wear resistance of these materials remains questionable.

Silver-cermet composite resin laminate technique

The development of tight contacts in the posterior composite resin restoration always poses a problem. To overcome this it is possible to use a silver-cermet cement, such as Ketac-Silver,* as the main

*ESPE GmbH, Seefeld/Oberbay, West Germany, and Valley Stream, N.Y.

bulk of the restoration and to replace the occlusal enamel with composite resin. It is essential to allow a minimum thickness of 2 mm bulk composite resin occlusally, and 3 mm approximally, to prevent breakage (Fig. 16-15).

After placement of the matrix band (Fig. 16-16), the silver-cermet cement may be injected into the proximal box (Fig. 16-17) and adapted with amalgam pluggers. At this stage it is easier to maintain the matrix band in tight contact with the adjoining tooth with the plugger. After setting, any excess cermet cement can be removed with sharp excavators or a fissure bur to leave at least 1.5 mm space for the posterior composite resin.

After five minutes the cermet cement base is then etched with 37% phosphoric acid gel for 30 seconds (Fig. 16-18) and a posterior composite resin inserted as described previously. Normally, it should not be necessary to pack the composite resin in increments, since the silver-cermet cement occupies the main bulk of the restoration (Fig. 16-19).

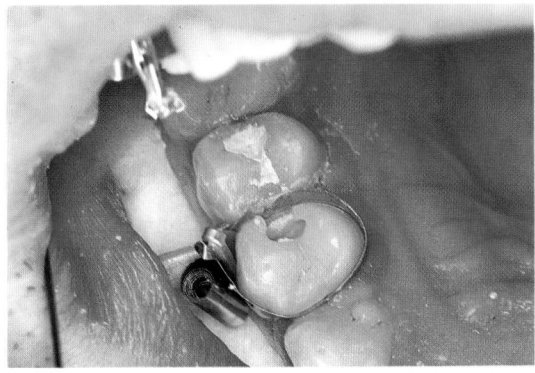

Fig. 16-16 Cavity preparation conditioned with poly(acrylic acid). Contoured matrix band applied in distal cavity in tooth 14. Distal cavity in tooth 15 has been treated via the internal occlusal fossa approach and filled with Ketac-Silver. Cavity in tooth 14 involved the marginal ridge. Patient is an epileptic with a high caries rate and gingival hypertrophy. A fluoride-leachable cement is ideal in this case.

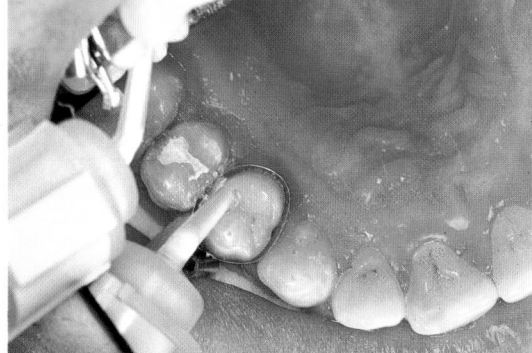

Fig. 16-17 Ketac-Silver injected into cavity and adapted with amalgam pluggers. When using cermet ionomers it is not necessary to apply a rubber dam.

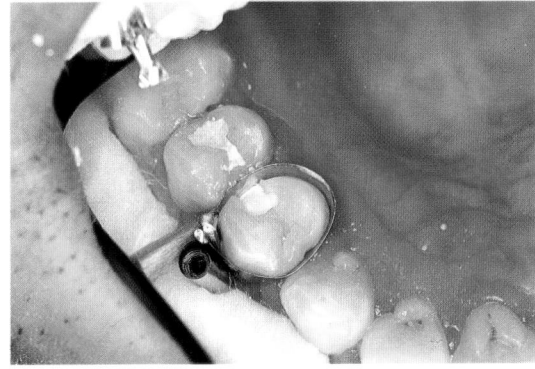

Fig. 16-18 Ketac-Silver removed from occlusal surface to leave a space of at least 1.5 mm for the composite resin. Providing the cavity is not too large, the composite resin can be reduced to 1.5 mm. Larger cavities would require 2 mm of composite resin. The cermet-ionomer cement and enamel are etched for 30 seconds with 37% phosphoric acid, and washed and dried. In this case the Ketac-Silver is occupying approximately 2 mm of the cervical box.

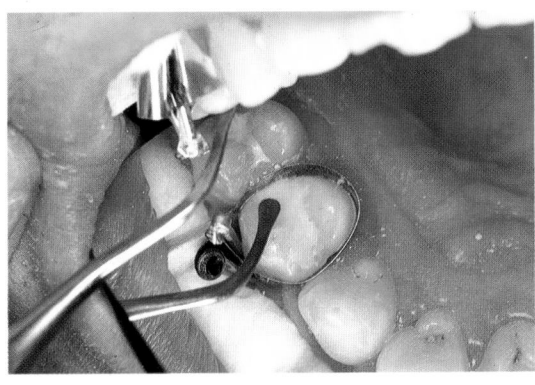

Fig. 16-19 After application of bonding resin the Occlusin posterior composite resin is adapted and light cured in one operation. The reduced bulk of material minimizes shrinkage.

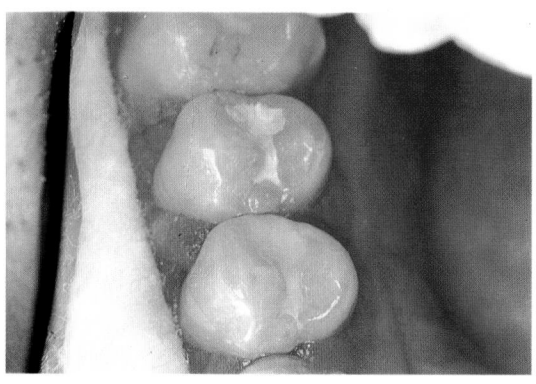

Fig. 16-20 Completed Ketac-Silver/Occlusin laminate restoration in tooth 14.

Sealing the cervical margin with silver-cermet cement reduces the problems of future microleakage, and the leaching of fluoride will protect the surrounding enamel. Elimination of cervical composite resin makes the technique much simpler since bonding of composite resins to cervical enamel can be very difficult. If only dentine and cementum are present, then the use of the silver-cermet cement/composite resin laminate technique should be the procedure of choice. Objections have been raised with regard to the colour of Ketac-Silver. However, the current material is considerably improved in colour, and unless the enamel is very thin, no shine-through should occur (Fig. 16-20). Even in these cases, a thin wash of Ketac-Bond can be applied against the dentine as a colour background. Ketac-Silver, being more abrasion resistant, will not wear during cleaning with dental floss.

Core buildup using silver-cermet-ionomer cements

The metal-reinforced glass-ionomer cements are preferred as core buildup materials. However, it should be clearly understood that glass-ionomer cements are not suitable for use in high-stress-bearing areas. Anterior tooth buildup is a risky procedure unless at least two thirds of the remaining coronal dentine is present. Glass-ionomer cements are weak in tension and their flexural strength is inadequate for support of complete porcelain crowns on anterior teeth; cast gold posts and cores are more suitable. Even composite resin materials lack rigidity and flexural strength where high stresses are involved (see Table 13-1).

The use of silver-cermet ionomer cements in the posterior teeth should also be done with discretion. Whenever possible, the maximum amount of sound tooth structure should be conserved and retention supplemented by drilling small holes in the dentine. Reliance on adhesive bonding as the sole means of retention is not advised. As a general rule, at least 2 mm of supporting coronal dentine should be left for circumferential retention. Where this requirement cannot be met, cast gold posts and cores are preferred. However, glass-ionomer cements reinforce teeth and may assist in preventing root fracture where root canals have been overwidened.

Restoring vital teeth

After removal of all caries, the deepest portion of the tooth should be covered with a thin layer of setting calcium hydroxide liner. Do not cover more than the immediate pulpal area since it is vital to retain as much exposed dentine as possible for bonding of the glass-ionomer cement. In cases where there is minimal coronal dentine, accessory pin anchorage must be used. Pins should be placed at converging angles and to a depth of 2 mm in the dentine. The pin length should extend right through the core buildup (Fig. 16-21).

The tooth surface should be cleaned for ten seconds with a 25% solution of poly(acrylic acid), and the acid should be dispersed with clean, warm air. Do not wash off all the acid, because a thin film is necessary for adhesive bonding when cermet-ionomer cements are used (see chapter 6). Inject a mix of Chelon-Silver* into the tooth using a Centrix syringe. The hand-mixed Chelon-Silver can be mixed in greater bulk and is often preferable to the smaller dosage of the capsulated Ketac-Silver. Additions of cement may be made to existing material and the core buildup smoothed in place with plastic or metal instruments (Fig. 16-22). Crown preparation may be commenced immediately after setting (five minutes), but in heavily infected teeth it is often preferable to leave the cermet cement as a provisional restoration for a few months to assess pulp vitality and allow secondary dentine formation (Fig. 16-23). Immediate preparation of infected teeth can tip the balance and result in an irreversible inflammation of the pulp. Old amalgam restorations often exhibit microleakage with bacterial penetration into dentine. By sealing the tooth with a silver-cermet-ionomer cement, the toxic onslaught of these bacteria can be arrested, in much the same way as fissure sealing works.

When trimming the cermet-ionomer cement, use sintered diamond stones or microdiamonds running under water spray. Do not use heavy pressure—otherwise, overtrimming can easily occur (Fig. 16-24). If care is taken, the final preparation becomes a monolithic structure with the cermet-ionomer cement forming a permanent seal at the tooth interface (Fig. 16-25). A clinical case is shown in Fig. 16-26. Cermet-ionomer cements are strongly preferred to composite resin core buildup materials in vital teeth and where secondary caries is likely to occur.

Restoring devitalized teeth

Where root canals have been filled with gutta-percha points, the canals can be slightly widened and fitted with endoposts.* First, all gutta-percha should be removed from the pulp chamber and a Gates-Glidden drill used to remove up to 4 mm of the root canal filling. It is then a simple procedure to insert the appropriate endopost drill and widen the canal. The endoposts are cut to length and cemented in the canal (Fig. 16-27). For cementation of posts, a water-hardening glass-ionomer cement such as Ketac-Cem is recommended because of its low viscosity. The coronal dentine should be surface conditioned with poly(acrylic acid) prior to injecting the main bulk of Chelon-Silver. Shaping and finishing should follow the same procedure as described for the restoration of the vital tooth (Fig. 16-28).

*ESPE GmbH, Seefeld/Oberbay., West Germany, and Valley Stream, N.Y.

*Paraposts, Whaledent International, New York.

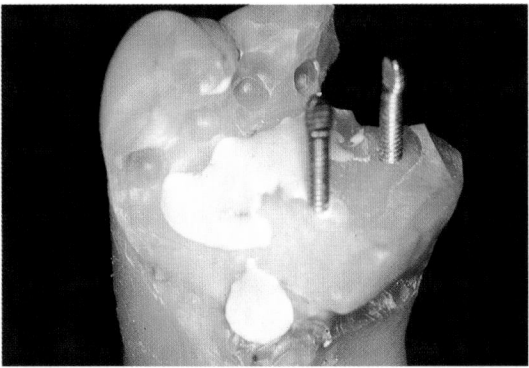

Fig. 16-21 A maxillary molar ideally suited for restoration with a cermet-ionomer cement core. The tooth is heavily decayed subgingivally and would present a great problem if amalgam or composite resin cores were used. A composite resin core would also not seal the dentine area. Two pins have been inserted buccally, extending through the core. Retention holes have been drilled in the lingual dentine and setting calcium hydroxide applied to the pulpal dentine floor. Do not allow the calcium hydroxide to encroach on the margins.

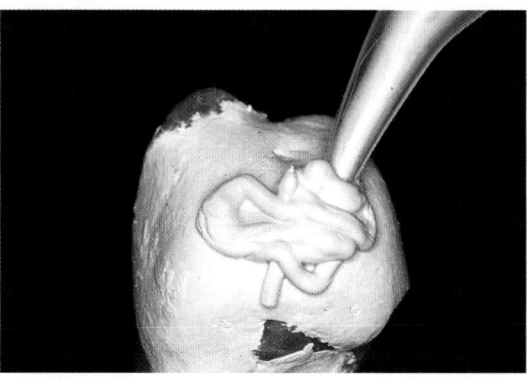

Fig. 16-22a Chelon-Silver is injected into tooth with Centrix syringe and additions made to the occlusal surface. Provided these are done prior to setting, good bonding will be achieved.

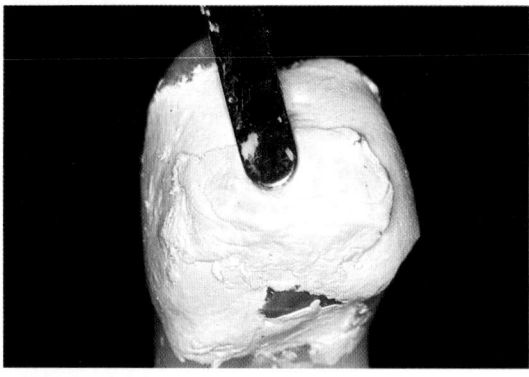

Fig. 16-22b Flat plastic used to contour cement.

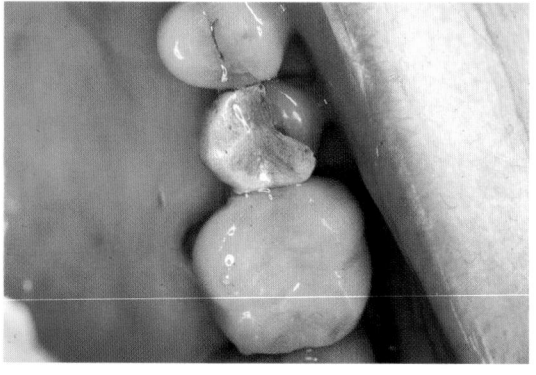

Fig. 16-23 Cermet-ionomer cement core inserted in tooth 25 prior to veneer crown preparation. If left for a few months, tooth can effect pulpal repair.

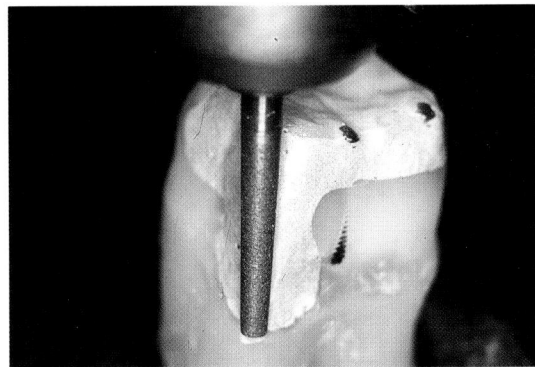

Fig. 16-24 Core trimmed with sintered diamonds under water spray.

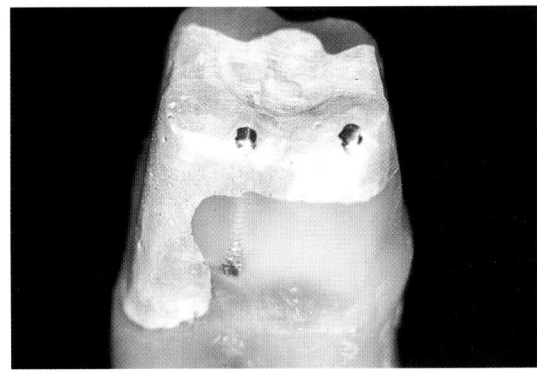

Fig. 16-25 Completed molar veneer crown preparation. The core has become a monolithic structure with the tooth and will strengthen the root.

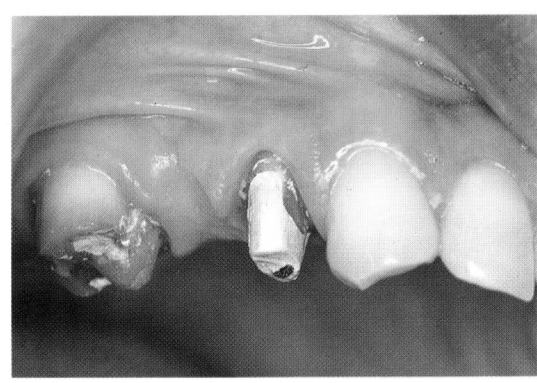

Fig. 16-26a Clinical case illustrating the use of Chelon-Silver to restore crown of tooth 14.

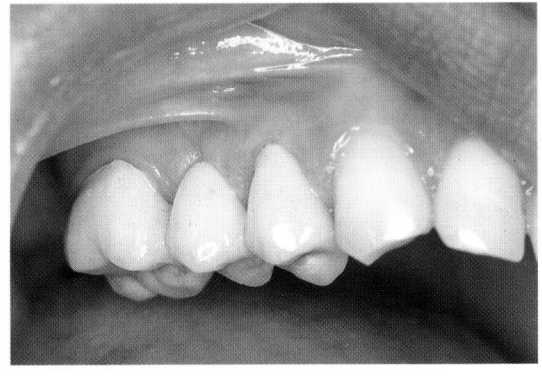

Fig. 16-26b Metal-ceramic bridge cemented.

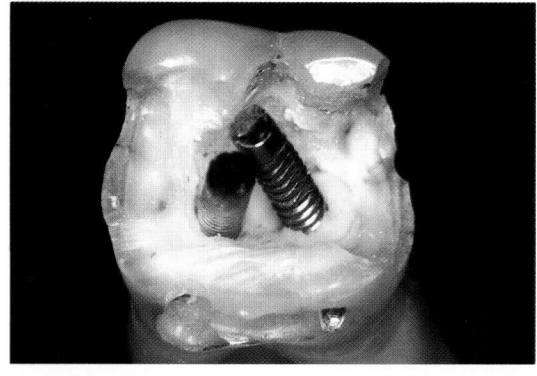

Fig. 16-27 Gutta-percha removed from root canals and endoposts fitted using glass-ionomer luting cement. Surface conditioner should be used prior to injecting cermet-ionomer cement.

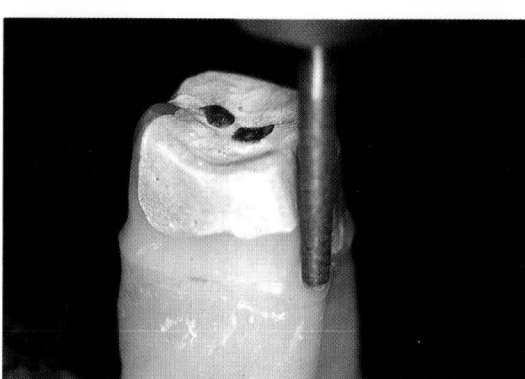

Fig. 16-28 Chelon-Silver core built up and prepared for full-veneer crown. Endoposts should extend through the core.

Miscellaneous uses for cermet-ionomer cements and glass-ionomer cements

Cervical lining for amalgam alloys

Amalgam alloy restorations fail more through microleakage and secondary caries than through mechanical failure (Mjör, 1985). Silver-cermet-ionomer cements can be useful in sealing the critical cervical floor, since they are chemically adhesive and possess cariostatic properties. The technique is simple: a matrix band (e.g., Caulk Auto-Matrix*) is ap-

plied and firmly wedged (Fig. 16-29), and the cement is injected into the Class II cavity to restore approximately 2 mm in height of the proximal box. The cement can be spread over the occlusal floor and burnished to a thin film over all the dentine and enamel walls (Fig. 16-30). At this stage the cervical floor is restored with silver-cermet cement, which also totally seals the dentine/matrix band junction, thus avoiding the risk of any amalgam alloy extruding into the gingival crevice (Fig. 16-31). After setting, the amalgam alloy is packed into the cavity by conventional techniques (Fig. 16-32). The radio-opacity of silver-cermet cements permits accurate monitoring with radiographs (Fig. 16-33), and the material can safely be cleaned with dental floss. The silver-cermet cement/amalgam alloy laminate is particularly useful in patients with a high caries incidence.

*L.D. Caulk Co., Milford, Del.

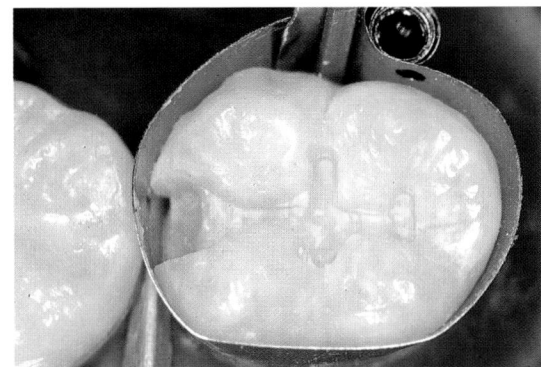

Fig. 16-29 Mesio-occlusal cavity in mandibular second molar with matrix band inserted and firmly wedged at cervical margin.

Fig. 16-30 After surface conditioning the tooth with poly(acrylic acid), Ketac-Silver is injected into the cavity and spread over the walls. The cervical box area should be filled with at least 1 to 2 mm of cermet-ionomer cement to act as a cariostatic seal.

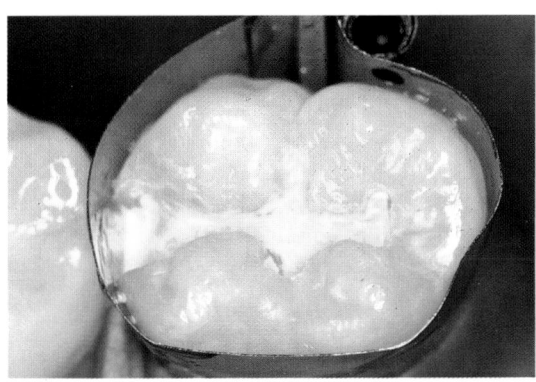

Fig. 16-31 *(below)* A Ketac-Silver/amalgam laminate.

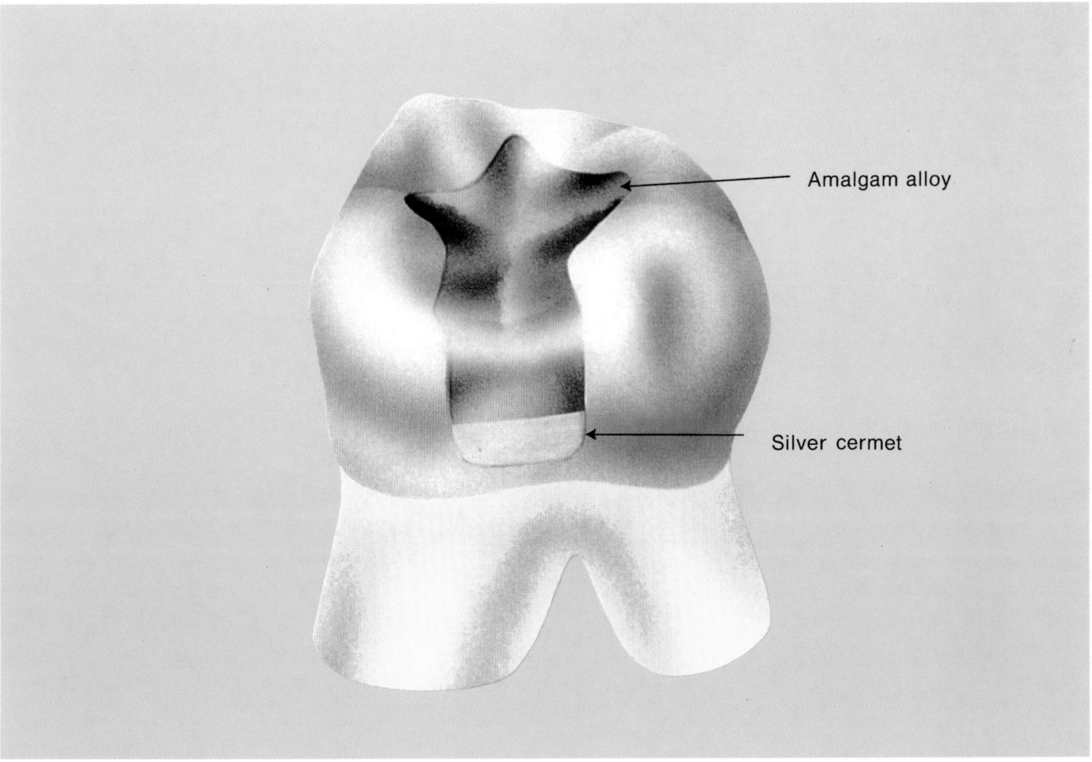

Amalgam alloy

Silver cermet

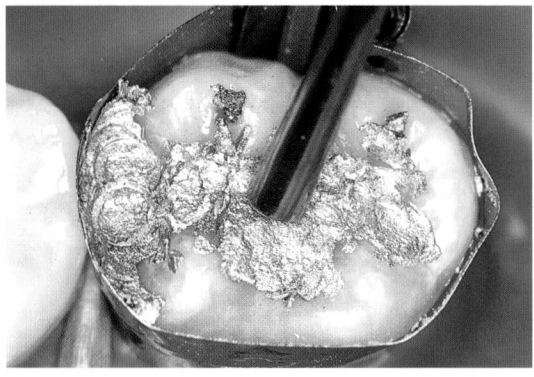

Fig. 16-32a Amalgam alloy packed into cavity using conventional technique.

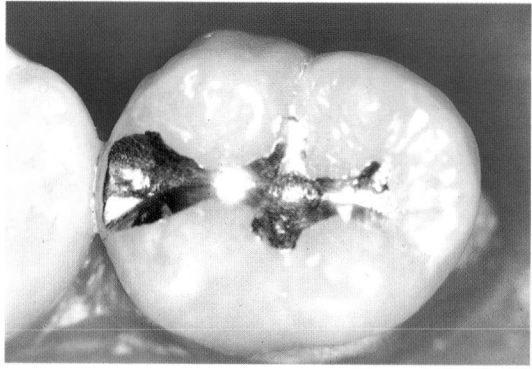

Fig. 16-32b Completed restoration after polishing.

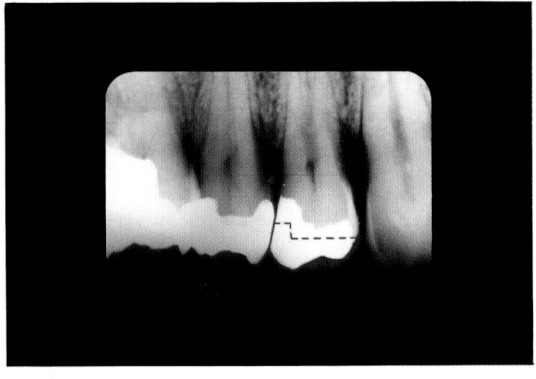

Fig. 16-33 Radiograph of a maxillary first molar. Ketac-Silver lining indicated by a dotted line.

Aesthetic repair of defective margins

Where open margins are detected around crowns and inlays (Fig. 16-34), glass-ionomer cements have proved excellent repair materials because of their aesthetic appeal. If caries is detected it should be removed with the smallest round bur, using magnifying loops. In many cases the marginal defects may be due to toothbrush abrasion over many years. Provided the margin is dry and clean, glass-ionomer cements are very easily injected into the space between crown and tooth. Surface conditioning with a 25% poly(acrylic acid) solution is also helpful.

Wherever possible, use a preformed

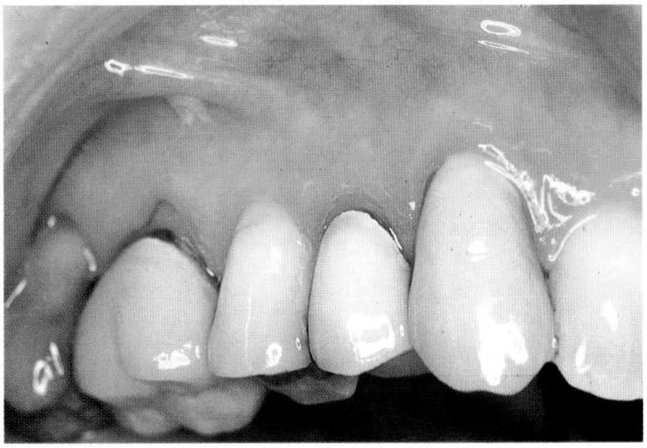

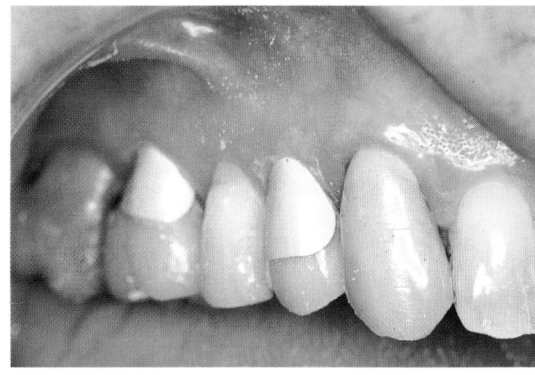

Fig. 16-34 Defective margins on metal-ceramic crowns inserted 15 years earlier on teeth 14 and 16.

Fig. 16-35 Any caries is removed with small round burs and the surface conditioned for 30 seconds with 25% poly(acrylic acid). Chem-Fil II* is injected into the cervical margin and a Hawe matrix obtains accurate contour.

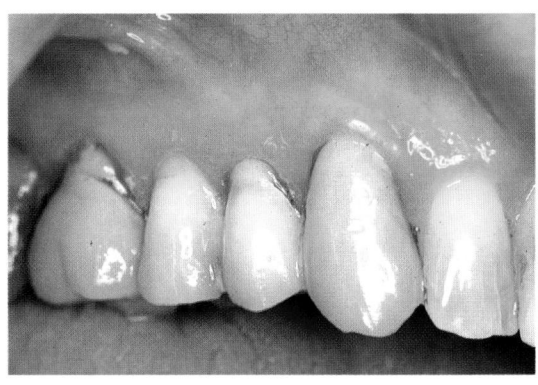

Fig. 16-36 Completed Class V Chem-Fil* restorations in teeth 14 and 16 after coating with light-cured bonding agent.

*Dentsply International, Inc., Weybridge, England, and York, Pa.

cervical metal matrix† to increase the pressure on the cement during adaptation (Fig. 16-35). On removal of the matrix, immediately apply varnish to the margins. Thin repair areas of cement are particularly susceptible to washout under saliva, and must be kept protected. After setting, remove any excess material with sharp excavators and apply light-cured bonding agent to the edges (Fig. 16-36).

†Hawe Matrices, Hawe-Neos Dental Co., Gentilino, Switzerland.

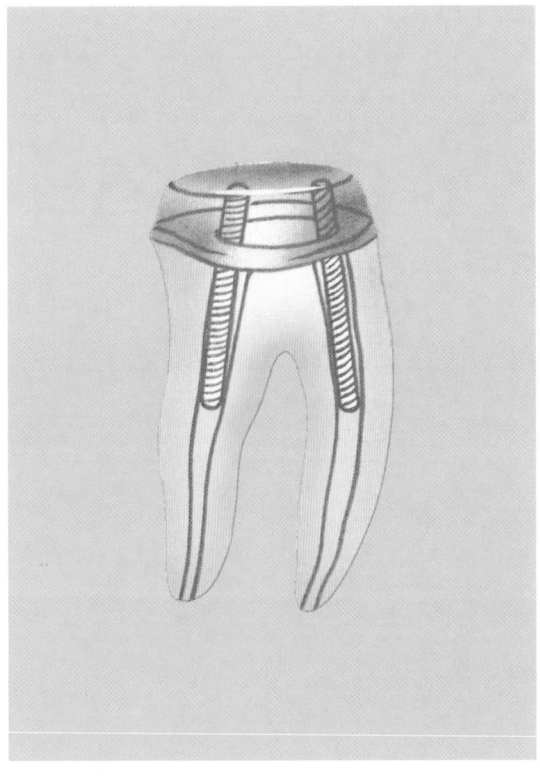

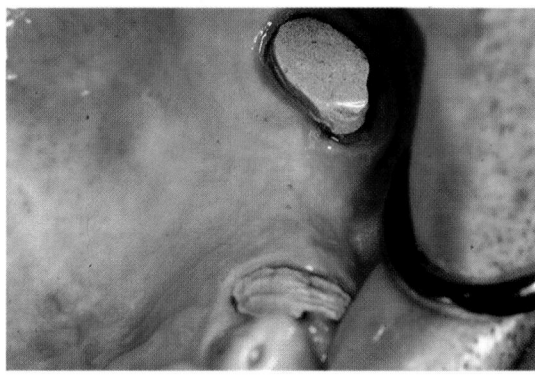

Fig. 16-38 Root cap in Ketac-Silver inserted in maxillary first premolar and second molar.

Fig. 16-37 *(left)* Use of cermet-ionomer cement for root capping prior to fitting over dentures.

Sealing root surfaces

Where teeth have been root-treated and prepared for the fitting of overdentures, silver-cermet cements are very useful for sealing the root surfaces. Ancillary pin anchorage may be used and a box cut in the root face (Fig. 16-37). After conditioning with a 25% poly(acrylic) acid solution for ten seconds, it is a simple procedure to inject a silver-cermet cement onto the root face and shape it as a small root cap (Fig. 16-38). After setting, the edges may be finished with microdiamond stones. This procedure is particularly useful in the older patient where oral hygiene may be poor and some cariostatic action is required.

Recementation of defective crowns and bridges

Cermet-ionomer cements are finding increasing application in the recementation of old crowns and bridges, where dentine has softened due to microleakage and secondary caries. Often patients are at an age where they find it difficult to afford a new construction. The rebuilding of internal tooth structure with cermet-ionomer cement can provide short-term relief.

A number of options are open to the clinician. Where caries is extensive, elective endodontics is probably the treatment of choice. Where retention is poor or the clinical crown is short, endodontics is also preferred. However, provided the tooth preparation is still retentive, any carious dentine should be removed and

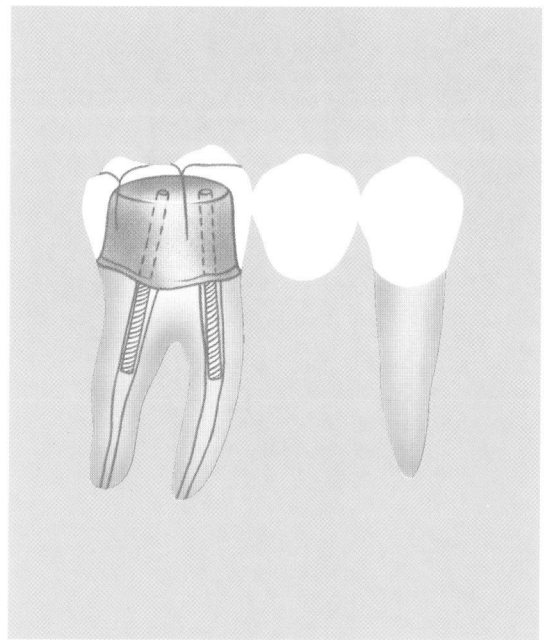

Fig. 16-39 Ideal height of endoposts in relation to retainer crown.

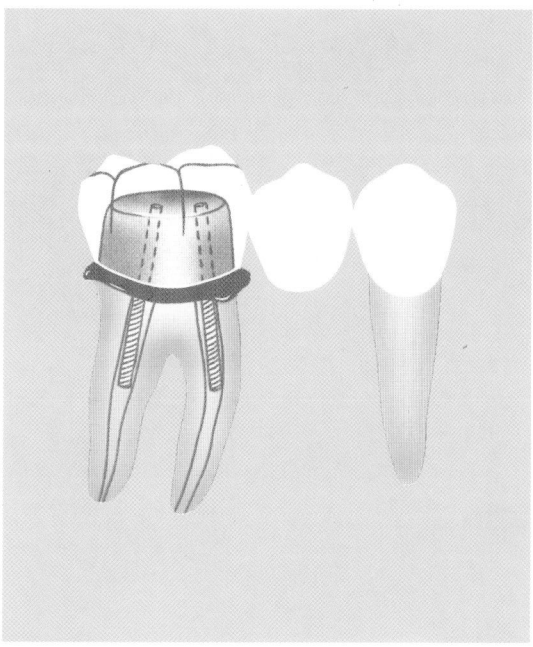

Fig. 16-40 The seating of the lubricated retainer crown onto the freshly prepared molar surface that has been injected with cermet-ionomer cement.

the crown or bridge recemented using a cermet-ionomer cement.

Recementation of existing crowns or bridges where caries is extensive or retention is poor

After endodontic procedures are complete, remove all the root filling from the pulp chamber and, where molars are being treated, ream at least two canals for fitting of endoposts (see Fig. 16-27). After cleaning the crown or bridge by internal sandblasting, check that the endoposts are short enough to allow easy seating of the retainer crown (Fig. 16-39). Make certain there are no undercuts in the crown and that it can allow release of

the cement core. Lubricate the internal surface of the crown with a thick film of oil or petroleum jelly and fill with either a hand-mixed or capsulated cermet-ionomer cement. Inject more material around the posts and onto the dentine interface, which should have been surface conditioned with poly(acrylic acid), and seat the abutment crown firmly into position (Fig. 16-40). Immediately cover with a sheet of soft wax to protect the edges, and ask the patient to bite firmly on the crown or bridge. It should now be possible to establish the original occlusion.

After five minutes of setting—providing the early check on undercuts has been made—the crown may be removed easily. Clean off the lubricant with a suitable solvent and thoroughly sandblast the interior with 30 μm aluminium oxide grit. The crown or bridge may be recemented

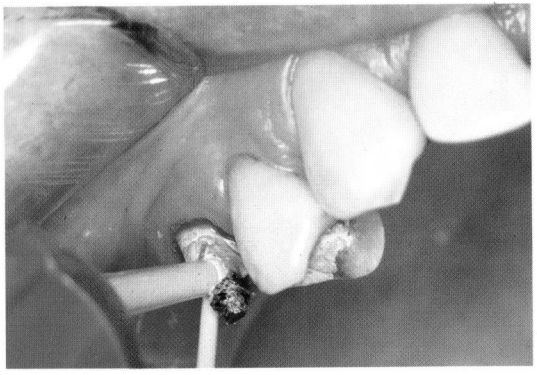

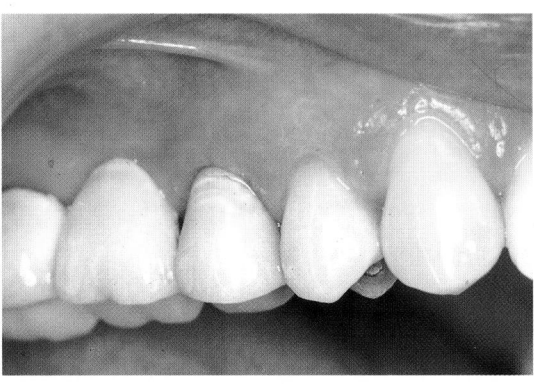

Fig. 16-41a Metal-ceramic bridge failed on tooth 15 due to death of pulp caused by root caries. Endopost inserted after root treatment in tooth 15, and Chelon-Silver injected around post to build up core. Existing retainer crown is then lubricated and seated over core.

Fig. 16-41b Metal-ceramic bridge recemented over core buildup with Ketac-Cem luting cement. Where root caries is present, new core acts as a metal collar. Bridge has now been functioning for nearly three and a half years.

with a water-based luting cement using standard procedures. A clinical case involving a second premolar is illustrated in Fig. 16-41.

In many cases where there has been extensive loss of dentine, it is possible both to inject a mix of silver-cermet cement (Chelon-Silver) into the crown and around the post retention and to recement the crown in one operation. Extrusion of the cement will be easier, since the open margins allow easy flow.

Recementation of existing crowns or bridges where the preparation is retentive and caries is minimal

This procedure is very easy because all that is required is ensuring clean surfaces on both dentine and metal. Any caries or softened dentine is removed. Where a near-exposure of the pulp is likely, cover with a small bead of setting calcium hydroxide. Surface condition the

dentine with 25% poly(acrylic acid) for ten seconds and remove excess with clean air spray. Do not wash off all the acid, but do not leave a thick film of it, either. Clean the internal surface of the casting by light sandblasting with 30 μm aluminium oxide grit.

Cementation

The mix of the silver-cermet cement should be of higher viscosity than standard luting consistency, but it should still exhibit easy flow so that it can be injected through a syringe nozzle. The crown is filled with cement and a thin coat injected over the tooth prior to seating the crown or bridge. Cover with wax and ask the patient to seat the restoration under pressure until the occlusion is comfortable. Any excess cement is then removed with sharp scalers after five minutes of setting, and the edges are lightly burnished.

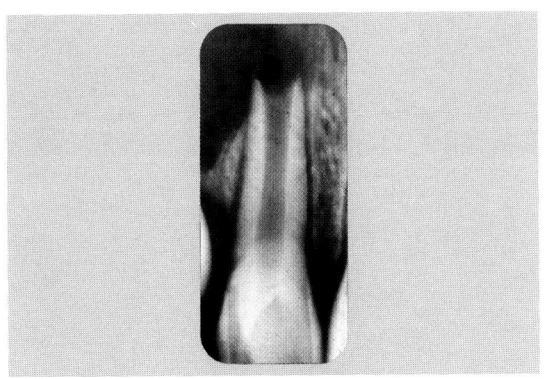

Fig. 16-42a Radiograph of acute apical abscess on tooth 12. Apical area was opened surgically, the abscess was drained and canal irrigated. Canal was dried and apex covered with Burlew's dry foil prior to injection with Ketac-Silver through coronal opening. Excess material burnished over at apex with dry foil and allowed to set prior to removing excess.

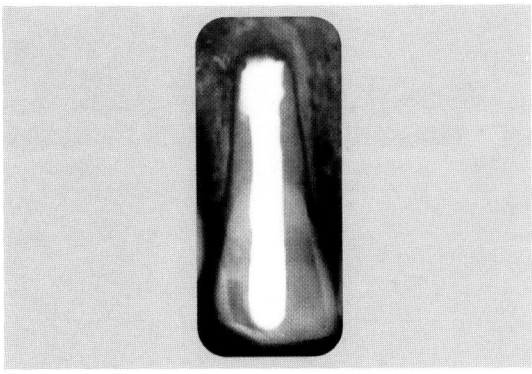

Fig. 16-42b Radiograph showing healing of bone area after one year. Courtesy of Richard Miller Yardley, O.B.E., L.D.S., M.G.D.S., R.C.S.

Cermet-ionomer cements will form a metal edge that will withstand toothbrush abrasion better than standard Type II glass-ionomer cements.

Where an abutment tooth at one end of the bridge is intact and only requires re-cementation, it is possible to cement both abutments simultaneously using cermet-ionomer cement for the defective tooth and a water-based luting cement for the sound abutment.

Bioactivity of glass-ionomer cement

Glass-ionomer cement has been shown to be bioactive and promote bone growth (Jonck, 1986). It is being used experimentally as a bone cement and also for retrograde root fillings or repair of perforated root canals. Clinical evidence is accumulating that indicates bone repair takes place within the first year, confirming the findings of Jonck (1986).

When used as a retrograde root filling,

clinicians have selected the cermet-ionomer cements for clinical trial. An interesting case illustrated in Fig. 16-42 shows that after root filling and sealing of a maxillary lateral incisor with an extensive apical abscess, complete healing of the bone occurred within one year. A further case illustrated in Fig. 16-43 shows the use of Ketac-Silver for retrograde root filling. The procedure for these cases is simple. Once the apex of the tooth has been opened or removed and the apical canal cleaned with a small round bur, Ketac-Silver can be injected via a small syringe nozzle directly into the canal. A small piece of Burlew's dry foil* can then be pressed over the apex to protect the cement during setting. After five minutes of setting, the excess material may be easily removed with a sharp excavator.

*Dentsply International, Inc., Weybridge, England, and York, Pa.

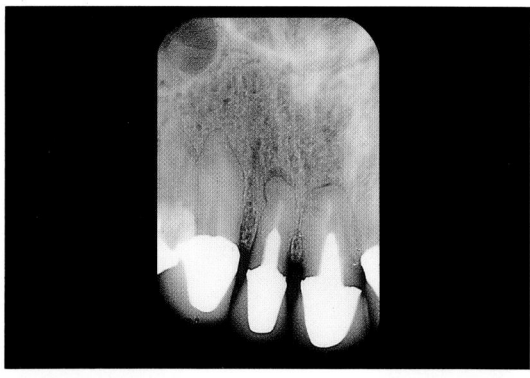

Figs. 16-43a to c Courtesy of R. W. Dinsdale, B.Ch.D., F.D.S., R.C.S.

Fig. 16-43a Radiograph prior to sealing apex.

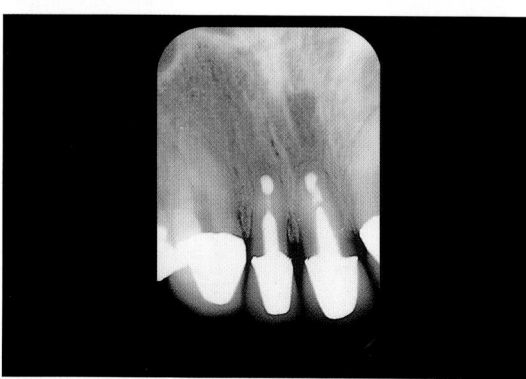

Fig. 16-43b Radiograph five months later showing bone healing after sealing with Ketac-Silver.

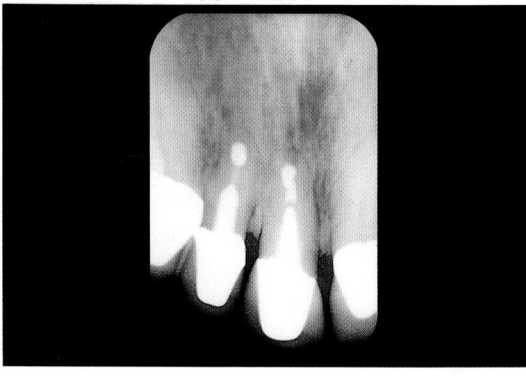

Fig. 16-43c Radiograph showing complete bone healing seven months later.

References

Albers, H.F. (1985) Tooth-Coloured Restoratives. 7th ed. Cotati, Calif.: Alto Books.

Hinoura, K., Moore, B.K., Swartz, M.L., and Phillips, R.W. (1987) Tensile bond strength between glass-ionomer cement and composite resins. J. Am. Dent. Assoc. 114:167–173.

Jonck, L.M. (1986) Personal communication.

McLean, J.W., and Wilson, A.D. (1977) The clinical development of the glass-ionomer cement. II. Some clinical applications. Aust. Dent. J. 22:120–127.

Miller, M.B. (1986) Reality. Esthetic Dentistry Research Group. Vol. I, no. 1. Houston: Reality Publ. Co.

Mjör, I.A. (1985) Frequency of secondary caries at various anatomical locations. Oper. Dent. 10:88–92.

Mount, G.J. (1986) Longevity of glass-ionomer cements. J. Prosthet. Dent. 55: 682–685.

Index